Neuropsychological Toxicology

Identification and Assessment of Human Neurotoxic Syndromes

Pergamon Titles of Related Interest

Goldstein & Hersen   HANDBOOK OF
PSYCHOLOGICAL ASSESSMENT
Frank   THE WECHSLER ENTERPRISE

Related Journals *

ARCHIVES OF CLINICAL NEUROPSYCHOLOGY
NEUROTOXICOLOGY AND TERATOLOGY
NEUROPSYCHOLOGIA
JOURNAL OF PSYCHIATRIC RESEARCH
NEUROSCIENCE AND BEHAVIORAL REVIEWS
CLINICAL PSYCHOLOGY REVIEW
BEHAVIOUR RESEARCH AND THERAPY ·
*Free sample copies available upon request

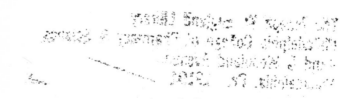

Neuropsychological Toxicology

Identification and Assessment of Human Neurotoxic Syndromes

by

DAVID E. HARTMAN, Ph.D.

Cook County Hospital
University of Illinois Medical Center
Chicago

PERGAMON PRESS

New York · Oxford · Beijing · Frankfurt
São Paulo · Sydney · Tokyo · Toronto

U.S.A.	Pergamon Press, Inc., Maxwell House, Fairview Park, Elmsford, New York 10523, U.S.A.
U.K.	Pergamon Press plc, Headington Hill Hall, Oxford OX3 0BW, England
PEOPLE'S REPUBLIC OF CHINA	Pergamon Press, Room 4037, Qianmen Hotel, Beijing, People's Republic of China
FEDERAL REPUBLIC OF GERMANY	Pergamon Press GmbH, Hammerweg 6, D-6242 Kronberg, Federal Republic of Germany
BRAZIL	Pergamon Editora Ltda, Rua Eça de Queiros, 346, CEP 04011, Paraiso, São Paulo, Brazil
AUSTRALIA	Pergamon Press Australia Pty Ltd., P.O. Box 544, Potts Point, N.S.W. 2011, Australia
JAPAN	Pergamon Press, 8th Floor, Matsuoka Central Building, 1-7-1 Nishishinjuku, Shinjuku-ku, Tokyo 160, Japan
CANADA	Pergamon Press Canada Ltd., Suite No. 271, 253 College Street, Toronto, Ontario, Canada M5T 1R5

Copyright © 1988 Pergamon Press Inc.

First edition 1988

Library of Congress Cataloging-in-Publication Data

Hartman, David E.
Neuropsychological toxicology: identification
and assessment of human neurotoxic syndromes
Bibliography: p.
Includes index.
1. Behavioral toxicology.   2. Neurotoxic agents.
I. Title. [DNLM: 1. Behavior--drug effects.
2. Cognition--drug effects. 3. Emotions--drug
effects. 4. Environmental Pollutants--poisoning.
5. Nervous System--drug effects. QV 76.5 H333n]
RA1224.H35   1987   616.89   87-14795

British Library Cataloguing in Publication Data

Hartman, David E.
Neuropsychological toxicology: identification
and assessment of human neurotoxic syndromes
1. Nervous system--Diseases 2. Neurotoxic
agents
I. Title
616.8   RC346
ISBN 0-08-034944-7

Printed in Great Britain by A. Wheaton & Co. Ltd., Exeter

Contents

Acknowledgments

This book is dedicated to my wife, Roberta Maller, and to my father, mother and sister: Harry, Marian and Deborah Hartman.

I am also grateful to two others who encouraged me to continue in the long development of this text: Charles Shaiova and Maryann Renzi.

Additional thanks go to Stephen Hessl, MD, Peter Orris, MD, Ann Naughton, RN, and the staff of the Occupational Medicine Clinic of Cook County Hospital. Their frequent requests for neuropsychological evaluation of their patients made this book necessary. Dr Jerry Sweet has a critical position in the development of this manuscript, not only for his invaluable editorial suggestions, but for obdurately insisting that I had collected far too much material for an article.

This book would not have been physically possible without the excellent library facilities at Cook County Hospital (special thanks to Ms. Grace Auer) and the University of Illinois Medical Center. Finally, completion of the manuscript was hastened by the support of my department chairperson, Dr Anne Seiden.

Preface

This book was originally written from personal need. As Director of Neuropsychology at Cook County Hospital in Chicago, Illinois, I began receiving a steady influx of patients from the hospital's Occupational Medicine Clinic who had been exposed to toxic substances in their place of work. It soon became apparent that conventional theories of neuropsychological dysfunction did not apply to patients whose subjective complaints were often the only available correlates of neurotoxic exposure. Thus, rules of diagnostic interpretation developed for diffuse, lateralized or localized dysfunction were not appropriate for this population. Neuropsychological interpretation strategies that worked for tumors, closed-head injuries, cerebrovascular disorders, etc., did not appear to fit patients with vaguely defined, diffuse, functional-sounding complaints; patients who had, nevertheless, been exposed to poisons capable of damaging the nervous system. These were patients for whom a conventional neurological examination was not diagnostic. For these patients a neuropsychological examination became the most fine-grained technique available to determine otherwise subclinical effects of neurotoxicity.

After becoming aware of the need for neuropsychological testing with this population, an attempt was made to find books on "neurobehavioral toxicology" that emphasized human clinical applications and diagnostic formulations. There were none written from a neuropsychological perspective. Futhermore, there were few easily available journal articles of any sort on the subject. I had to begin compiling a set of articles and books related to the field that would serve as a personal dictionary to aid in the assessment of these complex and puzzling cases.

My wish to assemble this information in a more accessible form led to the development of this book. It is my hope that *Neuropsychological Toxicology* will now serve others as my filing cabinet full of articles served me; as a "dictionary" of many human neurotoxic syndromes, as a review of human neurological and neuropsychological effects of common neurotoxins, and as a guide to testing and research.

Neuropsychological Toxicology is written for neuropsychologists, physicians and other health care providers. It is also intended for representatives of industry, government and the law with an interest in the cognitive, emotional, behavioral and neurological effects of neurotoxic substances. The first purpose of this book is to be a reference for clinical practitioners who must evaluate the history, symptoms, behavior and neuropsychological functioning of individuals whose occupation, hobbies or voluntary substance abuse exposes them to neurotoxic substances.

It is also written to provide information to members of the multi-disciplinary team who seek to unravel the diagnostic, psychological, legal and industrial complexities inherent to neurotoxic exposure evaluation. Thus, the book is focused on human psychological applications of toxicology research. Many active areas of toxicology could not therefore be included within this domain, including animal research, neurochemical investigations, and non-neuropsychological or neurological effects of toxic substances.

Finally, it is hoped that *Neuropsychological Toxicology* will provide resources and encouragement to those willing to undertake the research in this field that is so greatly needed.

I
Introduction

There is growing recognition that industrial and pharmacological agents affect the human nervous system and neuropsychological functions. Unfortunately most neuropsychologists, physicians and other health care professionals have had little training or experience in identifying the behavioral, cognitive and emotional patterns of nervous system dysfunction caused by exposure to toxic substances. The study of such patterns is so new that not even its name remains constant among researchers. It has been called *behavioral toxicology, neurobehavioral toxicology* or *psychological toxicology,* or simply *neurotoxicology,* but these distinctions probably have more to do with the profession of the researchers than objective differences in investigation. The researchers involved in the field come from diverse (and sometimes divergent) specialties, including neurology, neuropsychology, occupational medicine, psychiatry, public health administration, epidemiology, industry and pharmacology. Moreover, these researchers may conduct their studies *in vitro* or *in vivo;* all neurotoxin research, from the cellular to the sociological, can be considered branches of this field. Regardless of the name, this area of specialization explores clinical and theoretical aspects of "changes in behavior under the influence of certain natural or artificial substances" (Richelle, 1983, p.127). When additional inferences are made about the relationship between substance-induced behavior change and nervous system alteration or toxicity, the term "neurobehavioral" toxicology is often employed.

What's in a name? This book has been titled "Neuropsychological Toxicology", not because yet another name for this field is required, but rather to emphasize the relevance of neuropsychological theory and testing procedures to the understanding of overt and subclinical effects of toxins on the nervous system. For psychologists at least, it seems reasonable to substitute the more comprehensive "neuropsychological" in place of "neurobehavioral". "Neuro*behavioral*" connotes the restrictive limitations of directly observable action in an organism or the stimulus–response theories of Pavlov or Skinner. "Neuro*psychological*" recognizes the more global and holistic aspects of the human psyche; a domain that includes the

1

concepts of cognition, affect, *and* behavior, both subjectively experienced and objectively measurable. The psychology of the human organism, its cortical functions and objectively measured correlates of those functions, are well within the purview of clinical neuropsychology. So too is the assessment of toxic damage to those structures and functions. What is in a name, therefore, is the identification of a field where neuropsychological researchers may have a unique and valuable contribution; assessing observable alterations in human cognition, affect and behavior when the nervous system is exposed to toxic substances. To call that branch of neuropsychology concerned with toxic substances "neuropsychological toxicology" is to gather previously unrelated areas of investigation under a single conceptual banner. Thus, neuropsychological evaluation of alcohol, drugs (abused and prescription), toxic industrial substances, pesticides and as yet unresearched substances like biotoxins, allergens, etc. can all be considered part of the same field.

The value of the neuropsychologist's contribution to the assessment of neurotoxicity has been concisely summarized by Lezak (1984), who states that the "neuropsychological assessment probably offers the most sensitive means of examining the effects of toxic exposure, of monitoring for industrial safety, and of understanding the complaints and psychosocial problems of persons exposed to these toxins" (Lezak, 1984, p. 28).

DEFINITION OF NEUROPSYCHOLOGY

To appreciate Lezak's enthusiastic endorsement of neuropsychological methods in toxicological investigations, a brief definition and synopsis of modern neuropsychology may be helpful. Developed as a clinical science within the past 60 years, neuropsychology is the study of the relationship between brain structure and function. It attempts to understand patterns and variations of cognition, emotion and behavior in the context of cortical and subcortical neuroanatomical organization. Clinical applications of neuropsychology more specifically investigate the effects of brain dysfunction or damage on these same psychological and behavioral processes.

MODERN NEUROPSYCHOLOGICAL HISTORY AND THEORY

The major, theoretical precursors of modern neuropsychology were *localization* theory and *equipotentiality*, both formulated during the eighteenth and nineteenth centuries. There was spirited and occasionally acrimonious debate between those who believed the brain to be composed of a series of unconnected and arbitrarily assigned traits (localizationists or "faculty" psychologists) and those who understood the brain to function as a single unit (equipotentialists). Reductionistic arguments on both sides limited the utility of each theory. For example, simplistic application of localization theory produced "phrenology", a pseudoscience which assumed the brain to be composed of many "organs" or localized traits which could be palpated on the skull in a process called "cranioscopy" (Walsh, 1978). Popular books were published which instructed naive students how to recognize the ideal husband, wife, criminal type, etc. by the shape and the bumps on their skulls.

The actual term "neuropsychology" was apparently first used by Sir William Osler in 1913 at the opening address of the Phipps Psychiatric Clinic of Johns Hopkins Hospital (Bruce, 1985). However, modern neuropsychological understanding of brain–behavior relationships was dependent upon the development of an alternative to strict localization and equipotentiality. The English neurologist J. Hughlings Jackson created such a theory in the late nineteenth century, though his works were not published in the United States until 1958 (Golden, 1978). Jackson proposed that higher mental functions were not indivisible abilities but were themselves composed of more basic skills. The ability to write, for example, depends not on a "writing center" but rather a combination of interrelated functions including fine motor coordination, visual perception, spatial localization, kinesthetic–proprioceptive feedback,etc.

Jackson's theory combined the essential features of localization and equipotentiality. Brain function was considered to be a collection of basic abilities, and therefore localizable. However, since higher forms of behavior require these simple functions to interrelate, any higher cognitive ability must be considered as the product of the whole brain.

Alexander Luria has been the most recent and well-known proponent of a "dynamic localization of function model," where

> any human mental activity is a complex functional system effected through a combination of concertedly working brain structures, each of which makes its own contribution to the functional system as a whole (Luria, 1973, p 38).

Luria's functional systems are ever-changing interaction patterns of the basic brain functions necessary to complete a given behavior. With his extensive experience assessing the cognition, affect and behavior of brain-injured patients, Luria extended Jackson's ideas by positing the existence of "primary, secondary and tertiary" areas of interaction. Primary areas work as analyzers of rudimentary sensory and perceptual input; secondary areas perform integration and elaboration of the input from primary areas; and tertiary areas, in turn, integrate the output of secondary areas, resulting in the most complex forms of cognition (e.g. abstract reasoning).

The assessment of damage or recovery of these processing systems is accomplished by investigating patients' performance on standardized neuropsychological tests. While most modern neuropsychologists subscribe to a theory of brain–behavior relationships similar to Luria's, different strategies of assessment have been developed to elucidate these relationships.

NEUROPSYCHOLOGICAL TESTING STRATEGIES

During the past four decades several different neuropsychological testing strategies have evolved:

1. Standardized batteries

These are single tests or groups of tests for which norms and impairment indices are available to compare a patient against ipsative or population norms. These tests (e.g. the Halstead–Reitan, the Luria–Nebraska) typically attempt global assessments of neuropsychological functions, although there are also standardized batteries for more specialized functions (e.g. motor steadiness batteries).

2. Flexible batteries

This class includes standardized neuropsychological tests developed separately by various researchers but collected and presented together as part of a larger examination. Some flexible batteries provide global assessment of neuropsychological functions (e.g. Wysocki and Sweet, 1985). Others could be compiled to assess more specific functions or disorders. For example, a "dementia battery" might load more heavily on memory tests, while a battery for cerebrovascular disorders would more extensively tap language functioning.

3. "Contextual" and flexible test selection approaches

These may be somewhat less methodologically rigorous than the foregoing approaches. The advocate of flexible test selection chooses among tests to answer specific referral questions, and proposes that subjective "contextual" data obtained by the examiner are at least as important as, if not more important than, the statistical properties of the exam. The approach is valuable for its emphasis on understanding neuropsychological functions in the context of the patients' medical history, motivation for testing, educational level etc. (e.g. Walsh, 1985).

Conclusion

These clinical approaches, combined with ongoing theoretical advances in understanding neuroanatomical–behavioral relationships, have enabled neuropsychologists to compile valuable clinical information about the nature of damage and recovery of brain injuries, including open- and closed-head injury, cerebrovascular disorders, dementias and a variety of other impairments of brain function. The use of similar methods to trace the effects of nervous system poisons is only the most recent extension of this new, generative field.

HISTORICAL VIEWS OF NEUROTOXICITY

The recency of neuropsychology's entry into toxicological research parallels perhaps the very late development of a science of industrial medicine. In fact, the history of neurotoxic exposure, prevention and research has until recently been the province of informal literary anecdote coupled with formal medical neglect.

Anecdotal accounts of neurotoxins and their effects have been chronicled for centuries. Lead, perhaps the oldest human neurotoxin, was a subtle and ubiquitous poison for the Romans, who employed lead oxide to sweeten and preserve wine, cider and fruit juices (Fein *et al.*, 1983, p. 1189). In 1535, Anglicus Bartholomaeus wrote of mercury, "The smoke thereof is most grevous to men that ben therby. For it bredeth the palsey, and quaking, shakynge, neshynge (softening) of the synewes" (Bartholomaeus, cited in Goldwater, 1972, p. 91). Carbon disulfide, a solvent used in the cold vulcanization of rubber, has citations in the medical literature since 1856 (Wood, 1981).

Unfortunately, this long anecdotal chronology did not have the effect of increasing medical knowledge or curiosity, and even as late as the beginning of the twentieth century industrial medicine "did not exist" in the United States (Hamilton, 1985). Myths were allowed to stand without question, and body cleanliness was emphasized above environmental management of fumes and dust.

> I remember the head surgeon of a great Colorado smelting company saying in a public meeting: 'It is not the lead a man absorbs during his work that poisons him but what he carries home on his skin' (Hamilton, 1985, pp. 3–4).

It took detailed studies of lead's respiratory absorption (Aub *et al.*, 1926) to finally convince American physicians that workers required better advice than to "scrub their nails carefully" for protection against metallic poisoning (Hamilton, 1985, p.4).

Other misconceptions have remained until relatively recently. For example, medical disease models of symptomatology carried over from the previous century led researchers to assume that neurotoxins exerted their effects in an "all or none" fashion. That there was such a thing as "subclinical" toxicity did not become apparent until the Minamata methyl mercury poisoning incident in 1956 (Fein *et al.*, 1983) in which asymptomatic individuals contaminated by the output of a vinyl acetate plant continued to die from mercury poisoning long after the discharge was halted. Thus, these individuals were only *apparently* asymptomatic. Subtle signs of poisoning and continuing neuronal changes, which were initially invisible, continued to progress until they reached clinical threshold, without additional exposure (Fein *et al.*, 1983). Tragic events like Minamata redefined the domain of inquiry in industrial medicine, highlighting the need for research and tests of subclinical neurotoxicity.

TYPES OF NEUROTOXIC DAMAGE

Baker (1983 a;b) divides the damage caused by neurotoxic substances into three categories:

1. *Peripheral nervous system effects* including segmental demyelination and axonal degeneration;
2. *Central nervous system effects* caused by either direct toxic effects to CNS neurons, or disruption of neurotransmitter metabolism; and
3. *Combined CNS and PNS effects* with degenerative neuropathology in the central and peripheral nervous system.

Neuropsychologists will be sensitive to additional factors that cause impaired performance on neuropsychological tests. For example, *indirect structural* damage to the nervous system may occur via other organ systems, e.g. hepatic and vascular abnormalities. *Indirect reactive* components of affect and personality may substantially influence neuropsychological performance. The constellation of variables capable of affecting neuropsychological performance are further discussed in Chapter 2 (Evaluation of Neurotoxic Syndromes).

TESTING FOR SUBCLINICAL NEUROTOXIC EFFECTS

Diagnostic techniques that are currently available to monitor neurotoxic exposure can be divided into two basic categories: "internal dose indicators", which assay the chemical agents and their metabolites in the organism, and "indicators of effect", that "clarify the interactions between the external agent and the recipient organism" (Foa, 1982, p. 173). Since the "indicators of effect" provide greater information about the early (subclinical) effects of neurotoxic substances, than do internal dose levels (Lezak, 1984; Gamberale and Kjellberg, 1982; Foa, 1982) neuropsychological assessment may be considered a first-line diagnostic tool in the assessment of exposed patients.

THE DEVELOPMENT OF NEUROPSYCHOLOGICAL TOXICOLOGY

Psychological investigations of neurotoxic damage date back only about 40 years (Lindström, 1982). These studies detailing neurotoxic syndromes began with descriptive investigations of carbon disulfide (Raneletti, 1931; Pennsylvania Department of Labor, 1938). Research more clearly identifiable as neuropsychological in nature did not begin until about 1970.

Neuropsychological toxicology has had a very low profile in the United States scientific community, and is also little known among the general public, legislators and union representatives. A 1984 report sponsored by the National Toxicology Program reported that it was remarkable how few chemicals had been subjected to systematic behavioral analysis (Buckholtz and Panem, 1986). The same report identified the great need for neurobehavioral toxicology assessment of pesticides, cosmetics, food additives and other commercial chemicals. Landrigan *et al.* (1980) concur:

> More than 1000 new compounds are developed each year and are added to the approximately 40,000 chemicals and 2,000,000 mixtures, formulations and blends already in industrial use. Too frequently the neurotoxic or other toxic properties of new compounds have not been recognized before their introduction to the market" (Landrigan *et al.*, 1980, p. 43).

Other countries are somewhat ahead of the United States in recognizing the importance of neurotoxicity analyses. European and Scandinavian countries lead the U.S. in basic research, clinical application and legislative support of neuropsychological toxicity investigations. There are currently only about 700 occupational health researchers *including* neuropsychologists active in the United States, a country with over 60 million workers. These figures should be contrasted with those of Finland, a country with only 2 million people but which employs 500 occupational health researchers (Anderson, 1982). There are probably less than 50 full-time research and clinical practitioners of human neuropsychological toxicology in the United States at this time.

It is not surprising, given these statistics, to note that most of the basic neuropsychological research performed in the past two decades has been performed in European and Scandinavian countries and published there as well. In addition, Scandinavian countries have recognized the neuropsychological effects of one class of neurotoxic poisoning, "organic solvent syndrome", as a disability claim for over 30 years. Full compensation is awarded for symptoms of memory loss, lowered concentration and loss of initiative as a consequence of chronic solvent exposure. "In [the United States], we're still debating whether [solvent syndrome] exists" (Wood, in

Fisher, 1985, p. 14). Undoubtedly, differences in legal systems, insurance and employee health policies have contributed to such differences.

Fortunately, an increasing amount of attention is being paid worldwide to neurotoxicity and the psychological effects of toxic substances. Several journals now routinely publish neuropsychological investigations of toxic substance exposure. These include the *Scandinavian Journal of Work Environment and Health*, the *American Journal of Industrial Medicine*, the *British Journal of Industrial Medicine*, the *International Archives of Occupational and Environmental Health, Neurotoxicology and Teratology, NeuroToxicology*, and the *Journal of Occupational Medicine*. Occasional articles can be found in other related journals, including the *International Journal of Clinical Neuropsychology, Acta Neurologica Scandinavica, Acta Psychiatrica Scandinavica, Clinical Toxicology*, the *Journal of Neurology, Neurosurgery and Psychiatry* and others. It can be hoped that the other United States neuropsychological journals, including the *Journal of Clinical and Experimental Neuropsychology*, and the recently inaugurated *Archives of Clinical Neuropsychology*, will provide future forums for neuropsychological investigations of neurotoxic sequelae.

LEGISLATIVE ISSUES AND NEUROPSYCHOLOGICAL TOXICOLOGY

Individual issues

Neurotoxic syndromes are often closely tied to ongoing legal debates. Recent controversy about whether a pregnant woman should be held liable for drug abuse and subsequent harm to the fetus is just one example as to how voluntary individual exposure to neurotoxic materials may intersect with legislation (Morris and Sonderegger, 1984). Involuntary prescription drug use and industrial exposure to neurotoxic substances are two other areas where neuropsychological assessment and legal policy may intersect.

Environmental legislation

Legal and regulatory policy has directly encouraged neuropsychological research. A major spur to United States research interest in the psychological aspects of neurotoxic exposure was the 1970 Occupational Safety and Health Act, which attempted to "assure, so far as possible, every working man and woman in the nation safe and healthful working conditions" (Taft, 1974, p.8). The act further mandated NIOSH to "Conduct research into the motivational and behavioral factors relating to the field of occupational safety and health" (Fairchild, 1974, p.3).

Other recently enacted environmental legislation has further stimulated the field of neuropsychological toxicology in the United States by calling for regulation of toxic materials and the evaluation of toxicity. These acts include the Clean Air Act of 1970, the Resource Conservation and Recovery Act which regulates land disposal of toxic materials; the Marine Protection Research and Sanctuaries Act, which does the same for marine disposal of toxic wastes; the Clean Water Act and Safe Drinking Water Act; the Federal Insecticide, Fungicide and Rodenticide Act, and especially the Toxic Substances Control Act of 1976 (TOSCA); all implicitly or explicitly mandate research to support the development of safety regulations (Reiter, 1985).

Currently, however, such mandates do not customarily include neuropsychological assessment. In fact, with the exception of organophosphate pesticides, there are no requirements for routine neurotoxic assessments *of any kind* in the development of new environmental regulations (Buckholtz and Panem, 1986). Present-day statutes require special justifications to conduct such investigations, and there are no clear criteria for determining how behaviors or functions should be studied (Buckholtz and Panem, 1986).

While regulatory agencies have been somewhat slow to elicit neurotoxicity data, public health researchers are beginning to recognize neurotoxic syndromes as diagnostic entities, and to realize their importance to the quality of life. A background paper at a conference on long-term environmental research and development concludes:

> Even small degrees of central nervous system dysfunction are not for moral, ethical, and health reasons to be tolerated. The loss of five points in I.Q., fatigability, irritability, or lethargy or slowed reaction times are significant losses. These are areas of human function that make life enjoyable and worth living (Robins, Cullen, and Welch, 1985; cited in Buckholtz and Panem, 1986).

There are many potential places where neuropsychological research could interface with regulation. Neuropsychological data collection could occur at either the beginning or the end of the long chain of scientific and legislative actions that culminate in regulation. In the realm of industrial toxins, for example, individual neuropsychological studies could be used by the American Conference of Governmental Industrial Hygienists (ACGIH), the primary United States source of industrial exposure limit recommendations. A subcommittee of ACGIH representatives from government, academia, the National Institute for Occupational Safety and Health (NIOSH) and labor could incorporate the findings of neuropsychological research to influence their recommendations on toxic exposure effects (Anger, 1984).

ACGIH could then include neuropsychological data in its recommendations for what are called "threshold limit values".

Threshold limit values

Threshold Limit Values (TLVs) are an estimate of allowable toxic exposure level. Anger (1984) describes three types of TLV, of which the first and second are probably most relevant to neuropsychological research.

1. The TLV–TWA (time weighted average) which is the limit of exposure for an 8-hour day / 40-hour work week.
2. The TLV–STEL (short-term exposure limit) which is the highest level that should be not exceeded for a specified time limit (a 15-minute time weighted average as of 1982).
3. The TLV–C or "ceiling" concentration that must *never* be exceeded, even for an instant.

While ACGIH's recommendations are voluntary, when OSHA (the Occupational Safety and Health Administration) adopts ACGIH's regulations they can be considered as a basis for federal regulation (Anger, 1984). Regulations, once in place, could serve as stimuli for further neuropsychological investigations.

Advantages of neuropsychological toxicology assessment

Neuropsychological measures may be especially useful in providing the research validation required by TOSCA and other environmental regulations. The use of neuropsychological measures has several advantages in this regard:

1. Concurrent and predictive validity

It is commonly accepted that neurotoxic exposure symptoms may be validly assessed with psychometric techniques, and that neurotoxic symptoms may occur prior to the occurrence of other objective neurological sequelae (Gamberale and Kjellberg, 1982). Further, these disruptions may not be detectable *without* neuropsychological methods since subjects may develop alternative processing strategies to compensate for acquired neuropsychological deficits. Since neuropsychological tests are more demanding, and can isolate elementary components of cognition and behavior, obfuscating effects of compensation can be minimized and specific impairments can be measured.

2. Safety

Neuropsychological tests are safe and non-invasive. There is no risk to the participant. Unlike certain medical tests, neuropsychological evaluation is neither painful (i.e. nerve conduction studies), nor potentially dangerous (i.e.

CT with infusion). Tests may also be repeated to provide longitudinal data without harm to the patient. As Weiss (1983) succinctly states, "subjects' livers need not be fed into a blender to quantify damage" (p. 1174).

3. Comprehensiveness and flexibility

Neuropsychological evaluations can assess a wide variety of cortical and subcortical functions; tests may be employed to assess both global and local brain abnormalities. The neuropsychologist may choose among an array of assessment devices, from those which isolate specific nerve, muscle and cortical connections (e.g. Finger Tapping) to those designed to measure overall intellectual, neuropsychological or emotional abilities (e.g. Wechsler Intelligence Scales; Halstead–Reitan Neuropsychological Battery, Minnesota Multiphasic Personality Inventory).

4. Objectivity and replicability

Unlike more subjective forms of mental status examinations, neuropsychological tests can be made reliable; allowing for precise replication within or across individuals or patient populations. Standardization of patient variables, test administration, content and scoring allows replication and validation attempts by other researchers unconnected with the original study.

5. Cost

Compared to medical and neurological workups, neuropsychological measures generally do not require elaborate or expensive facilities to provide assessment results. Professional time spent in the assessment rather than equipment is the main cost. There are usually no special facilities needed; examination is not limited to the laboratory, but requires only a single, relatively quiet room without distractions.

6. Portability and convenience

A valid and complete neuropsychological test battery for neurotoxic assessment can be carried in one or two small suitcases. Recent trends in computerized neuropsychological toxicology batteries (e.g. Baker *et al.*, 1985a) may eventually result in further convenience by automating test administration, data acquisition and scoring procedures.

7. Complementarity

Neuropsychological evaluation can provide complementary information to conventional medical screens. For example, abnormal nerve conduction studies can be quantified in terms of behavioral dysfunction by employing neuropsychological tests of sensorimotor abilities. The meaning of CT-scanned cortical atrophy for the patient's real-world functioning can be quantified using neuropsychological measures that provide a comprehensive picture of cognitive, behavioral and emotional status.

8. Early warning

Because neuropsychological methods have the sensitivity to detect very early neurotoxic dysfunction, early testing can prevent lasting brain damage. In addition, neuropsychological examination could serve to identify workers already impaired from toxic exposure and suggest transfer to less hazardous employment.

UNSOLVED CHALLENGES IN ASSESSMENT OF NEUROTOXIC SYNDROMES

There are some unique complications inherent to the neuropsychological evaluation of patients with possible neurotoxic syndromes. Several of these difficulties are related to diagnostic limitations in the field of neurotoxicology itself, and are thereby transferred onto the neuropsychologist whose service is requested.

Problems inherited by the neuropsychologist

1. Neurophysiological and neurochemical uncertainties

There are few well-developed neurochemical or neurophysiological models of neurotoxic effects. While the neurotoxic effects of certain substances are fairly clear (e.g., *n*-hexane), these substances are the exception. Very little definitive research, especially regarding central nervous system toxicity patterns, is available to guide the neuropsychologist in test selection or localization.

2. Application and generalizability of animal models

Current research with animal subjects, while providing information unobtainable from human subjects (e.g. lethal dose estimates, autopsy results) suffers from limitations when extrapolated to human effects. First, animal models of neurotoxicity have not generally addressed behaviors of interest to human neuropsychological toxicologists, and have typically been limited to reinforcement paradigms. Functions often found to be impaired in humans — including vigilance, reaction time, complex psychomotor skills, memory and emotion — do not yet have testable analogues in animal research (Cranmer and Golberg, 1986).

A second problem in the use of animal models is the difficulty generalizing from lower mammals to humans. Species-specific effects may mislead researchers who wish to extrapolate human neurotoxic sequelae from the results of animal tests. Primate experimentation might allow better extrapolation to human effects; however, such studies have rarely been performed.

3. Exposure ambiguities

In industrial settings at least, individual exposure data are often difficult to obtain. Often, measurements are simply not available. When single-exposure measurements are taken in the environment these measures may not always reflect exactly where the individual has worked, or the variations of exposure intensity at any single site.

Thus, the incomplete state of the art in neurophysiological, neurochemical and relevant animal models of neurotoxicity, may come to haunt the neuropsychologist interested in human exposure effects by increasing diagnostic uncertainty. In addition, neuropsychological diagnosis of toxic exposure is complicated by the following factors.

Challenges to the neuropsychologist

Acute versus chronic effects

Since an exposed individual may present for evaluation while remaining in contact with noxious substances at the workplace, acute and chronic effects may require partialing out. The task of neuropsychological evaluation is correspondingly more difficult than when the injury is discrete and localizable in time.

Difficulties assessing premorbid function

Assessing neurotoxic damage to the nervous system may be difficult in some neurotoxic exposure victims because of job selection factors. Patients who are hired for unskilled factory employment may show premorbid deficiencies in education or other areas. Test interpretation may suffer without adequate records of such premorbid difficulties. Since many factory employees perform well-learned repetitive tasks that do not require high levels of verbal ability, memory or fine motor dexterity, low functioning on screening measures of neuropsychological toxicity may reflect premorbid abilities rather than recent, job-related impairment.

In our clinical experience it has been an unfortunate fact that the workers with the poorest premorbid educational or intellectual functioning are often the same individuals who suffer the most severe neurotoxic exposure. Job market pressures force unskilled or marginally skilled individuals into high-risk occupations; performing menial occupations in small, unregulated cottage industries (e.g. battery or metal reprocessing operations). When these individuals are finally evaluated for neurotoxicity, the neuropsychologist may find differential diagnosis particularly difficult.

Paucity of relevant test norms

Further complicating diagnosis is the lack of neuropsychological test norms for individuals most likely to have been exposed to neurotoxic substances. Few neuropsychological tests have been normed on the most common high-risk groups: factory employees and drug-abusing populations (i.e. glue-sniffers). While there is some generalization possible for tests normed on individuals with comparable educational levels, more appropriate validation on relevant population groups would be preferable.

Very low premorbid educational levels or premorbid IQ results can invalidate interpretation of current neuropsychological tests since such tests may assume average educational or intellectual abilities.

Lack of corroborating medical evidence

The ability of neuropsychological evaluation to provide early warning of toxicity effects necessarily implies that such data will not always be supported by medical test results. The neuropsychologist cannot always depend upon conventional medical diagnostic procedures (e.g. blood levels, CT and EEG) to validate neuropsychologically observable but medically subclinical impairments.

Differential diagnosis

The neuropsychological toxicologist will probably experience frequent diagnostic ambiguities in terms of classifying symptoms on the continuum of purely physical to mixed physical and psychological to purely psychological. For example, patients with acute industrial solvent exposure may suffer from cerebral atrophy and other structural brain damage (Hane and Ekberg, 1984, p. 8). They may also present with secondary impairments in the ability to cope with stress because of neurologically-based fatigue, headache, decreased nerve conduction, etc. and so display maladaptive reactions to normal stressors (Fig I.1). Fear of brain damage itself may be a significant stressor, irrespective of actual toxic exposure. Psychogenic illness can occur without actual neurotoxic exposure if an individual or group simply believes it has been exposed to neurotoxins (Murphy and Colligan, 1979). Finally, exposure to human neurotoxins may provide predisposed individuals with opportunities to malinger or otherwise implement strategies of secondary gain.

NEUROPSYCHOLOGICAL INVESTIGATIONS OF TOXIC SUBSTANCES — OTHER ISSUES

Economic consequences

Neuropsychological methods of research and assessment have been implemented more slowly in the United States than in European and

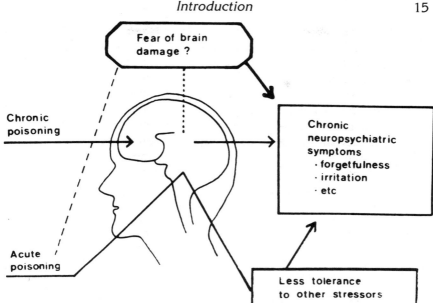

FIGURE I.1. Differential diagnostic possibilities in neurotoxicity evaluations. (Reprinted, by permission of the publisher, from Hane, M. and Ekberg, K. (1984). Current research in behavioral toxicology. *Scandinavian Journal of Work, Environment and Health,* Suppl. 1, 8–9.)

Scandinavian countries. The reasons for American caution in entering the field may be as much sociopolitical as scientific. Neuropsychological toxicology cannot be considered a "value-free" scientific enterprise. Definitive research involving nervous system effects of workplace toxins could potentially generate profound economic consequences for industry and insurance companies. First, new and stricter regulations based on such research could mandate costly reengineering and renovation of the physical plant. Second, the expense of implementing preventive medical care may prove prohibitive. Costs could be substantial, in terms of worker/management education as well as in monies allotted for testing and treatment. If not subsidized in some manner, the expense of such outlays might discourage employers from vigilant monitoring of chemical exposure. Smaller companies could be placed in the position of choosing between safety and solvency — a position that workers may find difficult to resolve.

Legal consequences

A third costly outcome of neuropsychological toxicology studies in our litigious society could be expensive legal judgments awarded for neurotoxic exposure. With 20 million American employees exposed to neurotoxic substances in the workplace (Anderson, 1982), legally and scientifically valid neuropsychological methods could stimulate litigation that results in numerous and extremely large damage awards.

Political impediments

Political as well as economic factors may influence the development of neuropsychological research. For example, recent executive branch decrees have increased the power of the Office of Management and Budget to limit toxic chemical regulations to those which meet stringent "cost–benefit" criteria. There is concern that the Environmental Protection Agency and OSHA under the Reagan administration have shown less motivation to implement more stringent exposure standards (Anderson, 1982). These factors, in turn, probably dampen the development of new regulations.

Limited numbers of researchers and clinical practitioners

Another limiting factor is simply the short supply of skilled professionals who could conduct research and administer clinical service. These professionals include physicians and neuropsychologists skilled in the biological and behavioral monitoring and treatment of neurotoxic illness, and health care workers able to work as a team with employees for prevention and detection of neurotoxic exposure. Unfortunately, previously cited limitations in the number of available occupational health researchers suggest that clinical demand far outstrips the supply. Increased support for training in occupational medicine and neuropsychological toxicology would be a prerequisite; however, graduate-level training in neuropsychological toxicology, at least, is very difficult to find.

Barriers to worker and patient acceptance

Finally, even if the political, professional and economic repercussions of neuropsychological toxicology research could be resolved, it is far from clear that basic research or neuropsychological monitoring will be particularly welcomed in the workplace. Confidentiality and privacy may not be easily maintained, and assurances may be viewed with skepticism in an adversarial labor–management climate. Many workers might perceive occupational health monitoring as a harmful intrusion into privacy, particularly since tests which screen for workplace toxins are also sensitive to effects of alcohol or drugs. An employee who is frequently monitored may be more quickly seen to demonstrate subclinical impairment, whether from neurotoxic exposure, alcohol abuse, psychological difficulties, aging or unrelated illness. Without proper safeguards it is conceivable that positive findings on biological or behavioral tests could result in temporary or permanent loss of employment.

THE ROLE OF AND NEED FOR NEUROPSYCHOLOGY IN TOXIC SUBSTANCE RESEARCH

Neuropsychological investigation of toxic exposures occurs within a large, overlapping, multidisciplinary context. Neuropsychologists and other professionals who examine patients with toxic exposure histories will find themselves cooperating with specialists in medicine, psychology, labor, management, epidemiology, government and the law; each investigating relevant aspects of nervous system and behavior alterations induced by exposure to poisonous or toxic substances.

Neuropsychologists who become occupational health advocates may also find themselves embroiled in legal, political, medical and scientific controversies. However, those clinicians and researchers who accept the multidisciplinary nature and impact of this somewhat controversial and exciting specialty may rightly consider themselves to be pioneers in a new form of clinical psychology. With special skills in psychometrics, research design and the identification of brain–behavior relationships, the neuropsychologist is in a unique position relative to other mental health professionals to contribute to industry and the private sector.

Currently, few neuropsychologists are trained to provide such contributions, but even if every practicing neuropsychologist were familiar with toxicology research, their combined numbers would be far too small to handle the sheer magnitude of the investigatory task. Human beings are exposed to over 53,000 different substances, including pesticides, drugs, food additives, cosmetics, commercial and industrial substances (Fisher, 1985). OSHA (Occupational Health and Safety Administration) sets standards for only 588 of these, and only 167 of these have been regulated for their neurotoxic effects. It is far from clear, however, that the remaining chemicals are free from risk, since a random sample of 100 chemicals revealed that almost none had actually been tested for neurotoxicity before being released on the market (Fisher, 1985).

The substances for which the American Conference of Governmental Industrial Hygienists (ACGIH) has recommended threshold limit values in the workplace, because of their neurotoxic potential, are listed in Table I. 1.

Since prescription drugs, many abused drugs and substances whose neurotoxicity is presently being researched (e.g. styrene, other pesticides) are *not* included, this list must be considered an *under*estimate of the substances presenting immediate neurotoxic danger. Unfortunately, available research lags far behind the need to assess these substances. The effects of toxic substances on the human nervous system are still largely unknown. Those

TABLE I.1. Chemicals for which ACGIH TLVs were set because of neurotoxicity. (Reprinted, by permission of Pergamon Journals, Ltd., from Anger, W. K. (1984). Neurobehavioral testing of chemicals: Impact on recommended standards. *Neurobehavioral Toxicology and Teratology,* **6**, 149–151.)

Abate (R)
Acetonitrile (methyl cyanide)
Acrylamide
Aldrin
Allyl alcohol
Anisidine
Barium
Baygon ®
Benzyl chloride
Bromine pentafluoride
n-Butyl alcohol
sec-Butyl alcohol
tert-Butyl alcohol
p-t-Butyltoluene
Camphor
Carbaryl
Carbon disulfide
Carbon tetrachloride
Chlordane
Chlorinated camphene (60%) (Toxaphene)
Chlorine trifluoride
Chlorobenzene
Chlorobromomethane
Chlorpyrifos (Dursban®)
Cobalt hydrocarbonyl
Cumene
Cyanides
Cyclohexylamine
Cyclopentadiene
Cyclopentane
Decaborane
Demeton
Diazinon
Diborane
Dibrom
Dibutyl phosphate
Dichloroacetylene
p-Dichlorobenzene
Dichlorodiphenyl-trichloroethane
2,4- Dichlorophenoxy-acetic acid (2,4-D)
Dichlorotetrafluoro-ethane (Freon 114)
Dichlorvos (DDVP)
Dicrotophos
Dieldrin
Diethanolamine
Diethylamine
Diethyl ketone

Ethyl amyl ketone
Ethyl bromide
Ethyl butyl ketone
Ethylene chlorohydrin
Ethylene glycol dinitrate
Ethyl ether (diethyl ether)
Ethyl mercaptan
N-Ethylmorpholine
Fenamiphos
Fensulfothion
Fenthion
Halothane
n-Heptane
Hexachlorocyclo pentadiene
Hexachloroethane
n-Hexane
Hydrogen cyanide
Hydrogen selenide
Hydrogen sulfide
Hydroguinone
Iron pentacarbonyl
Isoamyl alcohol
Isophorone
N-Isopropylaniline
Isopropyl ether
Lead, inorganic
Lindane
Manganese (and compounds)
Manganese cyclopenta-dienyl tricarbonyl (MCT)
Manganese tetroxide
Mercury, alkyl
Mercury, not alkyl
Mesityl oxide
Methomyl
4-Methoxyphenol
Methyl acetate
Methylacrylonitrile
Methyl alcohol (Methanol)
Methyl bromide (monobromomethane)
Methyl n-butyl ketone (MBK)
Methyl chloride (monochloromethane)
Methyl chloroform
Methylcyclohexane
o-Methylcyclohexanone
2-Methylcyclopentane-dienyl manganese tricarbonyl (Cl-2)

Naphthalene
Nickel carbonyl
Nitromethane
2-Nitropropane
Osmium tetroxide
Parathion
Pentaborane
Pentane
Perchloroethylene (tetrachloroethylene)
Phenyl ether
Phenyl mercaptan
Phenylphosphine
Phorate
Phosdrin
Phosphorus oxychloride
1 Propanol (n-propyl alcohol)
Propargyl alcohol
1,2-Propylene glycol dinitrate
Propylene glycol monoethyl ether
Propylene oxide
Pyridine
Quinone
Ronnel
Selenium (and compounds)
Selenium hexafluoride
Stoddard solvent (mineral spirits; white spirits)
Strychnine
Sulfuryl fluoride
Sulprofos
Tellurium
1,1,2,2-Tetra-chloroethane (acetylene tetrachloride)
Tetraethyl dithionopyrophosphate (TEDP)
Tetraethyl lead (TEL)
Tetraethyl pyro-phosphate (TEPP)
Tetrahydrofuran (THF)
Tetramethyl lead (TML)
Tetramethyl succinonitrile (TMSN)
Tetranitromethane
Tetryl
Thallium
Tin, organic

Difluordibromomethane (Freon 12B2)
Diisopropylamine
Dimethylanaline
1,1-Dimethylhydrazine
Dioxathion
Dipropylene glycol methyl ether (DPGME)
Diquat
Disulfoton
Dyfonate
EPN
Ethanolamine
Ethion

Methyl demeton
Methylene chloride
Methyl ethyl ketone (MEK; 2-Butanone)
Methyl mercaptan
Methyl parathion
Methyl propyl ketone
Methyl silicate
Metrizabin
Monocrotophos
Morpholine
Naphtha

Toluene
Tributyl phosphate
Trichloroacetic acid (TCA)
1,1,2-Trichloroethane (vinyl trichloride)
Trichloroethylene
Tricyclohexyltin hydrochloride
Trimethyl benzene
Trimethyl phosphite
Triorthocresyl phospate
Triphenyl phosphate (TPP)
Xylene

who survey the existing literature should therefore not be surprised by the number of questions which remain unanswered at each point on the continuum of neurotoxicological investigation, from the neuronal and neurochemical to the neuropsychological. Even the effects of lead (Pb), the most well-known metallic neurotoxin, have not been completely evaluated; only the peripheral nervous system effects have been adequately documented (Krigman, Bouldin and Mushak, 1980). Other metals, less commonly known to be neurotoxic (e.g. gold and manganese), have *no* neuropsychological studies available of their effects.

The situation is similar for other neurotoxins, including solvents and pesticides. Much basic research remains to be done to elucidate physiological and psychological nervous system function disturbances from these substances. Biological neurotoxins (e.g. animal venoms, plant poisons) are even less well researched, with no neuropsychological studies of their effects available.

Numbers of neurotoxic substances and exposed individuals

The task of providing such basic research is an enormous one. Neurotoxic substances pervade our environment. The number of potentially neurotoxic chemicals in the workplace has been estimated as high as 850 (*Chemical Regulation Reporter*, 1986). Even this large estimate may not include neurotoxic prescription medications or abused drugs. Estimates of individuals exposed in their jobs to neurotoxic substances have ranged from a conservative 7.7 million (*Chemical Regulation Reporter*, 1986), to over 20 million (Anderson, 1982). Voluntary solvent inhalant abuse appears to be equally prevalent with estimates of up to 18.7% United States high school seniors having tried inhalants at least once (Giovacchini, 1985). The total number of individuals exposed to neurotoxic medications, and the total number of adults and children who voluntarily abuse other neurotoxic

TABLE I.2. Subjects at risk for neurotoxic exposure at the workplace

NEUROTOXIC SUBSTANCE	ESTIMATED NUMBERS AT RISK
Alcohols (industrial)	3,851,000
Aliphatic hydrocarbons	2,776,000
Aromatic hydrocarbons	3,611,000
Cadmium	1,400,000
Carbon disulfide	24,000
Carbon tetrachloride	1,379,000
Dichloromethane	2,175,000
Lead	
(In children — from inorganic paint exposure)	45,000
Lead oxides	1,300,000
Lead carbonate	183,000
Lead naphthenate	1,280,000
Lead acetate	103,000
Metallic lead	1,394,000
Manganese	41,000
Mercury	
Mercury sulfide	8,900
Mercuric nitrate	10,100
Mercuric chloride	51,000
Metallic mercury	24,000
Organic mercury	280,000
N-hexane	764,000
Perchloroethylene (tetrachloroethylene)	1,596,000
Styrene	329,000
Thallium	853,000
Toluene	4,800,000
Trichloroethylene	3,600,000
Styrene	329,000
Xylene	140,000
Pesticides (1979)	1,275,000
Rubber solvents (benzene and lacquer diluent)	600,000

substances, have never been tallied. There are some exposure data compiled for industrial workers. Table I.2 has been compiled from various Center for Disease Control documents and other sources (e.g. Anderson, 1982) and suggests the magnitude of neurotoxic exposure in the United States alone.

WHO IS AT RISK?

Workers in many different blue-collar, white-collar and professional occupations are at risk for exposure to neurotoxic substances. The risk of exposure varies according to the occupation and the particular neurotoxin. Risk also varies with age (children are more susceptible than adults), amount of activity (higher activity increases respiration which increases airborne toxin intake) and individual differences in susceptibility that are not currently understood.

Sex differences

Gender may impact upon risk in two ways. First, insofar as many occupations still employ predominantly either male or female workers, toxic exposures may be expected to impact on the sexes differently depending upon the particular job's sex distribution. For example, the painting and plumbing trades remain predominantly male preserves, while the electronics industry employs many more women in occupations with high exposure to neurotoxic substances.

Second, there is growing evidence for biological differences in toxic susceptibility as a function of gender. A Soviet study, for example, exposed volunteers to minimally toxic levels of a cholinesterase-inhibiting pesticide. Females showed 20% greater decreases in blood cholinesterase than males, and experienced longer duration and higher intensity neurological and gastrointestinal symptoms (Krasovskii *et al.*, 1969, cited in Calabrese, 1985). Many pharmacologic agents also show sex-related differences, including Lithium, Lorazepam, Nortriptyline and Oxazepam (Calabrese, 1985).

There is no corpus of neuropsychological studies on the effects of either industrially or pharmacologically neurotoxic substances as a function of gender. Ethanol, one of the few neurotoxins for which this sort of data has been collected, has failed to yield definite gender effects (see Chapter V). However, Calabrese (1985) has identified almost 200 toxic substances which (at least in animal models) exhibit experimental sex differences. It seems possible that human neurotoxins may eventually be shown to impact differently on the neuropsychological performance of males and females.

Occupational risks

Table I.3 is a partial listing of occupations along with neurotoxic substances potentially encountered in each.

Considering the variety of occupations, the large numbers of unresearched neurotoxic chemicals and the even larger number of affected individuals, it is clear that the few psychologists currently engaged in this type of research can only begin to serve potential needs. While Weiss's (1983) call for "25,000 behavioral toxicologists" seems exaggerated, there is nevertheless a need for greatly expanded neuropsychological services in the industrial and private sector.

MECHANISMS OF SUBCLINICAL TOXICITY

Current understanding of neurotoxic mechanisms suggests that the nervous system can be damaged in several ways by toxic materials. *Anoxia* may cause cell death within minutes, either by decreasing the amount of oxygen carried in the blood, slowing the blood flow or by blocking the

TABLE I.3. Occupations and activities at risk for neurotoxic exposure

OCCUPATIONS AT RISK FOR NEUROTOXIC EXPOSURE	NEUROTOXIC SUBSTANCE
1. Agriculture and farm workers	Pesticides, herbicides, insecticides, solvents
2. Chemical and pharmaceutical workers	Industrial and pharmaceutical substances
3. Degreasers	Trichloroethylene
4. Dentists and dental hygienists	Mercury, anesthetic gases
5. Dry-cleaners	Perchloroethylene, trichloroethylene, other solvents
6. Electronics workers	Lead, methyl ethyl ketone, methylene chloride, tin, trichloroethylene, glycol ether, xylene, chloroform, freon, arsine
7. Hospital personnel	Alcohols, anesthetic gases, ethylene oxide (cold sterilization)
8. Laboratory workers	Solvents, mercury, ethylene oxide
9. Painters	Lead, toluene, xylene, other solvents
10. Plastics workers	Formaldehyde, styrene, PVCs
11. Printers	Lead, methanol, methylene chloride, toluene, trichloroethylene, other solvents
12. Rayon workers	Carbon disulfide
13. Steel workers	Lead, other metals
14. Transportation workers	Lead (in gasoline), carbon monoxide, solvents
15. Hobbyists	Lead, toluene, glues, solvents

utilization of oxygen. Other agents (e.g. lead, thallium, triethyltin) may produce neurotoxic damage by interfering with or destroying the myelin sheath (Williams and Burson, 1985). Still other substances may produce direct damage to the peripheral nervous system, (e.g. hexane, *n*-methyl butyl ketone) or central nervous system (e.g. mercury, manganese, organophosphate pesticides, lead). These effects will be discussed further in later chapters.

Symptoms of concern

Clinically, the types of subtle and gross damage described above will produce cognitive, emotional and behavioral dysfunction. Anger (1984) has compiled the reported neurotoxic effects from ACGIH documents through 1982 (Table I.4). From a neuropsychological point of view reported symptoms are somewhat unsystematically categorized; however, the list does suggest symptoms amenable to neuropsychological analysis.

A different way to categorize neuropsychological symptoms found in patients exposed to neurotoxins is contained in Table I.5. The list is not meant to be exhaustive, but rather to suggest the major groupings of dysfunctions that can be testable with neuropsychological methods. Exact patterns of neuropsychological impairment will be dependent upon the

TABLE I.4. Neurotoxic symptoms compiled from ACGIH documents. (Reprinted, by permission of Pergamon Journals, Ltd., from Anger, W. K. (1984). Neurobehavioral testing of chemicals: Impact on recommended standards. *Neurobehavioral Toxicology and Teratology,* **6,** 152.)

MOTOR		COGNITIVE		AFFECTIVE/PERSONALITY	
General motor		Alertness loss	1	Substance abuse	1
Activity changes	3	Impaired judgement	1	Anxiety	4
Incoordination	10	Memory loss	3	Asthenia/neurasthenia	2
Paralysis	9	Slurred speech	1	Belligerence	1
Performance changes	4			Delirium	2
Pupil constriction	2	*General changes*		Delusions	1
Rigidity	3	Analogy with other chemicals		Depression	4
Weakness	12		25	Disorientation	1
		Anorexia	15	Excitability	3
Abnormal movement		Behavioral changes	3	Exhilaration	1
Ataxia	4	Cholinesterase inhibition	26	Giddiness	6
Chorea	1	CNS depression	10	Hallucinations	2
Convulsions/spasms	18	CNS edema	1	Inebriation	1
Gait, spastic	1	CNS stimulation	4	Insomnia	4
Movement disorders	1	Encephalopathy	1	Irritability	4
Nystagmus	2	Narcosis/stupor	28	Lassitude/lethargy	7
Tremor	19	Neuropathy/neuritis	6	Laughter	1
		Neurophysiological/		Malaise	2
Sensory		electrophysiological		Nervousness/nervous	
Auditory disorders	4	changes	10	disorders	11
Equilibrium disorders/vertigo/		Neurotoxicology	5	Psychological/mental	
dizziness	20	Operant behavior changes	1	disorders	4
Gustatory changes	5	Pathology, CNS/PNS	15	Psychosis	2
Olfactory changes	2	Psychic disturbances	2	Restlessness	1
Pain disorders (incl. anesthesia)		Unpleasant taste/smell	12	Sleepiness	5
	7	Weariness/fatigue lethargy	8	Viciousness	1
Pain, feeling of	2				
Sensation deficits	1				
Tactile disorders	5				
Vision disorders	12				
Visual sense organ pathology					
	21				

particular neurotoxic exposure, severity of exposure, individual susceptibility and other factors. More information on these diagnostic factors will be contained in succeeding chapters.

SUMMARY

In conclusion, neuropsychological toxicology is the newest branch of the field of neuropsychology, a clinical discipline concerned with understanding the relationship between brain damage and behavioral alteration. Neuropsychological toxicology, then, applies neuropsychological testing methods to assess the subtle but definite brain dysfunctions produced by neurotoxic substances.

The relatively recent development of neuropsychological toxicology reflects the youth of its founding fields, industrial medicine and

TABLE I.5. Common neuropsychological symptoms of neurotoxicity

General Intellectual Impairments
Intelligence (IQ)
Attention
Concentration
Abstract reasoning
School learned skills (including arithmetic, spelling, writing)
Cognitive efficiency and flexibility
Global impairments (dementias)

Motor impairments
Fine motor speed
Fine motor coordination
Gross motor coordination
Gross motor strength

Sensory impairments
Visual disturbances
Auditory disturbances
Paresthesias/anesthesias
Tactile disturbances (PNS or CNS disorders)

Memory and learning impairments
Short-term memory (verbal and nonverbal information)
Learning (encoding of new information—verbal and nonverbal)
Long-term memory (verbal and nonverbal)

Visuospatial impairments
Constructional apraxias

Personality impairments
Anxiety, depression, delirium, organic brain syndrome, organic affective disorder, other psychotic disorders, anger, tension, fatigue, irritability, other symptoms

neuropsychology. There remain many unanswered biochemical, anatomical, psychological and behavioral questions that must be addressed before the field can deliver definitive pronouncements about the effects of toxic substances on the nervous system. In addition, the legal, political and economic complexities of this field have yet to be resolved. The number of multidisciplinary specialists in the field will likely have to increase significantly before such answers can be expected.

Despite current ambiguities in the field, the need for clinical service and research experimentation is immediate. Millions of workers, and an unknown number of other individuals, are exposed to neurotoxic substances as a byproduct of their jobs, hobbies, prescription drug use or voluntary substance abuse. The neurotoxic syndromes that result from this exposure can run the gamut from mild emotional disorder or other functional-seeming illness to complete and irreversible dementias.

American neuropsychologists have lagged far behind their Scandinavian and European colleagues in expanding the frontiers of this multidisciplinary field. Current trends, however, are in the direction of greater worldwide participation in research and clinical service. The huge number of potential neurotoxins and exposed individuals suggests an immediate need for clinical and research programs in all phases of toxicology research. Hopefully, the entire field of toxicology in all of its clinical, legislative and legal branches will see greater future growth. However, the need for neuropsychological research is particularly great. "Neuropsychological toxicologists" could provide immediately useful input to medicine, industry and regulatory agencies; all those concerned with providing safe working and living conditions. Neuropsychological toxicology, as a conceptual entity, is the banner under which an entirely new area of research can be conducted and clinical services can be performed. The niche is there and the need is great.

Note:

Many of the industrial toxins presented in the following chapters are preceded by general industrial hygiene information collected by the National Institute for Occupational Safety and Health (NIOSH), in their *Pocket Guide to Chemical Hazards*. Unless specifically noted otherwise, all OSHA exposure limits are for 8-hour time-weighted average (TWA) concentrations. Ceilings cited by the Occupational Safety and Health Administration (OSHA) "shall not be exceeded at any time, unless noted otherwise" (NIOSH *Pocket Guide*, 1985, p. 13).

Other abbreviations listed by the *Pocket Guide* include:

ppm	parts per million.
ACGIH	American Conference of Governmental Industrial Hygienists.
TLV	threshold limit value.
IDLH Level	Immediately Dangerous to Life or Health — a "maximum concentration from which one could escape within 30 minutes without any escape-impairing symptoms or any irreversible health effects" (NIOSH *Pocket Guide,* 1985, p. 14).

II
Evaluation of Neurotoxic Syndromes

INTRODUCTION

Diagnosis and management of patients with neurotoxic syndromes can best be carried out by a specialized team of health care professionals. The respective contributions from physicians and neuropsychologists will obviously depend upon the circumstances of toxic exposure. Individuals exposed to high concentrations of acutely toxic materials require immediate medical management to sustain life and, if possible, eliminate the toxin from the body. In such a situation, neuropsychological evaluation can be a valuable follow-up procedure to assess recovery of cortical function. Alternatively, when the diagnostic issue is one of subclinical effects and/or low-level, chronic exposure, then neuropsychological evaluation can proceed in tandem with medical tests and become an important *initial* contribution to final diagnosis and subsequent management.

Because more individuals are *chronically* exposed to neurotoxins, either at work, or via prescription or "street" drug use, than are in danger from high-concentration *acute* effects, and because available neuropsychological literature has concentrated on initial diagnosis rather than follow-up, the remainder of the chapter will chronicle the types of health questions and neuropsychological procedures that may typically be performed in such an initial evaluation.

INITIAL MEDICAL EVALUATION

Somewhere in their evaluation history, patients with verified toxic exposure should receive basic medical and neurological evaluation; toxicology screens of blood or urine and other tests may be initiated according to the types of substances to which the patient has ingested or been exposed. Clinical neurological examination of cranial nerves I through XII is recommended. "Assessment of optic (II) and trigeminal (V) nerves is particularly useful in suspected neurotoxic conditions" (Spencer, Arezzo and

26

Schaumberg, 1985, p. 12). Spencer *et al.* (1985) also recommend examination of the ocular fundi, motor and sensory systems, reflex examination and, in certain cases (e.g. anticholinergic drugs, pesticides) evaluation of the autonomic nervous system. While most patients receiving subclinical exposures of toxic substances will present with negative neurological findings, alternative medical or neurological illness occurring coincidentally with exposure should be ruled out.

A diagnostic decision tree of the typical sequence of clinical evaluation for neurotoxic syndromes at Cook County Hospital, Chicago, Illinois, USA, is illustrated in Fig II.1. While the flowchart is specific to industrial neurototin evaluations, its principles may be applicable to the diagnosis of other types of neurotoxic syndromes. The multidisciplinary, cooperative effort involved in diagnosing and treating these syndromes can be easily seen.

NEUROTOXICITY HEALTH QUESTIONNAIRES

Clinical questioning can often be facilitated with administration of structured interviews or symptom checklists. In addition, the systematic collection of basic demographic, medical and neuropsychological data allows for present or future research comparisons, an important consideration in any developing field.

Questionnaire construction and administration

Questionnaires may be designed to be self-administered or given in structured interview by an examiner. Which type of questionnaire is chosen depends upon many factors, among them the ability of the patient to work alone, the wish of the examiner to observe the patient's responses, and whether "in-depth" follow-up questions or elaborations are needed. Questionnaires may be constructed to acquire general information or they may be tailored to the specific substances under investigation. Hogstedt's questionnaire designed to assess solvent exposure symptoms is an example of the latter.

Solvent Exposure Questionnaire (Hogstedt, Hane and Axelson, 1980)
1. Do you have a short memory?
2. Have you ever been told that you have a short memory?
3. Do you often have to make notes about what you must remember?
4. Do you often have to go back and check things that you have done, such as turned off the stove, locked the door, etc?
5. Do you generally find it hard to get the meaning from reading newspapers and books?
6. Do you often have problems with concentrating?

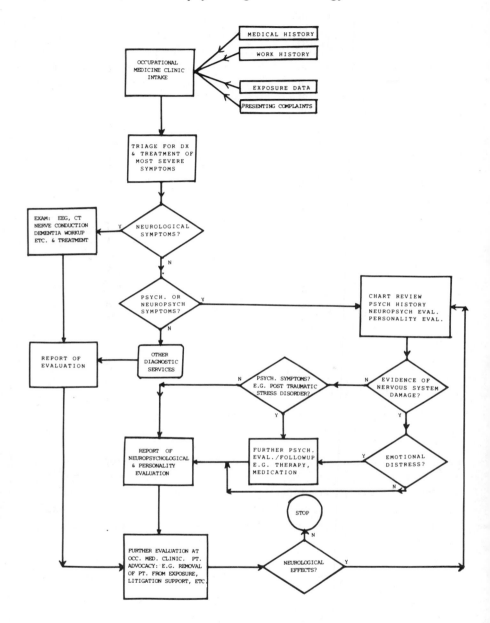

FIGURE II.1. Patient referral sequence through the occupational medicine clinic at Cook County Hospital: multidisciplinary process. (The author thanks Stephen Hessl, MD, Director of Occupational Medicine, Cook County Hospital, for his collaboration in the development of this flowchart.)

7. Do you often feel irritated without any particular reason?
8. Do you often feel depressed for any particular reason?
9. Are you abnormally tired?
10. Are you less interested in sex than what you think is normal?
11. Do you have palpitations of the heart even when you don't exert yourself?
12. Do you sometimes feel a pressure in your chest?
13. Do you perspire without any particular reason?
14. Do you have a headache at least once a week?
15. Do you often have painful tingling in some part of your body?

Beckmann and Mergler (1985) propose consideration of what might be considered "human factors" when designing and administering a questionnaire. These factors include:

1. Determining a "fatigue factor" for both examiner and patient in the administration of the questionnaire. Will exposed patients tire more easily than controls?
2. Will various forms of biases enter a patient's response set? Might there be differentially biased responding between exposed patients and controls? For example, will subjects be unwilling to accurately catalogue their alcohol intake for fear that such information will be made part of their personnel files?
4. How will impairment, if it exists, affect response quality?
   In addition, the authors suggest that questions be as specific as possible. Questions which are tied to independently observable behaviors rather than purely subjective data are preferred (Beckmann and Mergler, 1985).

Areas of inquiry

At least three areas of inquiry are relevant to neurotoxicology evaluation: medical history and current symptoms in major organ systems, occupational history and psychological information. These data can be garnered from questionnaires specially designed for a particular patient or research population, or they may be collected via careful selection and use of available surveys.

Medical history

Existing questionnaires, like the Cornell Medical Index, may be an aid to the diagnostic assessment of neurotoxic syndromes. A physical symptom questionnaire also can be constructed for specific target symptoms with specialized questions addressing common neurotoxic complaints, e.g. dizziness, headache, incoordination, paresthesias, etc. Any prior or current medical condition potentially capable of interfering with neuropsychological performance requires special inquiry. These conditions include, but are not limited to:

1. Central nervous system pathology, e.g. head injury, high fever, seizure disorder, periods of unconsciousness; diseases capable of affecting the nervous system, including lupus erythematosus, syphilis, AIDS or ARC, diabetes, etc., hereditary degenerative disease.
2. Peripheral nervous system (PNS) pathology, e.g. peripheral neuropathies, diabetes, carpal tunnel syndrome, PNS injury, chronic pain.
3. Non-neurological medical problems capable of affecting neuro-psychological functioning: arthritis, liver disease, infectious or metabolic disorder, orthopedic/muscle injury in upper body producing motor impairment.
4. Drugs and medications: alcohol, drug abuse, caffeine intake, prescription drugs with neuropsychological effects (e.g. benzodiazepines).
5. Psychological/psychiatric problems (see Psychological History Questionnaire)
6. Other factors: recent sleep history, nutritional status (e.g. dieting, recent unusual weight loss or gain).

Occupational history

For workplace exposures, questions to be addressed include frequency, duration of and interval between exposures and the relationship between these variables and symptoms. A detailed job description is essential for two reasons. First, job analysis will clarify the nature of the patient's contact with neurotoxic substances and will aid the examiner in assessing the severity of symptoms. Second, a detailed history of present and past job responsibilities can be compared with neuropsychological test results for consistency. For example, mild visuospatial difficulties in an "engineer" who draws and interprets blueprints might be seen differently from those same difficulties in an "engineer" whose job it is to sweep the factory floor. A list of occupational symptoms, illnesses and injuries should also be included, either in the context of an occupational questionnaire or in another medical checklist. In addition, satisfaction with the work environment, relationships with fellow-employees and degree of work stress are important areas of inquiry to determine the influence of psychosocial stressors upon symptom production.

Psychological history

Since many neurotoxic symptoms, by themselves, are nonspecific, e.g. headache, depression, forgetfulness, etc., a psychological history will allow the clinician to consider alternative explanations for neurotoxicity complaints. There are four possible relationships of psychological symptoms to neurotoxic exposure:

1. Symptoms may be *primary* behavioral, cognitive or affective concomitants of structural or neurochemical lesion. "Depression" as a result of lead poisoning, or slowed, confused thinking from pesticide exposure are examples.
2. Symptoms may be *reactive* to increased stress as a *secondary* consequence of real neurological disability. For example, if an architect were exposed to toxins that caused peripheral neuropathy, ensuing depression could be the psychological reaction to loss of fine motor control and subsequent inability to perform career duties. Similarly, an individual with carbon disulfide-induced cerebral vasculopathy may react catastrophically to perceived deficiencies in cognition. In both these cases, real neurological disability may coexist with, or be exacerbated by, affective components.
3. Symptoms may be *reactive* to the *psychosocial* stressors of exposure, rather than to structural or neurochemical abnormality. For example, an individual might develop neuropsychological symptoms after working in factory that has been found to be in violation of OSHA toxic exposure standards. Fears of possible exposure, job loss, non-neurological medical consequences of exposure (e.g. cancer), legal proceedings and financial hardships may produce "learned helplessness" and other reactive effects. These reactions, in turn, may produce abnormal neuropsychological test behavior.
4. Symptoms may be *unrelated*, linked to difficulties which existed prior to toxic exposure, or to stresses which occur coincidentally with toxic exposure, e.g. continuation of premorbid alcoholism or personality disorder, death of a parent or spouse.

Besides discrete symptom lists, psychological questionnaires may include the following items:

1. Social, marital, interpersonal adjustment (home and work adjustment).
2. Psychosocial stressors, e.g. a "Personal Problems Checklist" (e.g. Schinka, 1984).
3. Psychological history: prior or current history of mental health treatment, diagnoses; hospitalization and medication history; history of emotional functioning and psychological symptomatology.
4. Current behavioral and emotional adaptations/stressors. Representative questions might include queries pertaining to factors likely to interfere with neuropsychological test performance (e.g. alcohol, substance abuse, smoking, sleep, mood state, interpersonal adjustment).
5. Personality and affect inventories: questionnaires which assay personality

traits and current emotional state. Examples of the former include the Minnesota Multiphasic Personality Inventory (MMPI), or the Clinical Analysis Questionnaire (CAQ). Common inventories of current affect include the Beck Depression Inventory (BDI), the Profile of Mood States (POMS) and the Multiple Affect Adjective Checklist (MAACL). These are discussed in more detail later in the chapter.

Psychological questionnaire information may be obtained from family or collaterals if the patient is deemed to be an uncertain or inaccurate historian.

Other factors

A complete personal history will sometimes produce relevant information unrelated to job, social adjustment or psychosocial factors. Certain hobbies, for example, may include chronic exposure to neurotoxic substances, e.g. lead in stained-glass making, solder in electronic construction, toluene or *n*-hexane-based glues in plastic model construction.

CONSTRUCTION OF A NEUROPSYCHOLOGICAL TOXICOLOGY TEST BATTERY

Hänninen (1982), referring to the construction of neuropsychological toxicology batteries, stated that "not all neuropsychological assessment methods are good research tools" (p. 123). Similarly, neuropsychological instruments also vary in their clinical utility for toxicity diagnoses. Baker *et al.* (1983b) suggest the following criteria for the selection of a neurobehavioral toxicology battery. The evaluation must be *comprehensive*; it must be *adaptable* to field conditions; it must be free of, or at least able to factor out, extraneous influences (e.g. age and personal habits), and results must be reproducible.

To this, several additional criteria can be added. First, the battery should be psychometrically sound and experimentally validated, if possible among groups of patients with neurotoxin-related disorders. Second, while maintaining comprehensiveness, a battery of tests must also emphasize areas of neuropsychological functioning known to be correlated with subclinical changes in neuropsychological functioning.

Finally, it must be hoped that advances in the quantification and precision of neuropsychological toxicology batteries will proceed in tandem with similar advances in theoretical understanding and scientific vocabulary available to describe the syndromes. Letz and Singer (1985) believe the responsibilities of the scientific community should include:

1. A commonly agreed-upon categorization of neuropsychological functions,

an agreed-upon linking of specific tests to those functions, and a standard vocabulary for discussing those functions and tests should be established.

2. Rigid diagnostic criteria for clinical syndromes and specific definitions for subclinical effects associated with neurotoxicant exposure should be established.

Neuropsychological tests will be most useful when these recommendations are taken into account. A precisely defined scientific context for the use of these tests is a prerequisite for communication and advancement of knowledge.

CLINICAL USE OF NEUROPSYCHOLOGICAL TESTS IN ASSESSING NEUROTOXICITY

Several general recommendations can be made about neuropsychological toxicology testing. First, "blind" testing is inappropriate to clinical assessment of neurotoxicity. While well-designed research projects can justify isolating the neuropsychologist from information not collected during the actual test session, blind testing is almost never appropriate in a clinical context. Patients with neurotoxic exposure should have their evaluations interpreted within the larger context of any available medical, demographic, educational, psychological and sociological data that it is feasible to collect. Data from a period predating the patient's exposure to neurotoxic materials is a recommended context toward understanding the patient's current functioning. Developmental history, school records, premorbid personnel records detailing job performance and interpersonal adjustment are just a few of the data which may prove important to interpretation of the patient's current clinical behavior.

Second, neuropsychological toxicology batteries should, as much as possible, attempt to sample a *comprehensive* array of cognitive, affective and neurobehavioral functions. An overly narrow approach which limits test selection to one or two "sensitive" measures does not do the patient justice from a diagnostic viewpoint; every patient should be approached with the possibility that alternative, "rule-out" diagnoses may be required. Failure to administer a comprehensive battery will limit the validity of neuropsychological examination by restricting the data from which the neuropsychologist may make a diagnostic judgment.

NEUROPSYCHOLOGICAL TEST STRUCTURE

Hänninen (1982), discussing the use of test batteries in neuropsychological toxicology, suggests that European batteries constructed for this purpose have a similar structure; all test intellectual functions, memory, perceptual-motor speed and accuracy, and psychomotor abilities (p. 124). She notes several tests from these categories which have consistently proved to be sensitive to neurotoxicity. These include: the Benton Visual Retention Test, several tests of perceptual speed and accuracy (e.g. WAIS-R Digit Symbol Test), and the Santa Ana Dexterity Test, a pegboard task similar to the Minnesota Rate of Manual Dexterity Test. Cassitto (1983) provided an expanded list of functions to be tested in neuropsychological toxicology studies. These include: vigilance, focused attention, visual and auditory acuity, time and space orientation, motor abilities, eye–hand coordination, memory, verbal skills, perceptual abilities and abstract reasoning (p. 30). Summerfield (1983) additionally suggests that *reaction-time* tasks under time pressure or paced performance criteria may be more sensitive than unpaced tasks. He also advocates use of *parallel processing* or divided attention tasks that put the subject's neuropsychological functions under increased task demand, thereby increasing the likelihood that subclinical impairments will interfere with such complex processing and degrade performance.

Alternatively, certain tests do not appear to be sensitive to neurotoxic effects. Vocabulary tests and tests of school-learned facts are typical examples. These may function as "hold" tests; tests which "hold up" or are resistant to subclinical neurotoxic effects. Both types of tests can be usefully included in a neuropsychological toxicology battery. So-called "hold" tests can be used as a rough estimate of premorbid abilities to allow comparison with tests more sensitive to current function.

TESTING APPROACHES IN NEUROPSYCHOLOGICAL TOXICOLOGY

Neuropsychologists have tended to apply already familiar strategies of neuropsychological evaluation to the investigation of neurotoxicity. Thus, Lezak advocates an approach tailored to the effects of specific substances, stating that "different kinds of conditions have different behavioral manifestations and therefore call for different assessment programs" (Lezak, 1984). Christenson (1984) endorses the use of Luria's methods, while Bergman (1984) prefers the use of the standardized Halstead–Reitan neuropsychological battery. These camps may be loosely grouped into proponents of "fixed" batteries versus "flexible" approaches. Each has its advantages and disadvantages. Fixed batteries with a rigidly specified set of tests are advantageous to researchers because they allow for easy replication of testing conditions and materials, and thereby encourage validation attempts. Alternatively, fixed batteries may not adequately sample the types of functions known to be impaired with certain neurotoxic substances. For example, the absence of verbal memory and learning tasks on the

Halstead–Reitan would make that battery less than adequate for assessment of substances with documented effects on those functions, e.g. benzodiazepines or beta-blockers.

Flexible approaches that tailor examination procedures and materials for individual substances can emphasize certain neuropsychological functions over others, and thus under certain circumstances may produce a more "in-depth" analysis of particular impairments. On the other hand, an overly flexible approach may emphasize "in-depth" analysis at the expense of a comprehensive survey of neuropsychological function. Failure to test for a complete array of neuropsychological functions may limit the investigation of effects to what is already known, and can result in an incomplete neuropsychological profile. In addition, when flexible approaches become too "flexible" — that is, when they use unvalidated procedures, immediate clinical conclusions and future research validation may be compromised.

Recently, the World Health Organization (WHO) and the National Institute of Occupational Safety and Health (NIOSH) attempted to provide a compromise between fixed and flexible batteries by advocating what they termed a "core" battery of tests; tests selected for their known sensitivity to neurotoxicity effects, while not neglecting to provide a comprehensive survey of neuropsychological functions. The WHO battery includes the following tests (Baker and Letz, 1986):

1. Aiming (pursuit aiming).
2. Simple reaction time.
3. Santa Ana Dexterity Test.
4. Digit Symbol Test.
5. Benton Visual Retention Test.
6. Digit Span.
7. Profile of Mood States.

Such a "core" battery might be termed a "flexible battery" approach, combining the most powerful features of the fixed and flexible testing methodologies. Use of an internationally agreed-upon neuropsychological battery for neurotoxic research could potentially allow vast amounts of data to be collected and compared from all parts of the world. On the other hand, flexible "core" batteries are subject to limitations of both fixed and flexible strategies; once designed, they may fail to show generalized application to the range of substances they may be subsequently called upon to test. A "required" battery could also stultify creative research that deviates from the agreed-upon approach. Finally, if a core battery is not designed for comprehensive assessment, it may share limitations of overly flexible approaches.

Examples of the neuropsychological test materials from fixed battery and flexible battery approaches include:

Standard batteries

Two standard batteries have achieved international usage in neuropsychology: the Halstead-Reitan Battery (HRB) and the Luria-Nebraska Neuropsychological Battery (LNNB). The Halstead-Reitan may be the most commonly used standard neuropsychological battery (Bigler, 1984). It is composed of tests which were collected and introduced by Ward Halstead in 1947, and further developed by his graduate student, Ralph Reitan, who standardized the battery, eliminated some tests and added others. The present day HRB includes the following subtests: Finger Oscillation Test (Finger Tapping), Tactual Performance Test, Category Test, Seashore Rhythm Test, Speech Sounds Perception Test, Lateral Dominance Test, Grip Strength (Dynamometer), Trail-Making Tests A & B, Aphasia Screening Test (Reitan-Indiana) and the Reitan Klove Sensory-Perceptual Examination. One of the Wechsler Intelligence Scales is typically included as part of the HRB, originally the Wechsler-Bellevue, and currently the Wechsler Adult Intelligence Scale — Revised (WAIS-R). The Minnesota Multiphasic Personality Inventory is also often included.

Comparatively few neurotoxicology studies have used the full Halstead-Reitan battery, probably because of the time involved in administration and scoring (over 6 hours). Many researchers have utilized parts of the battery in neurotoxicology research, most frequently Finger Tapping, Trails, along with the Wechsler subtests of Block Design and Digit Symbol.

The Luria-Nebraska Neuropsychological Battery (LNNB) was developed by Golden, Hammeke and Purisch (1980) as a standardization of Russian psychologist Alexander Luria's methods. The authors used test items listed by Christensen (1975), included their own procedures and constructed 11 clinical scales, initially called Motor, Rhythm, Tactile, Visual, Receptive language, Expressive language, Writing, Reading, Arithmetic, Memory and Intelligence. The LNNB has had a somewhat controversial beginning; however, recent studies have demonstrated the LNNB to be statistically equivalent in diagnostic accuracy to the Halstead-Reitan (Golden *et al.*, 1981). While Luria's methods have been suggested to be useful in neurotoxicology research (Christensen, 1975), no research study has yet employed the LNNB with neurotoxic exposure patients.

Use of the LNNB for evaluation of neurotoxic syndromes may be problematic for several reasons. A major deficiency of the battery is the lack of complex, multi-component tasks, the same types of tasks which are most often found to be impaired in neurotoxic exposure patients. This limitation is carried over from Luria's original testing philosophy which emphasized the analysis of component abilities with systematic variation of simple tasks. Complex tasks were not given because their deficiencies could not be readily attributed to specific component abilities (Purisch and Sbordone, 1986). A second limitation in the LNNB is its relatively restricted investigation of memory, another neuropsychological function commonly impaired in neurotoxin-exposed patients. Given these limitations, it is not surprising that the LNNB is relatively insensitive to some types of alcohol disorders, the only major neurotoxin that has been investigated with this battery. Use of the LNNB in detecting early subclinical effects of other neurotoxins does not seem warranted at this time.

Intelligence tests

The revised Wechsler Adult Intelligence Scale (WAIS-R) is currently the most frequently used measure of "IQ" in the United States. Full-scale IQ scores computed from the Wechsler scales or other measures have not been found to be particularly sensitive to neurotoxic exposure effects. However, use of the WAIS-R may be important for neurotoxicology examinations for at least two reasons. First, IQ correlates with many neuropsychological functions; the necessity to control for IQ has become increasingly apparent to researchers wishing to make valid statements about neurotoxic effects irrespective of premorbid abilities (e.g. Gade *et al.*, 1985). Second, while overall IQ estimates from the WAIS-R are not diagnostic of neurotoxicity, several subtests appear to be sensitive to, and have been used quite frequently to test for, subclinical toxic exposure effects. These tests are Digit Symbol, Block Design, Similarities and Digit Span.

Flexible batteries

Most investigations of neuropsychological toxicology have used "flexible" batteries. These tests, like the WHO/NIOSH core battery, are typically constructed from existing neuropsychological tests whose diagnostic utility and validity have already been demonstrated. Use of existing tests saves research time otherwise spent on test construction and validation. It also allows researchers to tailor the focus of the battery to investigate the specific neurotoxic effects of a substance. There are a variety of neurotoxicity batteries that have been developed. Some attempt a comprehensive survey of functions, others are very minimal "screening" measures. A general recommendation to be made, regardless of the depth or breadth of the constructed battery, is that "every effort should be made to reduce the variance produced by unstandardized and subjective methods of administration and scoring" (Walsh, 1978, p. 301) by adhering to standardized instructions, methods of presentation and presentation orders. Standardization also benefits the research community in its attempt to replicate research findings.

Table II. 1 lists examples of the types of tests that can be used in neuropsychological toxicology research.

EXISTING NEUROPSYCHOLOGICAL TOXICOLOGY TEST BATTERIES

The following neuropsychological batteries have been developed by various researchers and put to use in neurotoxicology research. They should be considered "flexible battery" approaches.

1. Pittsburgh Occupational Exposures Test Battery (POET) Ryan et al. (1986)

WAIS-R Intelligence Subtests:
Information, Similarities, Digit Span, Digit Symbol, Picture Completion, Block Design

Visual Reproduction and Visual Memory:
Immediate reproduction, direct copy and 30-minute delayed recall of Wechsler Memory Scale Form I design cards.

Verbal Associative Learning:
10 pairs unrelated nouns simultaneously read and visually presented for 2 seconds. First word of each pair was retrieval cue. Delayed verbal recall of 10 pairs assessed 30 minutes later using first word as retrieval cue.

Symbol Digit Learning:
Visual presentation of symbols on Kodak Audioviewer for 3 seconds. Symbols presented at end of list as retrieval cue for digits. Response followed by presentation of symbol digit pair for 3 seconds. Four test trials. 30-minute delayed recall after all four trials completed.

Incidental Memory:
Subject asked to recall nine symbols from the WAIS-R Digit Symbol Substitution Test immediately after test.

Recurring words:
Continuous recognition paradigm. Fifty four-letter words individually presented either once, twice or three times. Subjects determined whether they had seen each word before.

Other tests:
Boston Embedded Figures, Mental Rotation Test, Trail Making Test, Grooved Pegboard Test.

2. Baker et al. *(1983b).*
Wechsler Memory Scale
WAIS Subtests:
Vocabulary
Similarities

(continued on page 41)

TABLE II.1. Representative neuropsychological tests for use in neurotoxicology evaluations

---

Sensorimotor: fine motor speed and dexterity
These are tests of basic central and peripheral nervous system integrity of sensory and motor nerves.

Test	*Purpose*
Finger Tapping Test	Fine motor speed
Two Plate Tapping Test	Fine and gross motor speed
Foot Tapping Test	Fine and gross motor speed
Motor Steadiness Test	Motor control
Purdue Pegboard Test	Fine motor speed and coordination
Dynamometer (Grip Strength)	Gross motor strength

Visual-motor-spatial tests
Tests which require integration of spatial information with visual and/or kinesthetic feedback.

Reitan–Klove Sensory Perceptual Examination

Grooved Pegboard Test	Fine motor speed, dexterity, irregular pegs and holes have spatial component
Minnesota Rate of Manipulation Test	Large circular pegs must be rotated by fingers and wrist; requires fine motor speed, dexterity and coordination
Santa Ana Test	Similar to above. Frequently used in Scandinavian neurotoxicology studies. Not commercially available in the U.S.

Abstraction
Tests which require reasoning processes (e.g. induction, deduction, verbal reasoning).

Halstead Category Test (Halstead, 1947)	Part of Halstead–Reitan Battery. Requires induction of categorization rules in geometric figure sequences.
Wisconsin Card Sorting Test (Grant and Berg, 1948)	As above, requires inductive identification of categorization by shape, color, or number and ability to change sets. Linked to pre-frontal lobe functions.
Shipley Institute of Living Test	Part 2, verbal reasoning

Tests of planning, concentration, cognitive flexibility and efficiency

Trail-Making Tests A and B (Reitan, 1966)	Included in the Halstead–Reitan Battery — connection of circled numbers or alternating numbers and letters. Timed test.
WAIS-R Digit Symbol Subtest	Requires matching numbers with specified abstract designs and drawing in appropriate designs under each number; timed test.

Stroop Color–Word Interference Test:
A three-part reading and color-naming test. The first page requires speeded word reading; the second page, naming the colors of the ink; the third page asks the subject to name the ink color of a color–word the name of which is a contrasting color (e.g. asking the subject to say "blue" when presented with the word "red" written in blue ink). The third page is considered to require sustained attention in the presence of a continuous distraction, to test cooperation between hemispheres, and management of conflicting input by frontal lobe function.

Paced Auditory Serial Addition Test (PASAT):
The subject listens to a tape-recorded series of numbers and adds pairs of numbers continuously.

Digit Symbol Test

Spatial–constructional praxis tests
Tests which require identification and manipulation of materials in space (e.g. drawing, manipulation of objects, mental rotation).
WAIS-R Block Design
WAIS-R Object Assembly
Benton Visual Retention Test (BVRT) (direct copy)
Complex figure of Rey (Rey, 1959; Osterreith, 1944)
Canter Background Interference Procedure (BIP): Modification of the Bender Visual-Motor Gestalt Test which requires geometric card designs to be presented twice — once to be copied on plain paper, the second time reproduced on an "interference" sheet already printed with irregular, intersecting curves and lines.

Tactual Performance Test (TPT):
From the Halstead–Reitan Battery, the TPT requires a blindfolded subject to place geometric shapes in a Seguin–Goddard-style form board. Hands are first tested individually and then simultaneously. Memory for kinesthetic and spatial information is tested subsequent to test performance.

Memory tests
Wechsler Memory Scale [original and Russell (1975) modifications]
Rey Auditory Verbal Learning Test (RAVLT)
Buschke Selective Reminding Test
Benton Visual Retention Test
Complex Figure of Rey

Language processes
Aphasia Screening Test
Token Test (De Renzi and Vignolo, 1962)

Tests used to estimate premorbid abilities ("Hold" tests)
WAIS-R Vocabulary
WAIS-R Information
Shipley Institute of Living — Vocabulary (Part 1)
Nelson Adult Reading Test (NART)

Personality tests
While there is no evidence that particular patterns or profiles of affect or personality are indicative *per se* of organic brain disturbance, personality measures have their place in the neuropsychological battery insofar as they assay the direct and reactive emotional effects of neurotoxin exposure. A caveat has been noted by Reitan and Wolfson (1985), who warn that personality profiles generated from patients with medical disorders may not be interpretable with the same decision rules as might be used for patients with uncomplicated emotional disorders.

1. *Minnesota Multiphasic Personality Inventory* (MMPI):
Long in common use by American neuropsychologists, it will probably be equally widely applied to the evaluation of neurotoxic sequelae. While no scale of the MMPI has proven diagnostic of organic disturbance, the large numbers of individual scales compiled for the instrument provide the researcher with a comprehensive selection of states or traits that can be investigated. Disadvantages of the MMPI lie in the length of time to complete the instrument (1–3 hours), and the fact that the questions surveyed were not originally selected for evaluation of neurotoxic exposure symptoms.

2. *Rorschach's Test:*
The Rorschach "inkblot" test has been suggested by Lindström (1984) to be capable of distinguishing between solvent-exposed workers and controls, although the author admits that time, complexity and unclarity of dependent variables limit the utility of this

instrument. Moreover, as a group, neuropsychologists have not been staunch adherents of projective measures. It seems unlikely that this instrument will be widely adopted in future neuropsychological neurotoxicology studies.

3. *Profile of Mood States* (POMS):
The Profile of Mood States (POMS) (McNair, Lorr and Droppleman, 1971) exemplifies another approach to personality and toxicology testing in that it surveys *presently experienced affect* as a *state* rather than potentially more stable personality *traits*. The test requires about 10 minutes of subject time to survey a list of feeling-state adjectives and mark how much they currently experience each particular affect on a five position Likert-type scale. Different additive combinations of response scores are compiled from scaled responses to compute measures of anger, tension, vigor, depression, fatigue and confusion. The POMS has been widely used by international neurotoxicology researchers. A new version utilizing bipolar measures of affect (the POMS-BI) may likewise be widely adopted.

Another useful (although somewhat more narrowly focused) measure of affective state is the Beck Depression Inventory (BDI) (Beck *et al.*, 1961). It is probably the most extensively validated test of depressive affect in current use by psychological researchers. Other newer, related measures also show promise for neurotoxic evaluation of depressive affect, e.g. the Multiscore Depression Inventory (Berndt *et al.*, 1984).

Finally, adjective checklists such as the Multiple Affect Adjective Checklist (MAACL) may prove similar to the POMS in their utility for neuropsychological toxicology research.

(continued from page 38)

    Block Design
    Digit Symbol (modified — 4th row from memory)
Continuous Performance Test
Santa Ana Dexterity Test
Tapping Tests (unspecified)
Profile of Mood States

3. London School of Hygiene Battery (Cherry et al., *1984).*
Trail-Making Tests,
WAIS Subtests:
    Digit Symbol and Block Design
Grooved Pegboard Test
Dotting Test
Visual Search Test
Buschke Selective Reminding Memory Test
Simple Reaction Time
NART (Nelson Adult Reading Test) index of premorbid functioning

4. Institute of Occupational Health Battery (Hänninen and Lindström, 1979)
Wechsler Adult Intelligence Scale (WAIS) Subtests:
    Similarities
    Picture Completion
    Block Design: including time score for first seven times and number of incorrect reproductions after the time limit.

Digit Symbol
Wechsler Memory Scale Subtests:
    Digit Span (forward, backward and total scores)
    Logical Memory
    Visual Reproduction
    Associate Learning
Modified Finger Tapping Test (Thumb Taps)
Santa Ana Dexterity Test
Mira Test
Symmetry Drawing Test

5. Tuttle, Wood and Grether battery (1976)
Reaction Time: Simple, Choice
Santa Ana Dexterity Test
Critical Flicker Fusion
Neisser Letter Search
WAIS Subtests: Digit Span, Digit Symbol
Feeling Tone Checklist

6. Valcuikas and Lilis (1980)
Block Design
Digit Symbol
Embedded Figures
Santa Ana

7. Putz-Anderson et al. (1983)
Choice Reaction Time
Michigan Eye–Hand Coordination
Neisser Letter Search
Short-Term Memory Span
Digit Span
Profile of Mood States
MMPI — Mania Scale
Orthorater

8. Smith and Langolf (1981)
Memory Scanning
Short-Term Memory Span
Continuous Recognition Memory
Stroop Test
Figure Rotation

9. Williamson, Teo and Sanderson (1982)
Critical Flicker Fusion
Paired Associates

Simple Reaction Time
Memory Scanning
Vigilance
Iconic Memory
Long-Term recall of paired associates

10. The TUFF Battery (Hogstedt, Hane and Axelson, 1980)
Solvent Screening Questionnaire
Vocabulary — Synonyms and Antonyms
Figure Classification
Block Construction
Unfolding — operations on drawings of unfolded geometric figures and
  comparison with folded figures.
Visual gestalt test — identifying a picture from successively more complete
  fragments.
Digit Symbol Test
Dot Cancellation Test
Number Underlining Test
Bolt Test and Pin Test (tests of fine motor coordination & dexterity)
Cylinders (tests of fine motor coordination & dexterity)
Benton Visual Retention Test
Auditory Perception and Retention

Neurobehavioral tests used in NIOSH-supported worksite studies (from Anger, 1985)

Sensory tests
  Orthorater, Vernier Acuity, Central Visual Acuity/Glare, Central Visual
Acuity/Moving Target, Binocular Depth Perception, Peripheral Field
Sensitivity, Eye Movement Fixation, Accommodation, Ainmark Perimeter,
Farnesworth Color Vision Test, Audiometer, Tone Decay, Rail Balancing.

Motor tests
  Toe Pointing, Toe Tapping, Finger Tremor, Arm Tremor, Finger
Tapping, Michigan Eye-Hand Coordination, Pencil Flipping Speed, Santa
Ana Test, Dynamometer, Drop Reaction Time, Simple Reaction Time.

Cognitive tests
  Choice Reaction Time, Time Estimation, Arithmetic, Letter Recognition,
Critical Flicker Fusion, Dual Task, Divided Attention, Light Flash
Monitoring, Neisser Task, Pattern Comparison, Digit Span, Digit Symbol,
Block Design, Raven's Progressive Matrices.

Affect/Personality
Multiple Affect Adjective Checklist (MAACL)

Edwards Personal Preference Scale
Feeling Tone Checklist
Clinical Analysis Questionnaire (CAQ)
Marlowe-Crowne Lie Scale
Profile of Mood States (POMS)
Mania Scale/MMPI

MICROCOMPUTER BATTERIES IN NEUROPSYCHOLOGICAL TOXICOLOGY

Automated neuropsychological batteries designed for microcomputers have the advantages of being (at least fairly) easy to transport to the testing site, as well as being capable of accurately administering certain tests and recording large amounts of patient data. There are several batteries currently being validated that have been developed specifically for neuropsychological assessment of environmental or occupational exposure to neurotoxic substances. While computerized batteries are too new to have been completely validated, with continued testing on relevant patient population groups, microcomputer batteries show promise for research and clinical applications.

The following batteries are in various stages of development and validation, and as such, not all may prove useful or continue to be produced. These diverse offerings do suggest the potential creativity and promise of computerization.

Psychometric Assessment System (PAS)/Dementia Screening Battery (DSB) (Branconnier, 1985)

This system is designed for the Apple II+ microcomputer with monochrome monitor. Versions of the Nelson Adult Reading Test (NART) are presented, along with WAIS subtests of Information, Similarities and Vocabulary, to obtain an estimate of verbal IQ.

Memory is assessed with a selective reminding-type task, until five trials or two consecutive perfect trials have occurred. Subsequent recall is tested in the presence of distractor items and a signal detection paradigm is used to compute response criterion ("beta") and criterion-free estimate of sensitivity (d'). What the authors call "amnestic aphasia" is tested with a word fluency task, requiring the subject to name as many items as come to mind beginning with certain letters. Spatial disorientation is tested by the Money *et al.* (1965) Standardized Road Map.

The principal aim of this battery is the identification of dementias. Since its sole reported validation has been on patients with Alzheimer's disease, it is unclear whether the battery will prove differentially diagnostic for less severely impaired patients in the early stages of neurotoxic exposure. The battery uses several novel approaches to neuropsychological function which may prove useful with further validation.

MTS — Microcomputer-based Testing System (Eckerman *et al.*, 1985)

Another system using the Apple II series of microcomputers, the battery attempts to test a set of cognitive factors derived by Carrol (1980) using factor analysis and hypothesized to be basic elements of neuropsychological function. The current program is written in the PASCAL language and tests the following functions (the reader is referred to the article for more elaborate descriptions of individual tasks):

1. Perceptual Apprehension: tachistoscope-like presentation of letters and objects.
2. Reaction Time and Movement: simple and choice reaction time using auditory modality.
3. Evaluation/Decision: comparison of similar pictures.
4. Stimulus Matching: comparing length of lines, running recognition of words.
5. Naming, Reading, Association: Stroop task.
6. Episodic Memory: a "Simon-sez" task, digit span, supraspan digit learning, "which word came last" task, a "keeping-track" task. The authors correctly note that the current set of tests lack a longer-term 30-minute recall task, and recommend inclusion of such a task in the neuropsychological battery.

Initial validation with parts of the MTS battery, using experimental exposures to alcohol and carbon monoxide, suggests that MTS tasks are sensitive to acute neurotoxic effects of these agents. The battery does, however, require specialized computer equipment not generally a part of the Apple series, including a "touch screen" and a special reaction-time clock. This may limit its acceptance somewhat.

Naval Biodynamics Laboratory Battery (Irons and Rose, 1985)

This Apple II system is designed for individuals working in "unusual environments" (Irons and Rose, 1985, p. 395). The following tasks are included:

1. Sternberg Memory Scanning Task.
2. "Stroop-like" Task.
3. Pattern Comparison Task.
4. Math Test.

5. Code Substitution Test (like Digit Symbol using letters and numbers).
6. Choice Reaction Time Task.
7. Visual and Auditory Recognition Memory.
8. "Spoke" Task (using a light pen to "tap" from the center outward to a series of lighted circles around the screen).
9. "Manikin" Task — a "mental rotation" task which asks the subject to identify the hand in which a computer-generated figure holds a box. The figure may be rotated in a number of orientations toward the subject.
10. Visual or Auditory Serial Addition (similar to the PASAT).
11. Auditory Digit Span.
12. Maze Task (uses joystick).
13. "Logic Test" — requires subject to learn the correct numbered sequence of a set of 16 boxes drawn on the screen.

This battery is just beginning to be validated, and has several interesting tasks not found in other computerized batteries. It is hoped that future validating studies will include populations at risk for neurotoxic exposure.

The Walter Reed Performance Assessment Battery
(Thorne *et al.*, 1985)

The unique distinction of this battery is the authors' foresight to program equivalent versions for both the Apple and IBM- compatible disk operating systems. The programs are written in BASIC and are modifiable by the user. The following tasks are included in the battery:

1. Two-letter Search — identification of letters in a string of characters.
2. Six-letter Search — as above with six target letters.
3. Encoding/Decoding — letters to be translated to map coordinates.
4. Two-column Addition — mental arithmetic task.
5. Serial add and subtract — computer-paced — requires sustained attention.
6. Logical Reasoning — true–false decision after comparing a sentence describing letter order (B is followed by A) with a letter pair.
7. Digit Recall — short-term supraspan memory test.
8-9. Pattern Recognition I and II — spatial memory tasks of increasing complexity.
10. Visual Scanning — visual search task with minimal memory load.
11. Mood-Activation Scale — POMS-like adjective/Likert scale.
12. Mood Scale II — 36-adjective, 3-point scale of affective states.
13. Four-choice Serial Reaction Time.
14. Time Estimation I — identifies when a moving object will reappear from behind a barrier.

The Walter Reed Battery is available free of charge to agencies and professional users, on the conditions that users will exchange information about the battery, that it is not distributed to third parties without permission, and that published research will cite its source.

The Neurobehavioral Evaluation System (NES) (Baker *et al.*, 1985a)

The NES battery is perhaps the most extensively distributed of all microcomputer batteries used in neuropsychological toxicology studies. Baker *et al.* (1985) have NES work groups in a number of foreign countries and have wide distribution in the United States as well. Unlike most of the previous batteries, the NES tests have been implemented only for the IBM and Compaq (MS-DOS) computers. They may also run on other MS-DOS clones or compatibles but have not been so tested.

The tests employed by the NES system are, for the most part, more traditional extensions of conventional neuropsychological tests than have been developed for previously cited batteries. The authors have elected to stay close to the series of "core" tests recommended by the World Health Organization and NIOSH for use in the epidemiologic investigation of neurotoxic substances. Five of the NES tests are modified versions of WHO/NIOSH core tests and two others were recommended by the World Health Organization as supplemental tests. The NES battery consists of the following tests:

1. Continuous Performance Test: subjects press a button when a tachistoscopically presented "S" is projected on the monitor.
2. Symbol–Digit Substitution: similar to WAIS-R Digit Symbol Test.
3. Hand–Eye Coordination Test: Patient traces the cursor over a sine wave drawn on the monitor, using a joystick.
4. Simple Reaction Time.
5–9. Memory: Digit Span, Paired Associate Learning Test (with delayed recall), Visual Retention Test (like the Benton VRT), Memory Scanning Test, Pattern Memory Test.
10. Vocabulary Test.
11. Mood Scales.
12. Pattern Recognition Test.

Several preliminary validation studies exist for the NES. Baker, Letz and Fidler (1985b) found effects of age, education and solvent exposure for several of the tests in the battery. Another study (Greenberg *et al.*, 1985) examined NES performance under acute exposure to nitrous oxide. Significant decrements were found on the Continuous Performance Test, Symbol–Digit Substitution and Finger Tapping. The authors did not correct for the use of multiple *t* tests, but claim that the similarity in functions tested by these three tasks and known effects of nitrous oxide mitigate this methodological insufficiency.

Special issues with microcomputer batteries

The recent development of microcomputer batteries, both in neuropsychological toxicology and general psychometric testing, requires consideration of some special testing issues. These have been extensively covered elsewhere (Hartman, 1986a,b; Matarazzo, 1985) so only a short review of these issues is presented here.

Validation

Computer batteries, like all psychometric tests, must be validated on appropriate patient populations to provide meaningful clinical and research data. Demographic and cultural differences in subjects must be addressed if the battery is to be used with heterogeneous groups of patients.

Administration

Because a well-designed computer battery can essentially self-administer, care must be taken to assure that neuropsychologically trained clinical personnel administer the battery and observe the patient's actual behavior during test procedures. Test data are not meaningful without an observed context of test-taking behavior (Matarazzo, 1985). Subject cooperation, affect and behavior must be independently observed by the clinician.

A related problem in automated battery administration is the potential for misuse by personnel untrained in diagnosis or data interpretation. An even more serious possibility is that such users will apply a computer battery to situations for which it was never intended (e.g. hiring or firing of workers, "drug screenings"), and mass testing for the purpose of generating income for the tester rather than any useful medical–neuropsychological purpose.

Nonetheless, with proper validation and adherence to relevant ethical and methodological concerns, microcomputer batteries may greatly advance the science of measuring cortical function. Computerized test batteries allow assessment of complex cognitive paradigms heretofore confined to the laboratory, among them Sternberg memory tasks and signal detection paradigms. With adequate patient observation and test validation, batteries such as these may prove to be powerful additions to the neuropsychologist's armamentarium.

CHILDREN'S TESTS

Behavioral toxicology batteries for children have received comparatively little attention, which is unfortunate, since children are considered to be more at risk than adults for neurotoxic exposure to many substances (Winneke and Collet, 1985). Test selection strategies are similar to those of adults; a standardized battery may be used (e.g. the Young Children's and Older Children's versions of the Halstead–Reitan Batteries), or a flexible battery approach may be substituted. Winneke and Collet (1985) recommend that a children's neurotoxicology battery include tests of intelligence, language, memory, perception, attention and motor functions. They have found the following tests to be useful for the evaluation of childhood lead neurotoxicity: the WISC-R or WPPSI, the Bender–Gestalt, children's versions of the Trail-Making Tests, a delayed reaction time test and a complex reaction time test (i.e. the Wiener Test) (p. 47). Other useful tests might include the Lincoln–Oseretsky or the Bruninks–Oseretsky tests of fine and gross motor control, cancellation tasks, the "Continuous Performance Test", and the Benton Visual Retention Test, which has child norms.

SUMMARY

Reviewing neuropsychologists' testing recommendations, it is possible to see some commonalities, whether the authors favor standard or flexible battery approaches. All recommend measures of reaction time or motor speed. Fine motor coordination and finger dexterity testing is likewise required. Memory assessment is considered to be a mandatory part of these neurobehavioral batteries (e.g. Wechsler Memory Scale, Fig II.2). Tests of cognitive efficiency and flexibility (e.g. Trails, Digit Symbol) are included on most batteries, as are tests which can suggest premorbid function (e.g. the Vocabulary Subtest of the WAIS). Some batteries, but not all, include personality testing as part of the examination.

From this it is possible to make some recommendations concerning the construction of a neuropsychological battery to test for neurotoxic sequelae. Because nonverbal abilities tend to be differentially more affected by common neurotoxins, a neuropsychological toxicology battery should load more heavily on these functions.

Table II.2 can be considered a representative collection of commonly available tests to evaluate neurotoxic syndromes. Additionally, neuropsychologists might consider dusting off old psychophysics equipment, including rotary pursuit, graded weights, tachistoscopes, etc. This equipment, well-normed in experimental psychology for use with intact subjects, might be of renewed utility to neuropsychologists investigating peripheral and central nervous system impairment.

The scoring form used at Cook County Hospital (Table II.3) summarizes the results of the above-mentioned (and other related) tests. This collection has been expanded over several years, beginning with a basic "screening battery" developed by Wysocki and Sweet (1985). Not all tests are used for each patient.

TESTING CAUTIONS

The diagnosis of subclinical neurotoxic syndromes is a difficult and often ultimately ambiguous process. Neurotoxic syndrome presentations are

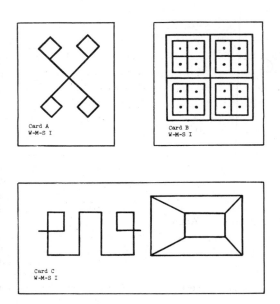

FIGURE II.2. Wechsler Memory Scale, Figural Memory Cards, Form I. Copyright © 1955, renewed 1974 by The Psychological Corporation. Reproduced by permission. All rights reserved. Cards have been photo-reduced.

complex and may interact with a variety of pre-existing medical and psychological difficulties which could mimic neurotoxic presentations. For example, patients may have unadmitted drug or alcohol problems that are capable of causing neurotoxic syndromes similar in appearance but unrelated to a primary toxic exposure substance. Stress can cause decrements in neuropsychological performance, and to further complicate diagnosis, such stress may be functional and unrelated to neurotoxic exposure, *reactive* to physical or emotional limitations caused by exposure, or *primary* as a direct result of neurotoxicity. Many seemingly unequivocal test results may be mitigated by factors completely extrinsic to toxic exposure. In many cases, current theory and test applications simply do not allow more definitive diagnosis. Neuropsychologists unused to ambiguity or complex multifactorial diagnostic questions may find it difficult to adjust to the specialized diagnostic problems presented by this new field.

COMPLEMENTARY APPROACHES

The field of neuropsychology exists in a complementary and mutually beneficial relationship with medicine. Medical examination provides basic

TABLE II.2. Representative neuropsychological testing battery for neurotoxicity evaluations

TEST	FUNCTIONS TESTED
Finger Tapping Test	Peripheral nervous system and central nervous system motor strip
Grooved Pegboard Test	Visual–motor–spatial coordination/dexterity
Minnesota Rate of Manipulation Test	Visual–motor–spatial coordination/dexterity
Grip Strength (Dynamometer)	Gross motor strength
Digit Symbol Test	Cognitive efficiency and flexibility
Trails A and B	Cognitive efficiency and flexibility
Stroop Test	Reading, color naming, sustained attention under continuous distraction
PASAT (Paced Auditory Serial Addition Test)	Auditory comprehension, processing of simple arithmetic problems under conditions of sustained attention
Block Design	Constructional abilities
Rey Auditory Verbal Learning Test	Supraspan verbal short-term memory and learning

Wechsler Memory Scale:
  Logical and Figural Memory
  Immediate and 30-minute delay
  (Russell modification)
	Verbal and nonverbal memory with immediate and long-term recall

WAIS-R Subtests:
  Vocabulary
  Information	

Shipley Institute of Living Test	As estimates of general intellectual function
Inventories: Medical	Complete clinical history, exposure data, drug and alcohol history, occupational and social functioning.
Psychological	Used to identify variables relevant to neurotoxic exposure and rule out alternative diagnoses.
Occupational	

physical data and quantified measures of neurological integrity. Medical examination also allows the health team to rule out other illnesses which may mimic neurotoxic effects. Alternatively, neuropsychological data benefit the physician by providing a fine-grained and comprehensive measure of neuropsychological function, information that may support medical diagnosis and clarify the severity of the patient's neuropsychological

TABLE II.3. Neuropsychological test battery – scoring sheet D. Hartman, Ph.D., 1987.

Name _____ Date:___/___/___ ___Testing Age:____

Address: _____

BD:___/___/___ Education:_____ Tested by: _____

Reason for Referral: _____

Place of Testing:_____

Referral Source:_____

[] 1. Finger tapping: RH mean:____   Russell____

      (Dom. hand:____) LH mean:____   Russell____

[] 2. Wechsler Memory Scale: Logical

      Immediate recall: A:___ B:___   Total:____   Russell____ AC____

      Delayed recall: A:___ B:___   Total:____   Russell____ AC____ %R____

                  Figural

      Immediate recall: A:___ B:___ C:___   Total:____   Russell____ AC____

      Delayed recall: A:___ B:___ C:___   Total:____   Russell____ AC____ %R____

[] 3. Trail Making Test: A:___(seconds)   Russell____ AC____

                 B:___(seconds)   Russell____ AC____

[] 4. WAIS-R Digit Symbol Test: Raw score:____ Scaled score:____ AC____

[] 5. Stroop Test: No. of words:____ + age corr.:____ Total:____ T score ____

              No. of colors:____ + age corr.:____ Total:____ T score ____

       No. of colored words:_____ + age corr.:____ Total:____ T score ____

[] 6. Luria-Nebraska Pathognomonic Scale:

       68.8 + Age value:____ – Education value:____ = Critical level ____

                     No. of errors:____   T score ____

[] 7. Spatial Relations: (Greek Cross) Best:____ + Worst:____ = ____ Russell____

[] 8. Associate Learning: 1) E____ H____ 2) E____ H____ 3) E____ H____

[] 9. Rey Auditory Verbal Learning Test (ALVT):

       1____ 2____ 3____ 4____ 5____ (IRL)____ (Recall)____ (Recog.)____

[] 10. Block Design: Raw score_____ Scale score_____ AC____

[] 11. Tactual   RH Time_____ No. of blocks____ Russell____ Memory____ Russell____

       Performance LH Time_____ No. of blocks____ Russell____

       Test   BH Time_____ No. of blocks____ Russell____ Location____ Russell____

      12. IQ Estimates:

[]   a) Kent EGY   Raw____   IQ est.:____

[]   b) SILS: V Raw____ T____ A Raw____ T____ Total____   CQ____

               Pred. Abs. from, Age, Ed. & Vocab. ____AQ Conversion   ____

               Estimated WAIS-R Full Scale IQ from Total SILS by Age   ____

[]   c) WAIS-R; Information   Raw____ Scale score____ AC____

                 Vocabulary   Raw____ Scale score____ AC____

[] 13. Category Test: No. of errors:____   Russell____

[] 14. Grip Strength: RH: 1____ 2____   LH: 1____ 2____

       (Lb/Kg)   Mean RH: ___ T___   Mean LH: ___ T___

[] 15. Pegboard: (Purdue/Grooved): RH:___ T___ LH:___ T___ BH:___ T___   [] 22.

                                                            WAIS-R

[] 16. Minnesota Rate of Manipulation Test: VIQ   ____

				1 Hand		2 Hand		
	Placing	Turning	Displacing	Placing & Turning		Placing & Turning	Info	____
							DSp	____
							Voc	____
P	R____ L____	____	R____ L____	R____ L____	____		Arit	____
							Comp	____
1	R____ L____	____	R____ L____	R____ L____	____		Simi	____
							Tot	____
2	R____ L____	____	R____ L____	R____ L____	____			
							PIQ	____
3	R____ L____	____	R____ L____	R____ L____	____		PCom	____
4	R____ L____	____	R____ L____	R____ L____	____		PArr	____
							BlkD	____
				2/3/4 Trial total			ObjA	____
							DSym	____
	R____ L____	____	R____ L____	R____ L____	____		Tot	____
SS	____ ____	____	____ ____	____ ____	____			
%R	____ ____	____	____ ____	____ ____	____		FSIQ	____
				2/3/4 Trial mean				
	R____ L____	____	R____ L____	R____ L____	____			

[] 17. Aphasia Screening Test:_____

[] 18. Fingertip Number Writing:

Finger	1	2	3	4	5
	4 6 3 5	3 5 4 6	6 5 4 3	5 4 6 3	6 3 5 4

Right   - - - - - - - - - - - - - - - - - - - -   R___

Left   - - - - - - - - - - - - - - - - - - - -   L___

[] 19. Rhythm errors _____   Russell___
[] 20. Speech errors _____   Russell___
[] 21. PASAT _____
23. Personality Tests:
[] MMPI: (T scores) ?___ L___ F___ K___ Hs___ D___ Hy___ Pd___ Mf___ Pa___
[] BDI:___   Pt___ Sc___ Ma___ Si___ A___ R___ Es___ MAC___
[] POMS (T Scores): T___ D___ A___ V___ F___ C___
[] Other tests: _____

[] Occupational Health Questionnaire
[] Psychological Social History

[] Personal Problems Checklist
[] Other _____

impairment. Medical tests which have suggested utility for neurotoxicologic investigations include:

1. *Conventional neurological and cerebellar examination* (Juntunen, 1982).
2. *Evoked potentials.* Sensory evoked potentials provide an index of the integrity of sensory pathways from the peripheral nervous system to the cortex. Damage from neurotoxins associated with peripheral nervous system dysfunction (e.g. *n*-hexane, methyl butyl ketone) may be quantified with evoked potential studies. While non-invasive, the electrical stimulus may be painful to some.

    Promising results obtained from animal studies using visual (flash) evoked potentials suggest that VEPs and especially pattern reversal evoked potentials (PREPS) may be of future use in human studies (Wennberg and Otto, 1985). Additionally, the authors enthusiastically recommend the use of brainstem auditory evoked potentials (BAEP) as the "most promising" sensory evoked potential test for neurotoxicity testing (Wennberg and Otto, 1985).
3. *Nerve conduction studies.* While slowed nerve conduction is characteristic of a number of neurotoxic substances, Bleeker (1984) is against using nerve conduction studies as a screening device, since "more than 50% of nerve fibers must be blocked or lost before the amplitude of evoked action potential is outside normal limits (p. 216). Present knowledge concerning exposure-effects on nerve conduction is too uncertain to currently

promote the use of nerve conduction studies for neurotoxicity screenings (Muijser *et al.*, 1985).

4. *Electroencephalography (EEG).* While the EEG has proven utility in the identification of neurological disorders — including epilepsy, tumors and other diseases — its utility for the detection of subclinical toxicity has not been demonstrated. EEG abnormalities have been detected in exposure to certain toxic substances, including pesticides and organotins, but other substances (e.g. solvents) have not been shown to consistently produce EEG changes. At this time, EEG findings may be more appropriate for ruling out alternative diagnoses than for accurate detection of subclinical toxicity (Wennberg and Otto, 1985).

5. *Other tests.* Bleeker (1984) suggests that other neurological tests are useful in neurotoxicology diagnosis, including tremometry and quantitative sensory testing (e.g. the Optacon Tactile Tester). Electromyography (EMG) has also been used to investigate potential cases of toxic neuropathy (Seppäläinen, 1982). Tests which show promise but which have not yet been validated for neurotoxicology research include tests of warm/cold perception, vibration sensitivity and autonomic nervous system function.

III
Neuropsychological Toxicology of Metals

HISTORY

Human contact with metallic substances is virtually coexistent with the development of civilization. It is likely, for example, that metallurgy accompanied the earliest cultures of the Tigris and Euphrates rivers around 6000 B.C. Metallic ornaments discovered at Ur in Babylonia suggest that "the casting of copper silver and gold . . . began around 3500 B.C." (Marks and Beatty, 1975, p. 5). The Egyptians were working with lead as early as 3400 B.C. (*ibid.*, p. 6).

Metals were also among the earliest neurotoxins produced by humans; their toxic effects have been chronicled for centuries. As early as 1473, Ulrich Ellenbog wrote a treatise on what today would be called industrial toxicology. It detailed some effects of occupational metal poisoning:

> This vapour of quicksilver, silver and lead is a cold poison,/ for it maketh heaviness and tightness of the chest, burdeneth the limbs and oftimes lameth them/ as often one seeth in foundries where men do work with large masses and the vital inward members become burdened therefrom (Ellenbog, cited in Bingham, 1974 p. 199).

Somewhat more recently, Weiss (1983) corroborates that "Excessive exposure to metals . . . has been implicated in a remarkable range of adverse signs and symptoms involving the central nervous system (CNS) and behavior" (p. 1175). Exposure to almost any metal can cause central nervous system dysfunction.

Metallic exposures are not restricted to industrial sites. Metal products are ubiquitous in the environment, and metallic byproducts of various industries have pervaded the atmosphere, been discharged into the water, and have entered world food supplies. Metals have been used as medicines, added to gasoline and used as insecticides and pesticides. While levels of certain metals have been declining in the environment, they may be replaced by others. For example, mercury and lead have been better regulated in recent years, and the number of exposure victims of these toxins has been decreasing (though they still number in the millions). However, as environmental levels of these metals decline, the newer "high technology" metals may take their place in the environment. The future may see increased poisonings from less well-known metallic toxins including nickel, cadmium and selenium compounds (Gossel and Bricker, 1984).

SITES OF NEUROTOXICITY

In addition to causing central nervous system damage, metals may also be toxic to other parts of the nervous system. Peripheral nervous system toxicity has been noted for a number of common metals (e.g. lead, arsenic). Several metals (e.g. iron) produce neurotoxic effects on the extrapyramidal system, damaging the caudate nucleus, putamen, globus pallidus and their connections to the thalamus, substantia nigra and cerebellum (Feldman, 1982a). Finally, a number of metals are capable of damaging both the central and peripheral nervous system.

VARIABLES AFFECTING NEUROTOXICITY

Substance

Some metals are more toxic to the nervous system than others. For example, mercury and lead are far more neurotoxic than iron or inorganic tin. Different forms of the same metal may be differentially toxic to the nervous system. In general, organic metal compounds both penetrate the brain more effectively and are absorbed more completely than inorganic metals. Thus, organometals may potentially cause greater neurotoxic damage than elemental forms of the same metals. Methylated mercury, for example, is far more damaging to the central nervous system than inorganic mercury. Elemental tin is another metal which poorly penetrates the nervous system in its inorganic state, but as an organotin is responsible for a wide range of neurotoxic and neuropsychological effects in humans.

Developmental influences

The degree of neurotoxic damage from metal exposure is also influenced by other factors. The age of the exposed individual may affect toxicity, with the highest risk to fetal and perinatal development. Young children are also at greater risk than adults for the development of certain toxic effects (e.g. lead-induced hyperactivity).

Weiss (1978) makes the useful suggestion that developmental effects should not be considered "a shorthand for youth" (p. 24). Thus, neuropsychological effects of toxic metals may also occur in older individuals whose nervous systems may lose plasticity and the ability to compensate for neurotoxic damage. Unfortunately, the question of human developmental neurotoxicity is largely unexplored at this time. One important question for this sub-field might include whether pre– or perinatal neurotoxic effects produce neuropsychological impairments in older adults when compensation mechanisms can no longer hide subclinical effects. Another question is whether chronic exposure to metal neurotoxins in older adults produces different neurotoxic symptoms in kind or degree, compared to younger adult exposure.

Acute versus chronic exposure

Certain metals (e.g. arsenic) may show one set of effects from acute dose, while chronic exposure produces other forms of neurotoxic damage. In industry there is increasing concern as to whether chronic exposure to low doses of metals can cause neurotoxic damage.

Individual variation

As is the case for all neurotoxins, there appears to be wide inter-individual variation in susceptibility to neuropsychological deficit. One cause of such individual variation may be the ability of the individual to eliminate toxins from the body. Aluminum compounds, for example, are not thought to be neurotoxic in healthy individuals. However, in persons with impaired renal functioning, aluminum has been cited as a cause of dementing syndromes.

The reasons for other inter-individual variations remain obscure. Certain individuals with chronic exposure to lead and with documented blood levels above 70 μg/dl may show only mild neuropsychological abnormalities, while other individuals with lower blood levels and shorter exposures can present with more severe forms of neuropsychological impairment. The causes of such variability are presently unknown, but may be related to differential ability to eliminate toxic substances, metabolic differences, or perhaps variations in brain susceptibility or permeability of the blood–brain barrier to these toxins.

NEUROPSYCHOLOGICAL TESTING OF METAL EXPOSURE

The value of neuropsychological testing for metal exposure has been described by Grandjean (1983), who states that

studies of [metal] exposures have been greatly advanced by the use of modern neuropsychological methods . . . . while such psychological tests may be influenced by other factors not related to neurotoxicity, they provide a useful and relatively accurate assessment of the degree and character of neurotoxic effects in humans (p. 331).

Despite clear endorsements and demonstrated value for individual cases, neuropsychological investigations of metal poisoning are difficult to locate in the research literature, perhaps due to the factors described in Chapter I.

Lead and mercury are the metals whose neuropsychological effects are the most completely explored, although their exact pathophysiology is far from completely understood. Other neurotoxic metals have been described in the neurological literature, but have little or no accompanying neuropsychological data. Iron, cadmium and tellurium are examples from this group. Because of the variety of neurotoxic effects capable of being produced, there is no general "metal encephalopathy" syndrome, even though some symptoms of poisoning are common to several metals. It is more informative to describe the unique neurological and neuropsychological features of exposure to individual metals. Accordingly, several of the more well-known effects of metallic neurotoxins are described in the following pages.

Where available, NIOSH and OSHA industrial safety levels precede each discussion.

ALUMINUM

History

Aluminum's use in medicinal compounds predates by thousands of years its isolation as a pure metallic ore. Salts of aluminum were used during the Roman empire for water purification. During the Middle Ages these aluminum salts were mixed with honey and employed as a treatment for ulcers (Crapper and De Boni, 1980, p. 326), a treatment not altogether different from current over-the-counter remedies.

Aluminum was discovered to be a CNS neurotoxin in the late 1800s and is of scientific value in this capacity; its oxide or hydroxide applied to the cortex of animal subjects produces a useful research model for studies of focal epilepsy (Ward, 1972).

Individuals at risk

Common routes of aluminum accumulation include industrial exposure as well as ingestion of processed food (e.g. pickles), with the average diet containing about 22 mg/day of aluminum (Shore and Wyatt, 1983). Despite such continuous environmental exposure, most individuals with normal renal function appear able to clear aluminum effectively. An exception may be patients with Alzheimer's disease (AD).

The relation between aluminum accumulation and AD is unproven, and AD patients do not show differential levels of aluminum relative to controls in serum, CSF or hair. In addition, the neurofibrillary tangles experimentally produced by aluminum differ from those which occur in AD (Shore and Wyatt, 1983). While both AD and aluminum intoxication have produced 10 nm neurofibrillary degeneration filaments, Alzheimer filaments are bundled pairs of filaments twisted in a helical array, while aluminum-induced neurofibrillary tangles are single 10 nm filaments (McLachlan and De Boni, 1980). It may be the case, however, that while aluminum does not *cause* AD, the damaged brain tissues of AD patients may be more vulnerable to this metal. It is also possible that the blood-brain barriers of AD patients may be damaged in the course of the AD process, rendering brain tissues increasingly vulnerable to aluminum accumulation from foods, antacids and buffered aspirin (McLachlan and De Boni, 1980; Shore and Wyatt, 1983).

Patients with impaired kidney function or chronic renal failure may be especially vulnerable to aluminum neurotoxicity. Body and brain accumulation of aluminum in renal-compromised patients has been linked to several factors. Dialysis using water that has not been deionized and/or which has been stored in aluminum tanks has been posited to cause aluminum accumulation (Crapper and De Boni, 1980). High aluminum concentrations can also be found in the tissues of some dialysis patients as a consequence of ingesting large amounts of antacids and phosphate binding gels (Sedman *et al.*, 1984), although it had been previously thought that oral aluminum was poorly absorbed and therefore not neurotoxic. Sedman *et al.* (1984) report progressive neuropsychological deterioration and dementia from brain aluminum accumulation in a child whose single kidney functioned poorly and was unable to adequately excrete prescribed doses of antacids.

Aluminum may also be neurotoxic to normal children when combined with exposure to other metals. A recent study suggests that combined exposure to aluminum and lead may synergistically affect visual-motor performance in children (Marlowe *et al.*, 1985).

"Dialysis dementia"

Clinically, some end-stage renal disease (ESRD) patients develop what appears to be a form of aluminum encephalopathy. Exposure to aluminum occurs via aluminum-containing dialysate and, probably somewhat less often, the chronic ingestion of aluminum-containing antacids, the latter being a usual concomitant of ESRD therapy. The disorder has been termed "dialysis dementia" and shows a rapid progression from personality changes to global intellectual impairment, accompanied by seizures, gait problems, asterixis, dysarthria, apraxia and myoclonus. Abnormal EEG or CT may be found (Sedman *et al.*, 1984). Since not all dialysis patients who take large quantities of antacids develop dialysis dementia, unspecified individual differences may interact with aluminum ingestion to produce the disease.

Onset of dialysis dementia is apparently subtle, and initial symptoms occur after a mean of 37 months from initial dialysis. Severity is correlated with brain aluminum concentration. Uncorrected, aluminum encephalopathy is progressive and potentially fatal. Brain aluminum concentrations of "15 to 20 times above control populations" have been found in patients with this disorder (Crapper and De Boni, 1980, p.326). While overall percentages of patients who develop dialysis dementia have not been tallied, it is thought to be a leading cause of mortality among patients undergoing chronic hemodialysis (Rosati *et al.*, 1980). It is not, however, an inevitable consequence of ESRD. Rosati *et al.* (1980) failed to find any significant neuropsychological deficits in a group of nine dialysis patients who *did* have significantly increased serum aluminum level. However, serum aluminum levels may have been too low to produce the syndrome.

Other diseases with possible links to aluminum

Other diseases have been linked to elevations in brain aluminum. These include Down syndrome, Parkinson dementia complex of Guam and striatonigral syndrome (Feldman, 1982a). Aluminum has also been linked to cerebellar Purkinje cell degeneration secondary to alcohol abuse (McLaughlin and De Boni, 1980). It is not clear at this time whether genetic variations exist in the ability to handle this metal, causing certain individuals to be at higher risk than others.

Occupational encephalopathy

Encephalopathic syndromes have also been reported as a consequence of industrial aluminum exposure. The first recorded industrial aluminum poisoning was in 1921 in a metal worker who developed memory loss, tremor, cerebellar signs and loss of coordination (Wills and Savory, 1983). A later case study verified a syndrome of rapidly progressive encephalopathy in an aluminum powder factory worker who had been heavily exposed to aluminum dust (McGlaughlin *et al.*, 1962). The worker developed left-sided focal epilepsy, became increasingly demented in the course of several months, and finally died of pneumonia. Brain aluminum concentration at autopsy was found to be 17 times greater than normal.

More recently, three patients who had worked for 12 years in the potroom of an aluminum smelter (which also included exposure to lithium) were discovered to have neurological and neuropsychological abnormalities

TABLE III.1. Neuropsychological performance of three aluminum workers. (Reprinted, by permission of the American Medical Association, from Longstreth et al. (copyright 1985). Potroom palsy? Neurologic disorder in three aluminum smelter workers. *Archives of Internal Medicine*, **145**, 1972–1975.)

TEST	SUBJECT NO.		
	1	2	3
WAIS-R:			
Full Scale IQ	93	71	87
Verbal IQ	97	67	91
Performance IQ	87	78	84
Wechsler Memory Scale (WMS):			
Memory Quotient	86	62	97
Problem Solving (unspecified)	Poor	Poor	Poor
Halsted-Reitan Impairment Index	1.0	1.0	0.6

(Longstreth, Rosenstock and Heyer, 1985). Neurological symptoms common to all three included joint pains, severe lack of energy and strength, and tremor. Neurological examination revealed bilateral hearing loss, incoordination, intention tremor and ataxic gait. Electrophysiologic studies were normal except in one individual who showed bilateral delays in visual evoked potentials and delays at the medullar level with somatosensory evoked potentials. Neuropsychological performance showed clear deficit (see Table III.1).

The exact etiology of these abnormalities cannot be verified. While results are consistent with known neurotoxic effects of aluminum, the patients' lithium exposure may have also contributed to the symptoms shown here. Furthermore, because blood or bone aluminum burden may not accurately reflect brain aluminum content, these patients' normal bone aluminum cannot rule out neurotoxic brain concentrations of the metal. The results are worth noting as an alert to possible human neurotoxic effects of prolonged aluminum exposure.

ARSENIC

OSHA exposure limit (inorganic)   10 $\mu g/m^3$, 8 hr TWA
NIOSH recommended exposure limit   2 $\mu g/m^3$ ceiling (15 min)
ACGIH   200 $\mu g/m^3$

As arsine (hydrogen arsenide or arsenic trihydride):
OSHA   0.05 ppm (0.2 $\mu g/m^3$) 8 hr TWA
NIOSH   2 $\mu g/m^3$, 15 min ceiling
IDLH level   6 ppm
(NIOSH, 1985)

History

Arsenic has the dubious reputation among metals as "historically the most important of the poisons used for criminal purposes" (Hamilton and Hardy, 1974, p.31). It was employed in the pharmacopoeia of the Assyrians where it is mentioned in a papyrus dated from about 1552 B.C. (Marks and Beatty, 1975). Like many other metals, arsenic had been tried as a cure for many illnesses, including cancer, fever, herpes, ringworm, eczema and ulcers (Marks and Beatty, 1975). A common treatment for syphilis over the past two centuries, arsenic was the cause of more injuries than cures, producing optic neuritis and encephalopathy as a consequence of its use (Windebank, McCall and Dyck, 1984).

With even less reputability, arsenic has been used in poison gases during wartime and as a method of homicide or suicide. The latter two uses account for most of the recently reported cases of arsenic poisoning.

Several mass poisonings related to accidental arsenic exposure have been reported, the first involving 40,000 individuals who became poisoned when arsenious acid was accidentally mixed with wine and bread. In another epidemic, sugar used in beer manufacture became contaminated with arsenic, poisoning 6000 people and resulting in 70 fatalities (Katz, 1985).

Current uses and individuals at risk

Currently, the main legitimate uses of arsenic are in the pharmaceutical and agricultural industries. Arsenic is a principal element in many insecticides, weedkillers and fungicides. Calcium arsenate, an insecticide used in fruit orchards, is the most toxic of the arsenic compounds.

Other industries where workers may be exposed to arsenic include any industry which adds acid to iron and steel. These metals both contain small amounts of arsenic, and their immersion in acid frees this available arsenic. Metal "pickling" (acid treatment) plants may be dangerous in this regard (Hamilton and Hardy, 1974). NIOSH (National Institute for Occupational Safety Health, 1975a) estimates that approximately 1.5 million workers are exposed to inorganic arsenic.

Neurological effects

Peripheral nervous system
Peripheral neuropathy is the principal finding associated with inorganic arsensic intoxication. Schaumberg, Spencer and Thomas (1983) report different profiles of neurotoxic damage, depending upon whether the exposure was high level and acute (e.g. a suicide attempt) or prolonged and

low level. Subacute, 3–10-day delayed neuropathy may develop in survivors of single high-level doses. Numbness, weakness in extremities and "intense" paresthesias develop with the eventual outcome ranging from mild sensory neuropathy to "severe distal sensorimotor polyneuropathy" (Spencer, Schaumberg and Thomas, 1983, p. 134).

Central nervous system effects

Bleecker and Bolla-Wilson (1985) speculate that central nervous system effects of arsenic may be similar to those found in thiamine deficiency, since arsenic prevents the transformation of thiamine into acetyl-CoA and succinyl-CoA. Validation for this hypothesis could potentially come from autopsy studies investigating neuropathological similarities between thiamine deficiency states produced by arsenic and those reported in the common alcohol-induced thiamine deficiency disorder, Wernicke–Korsakoff syndrome.

Neuropsychological effects

Assessing neuropsychological dysfunction in arsenic exposure cases has been difficult because of potential confounding effects of alcohol intake. Feldman *et al.* (1979) report that 92% of arsenic-exposed smelter workers are also moderate drinkers. Bleecker and Bolla-Wilson (1985) report the case of a 50-year-old engineer exposed to chronic low-dose inorganic arsenic who consequently developed severe and chronic verbal memory and learning impairment on the Rey Auditory Verbal Learning Test and the Logical Memory Subtest of the Wechsler Memory Scale. However, interpretation was complicated by a family history of rapid-onset dementia. Unfortunately, there do not appear to be any complete neuropsychological studies of arsenic intoxication that would validate the finding of low-dose arsenic-induced memory disorder. The suggestion that arsenic causes "unequivocal" damage to the central and peripheral nervous system (Windebank *et al.*,1984) implies that neurobehavioral evaluation could be employed as a useful index of damage and recovery.

Emotional effects

Organic arsenic-containing compounds may cause rapidly developing central nervous system symptoms, with progression from drowsiness to confusion and stupor. Organic psychosis resembling paranoid schizophrenia is a common result of organic arsenic intoxication and delirium may follow (Windebank, McCall and Dyke, 1984). Fluctuating mental state, agitation and emotional lability have been noted (Beckett *et al.*, 1986).

Case study

The following patient was accidentally exposed to arsenic compounds during his employment. Test results and case discussion clearly support the use of neuropsychological evaluation in arsenic exposure cases.

TABLE III.2. Neuropsychological test scores: Long-term consequences of acute exposure to arsenic

1. *Finger Tapping:* (Dom. hand: R)	RH mean: 39 LH mean: 39.8		Russell 3 Russell 2
2. *Wechsler Memory Scale:* (a) *Logical*			
Immediate recall:	A: 10.5　B: 0	Total: 10.5	Russell 4
Delayed recall:	A: 4.0　B: 0.5	Total: 4.5	Russell 4
(b) *Figural*			
Immediate recall:	A: 3　B: 2　C: 4	Total: 9	Russell 2
Delayed recall:	A: 3　B: 2　C: 3	Total: 8	Russell 2
3. *Trail Making Test:*	A: 43 (seconds)		Russell 2
	B: 131 (seconds)		Russell 3
4. *WAIS-R Digit Symbol Test:*		Raw score: 38	Scaled score 6
5. *Stroop Test:*			
No. of words: 108 + age corr.: 0		Total: 108	T score 50
No. of colors: 78 + age corr.: 0		Total: 78	T score 49
No. of colored words: 41 + age corr.: 0		Total: 41	T score 46
6. *Luria-Nebraska Pathognomonic Scale:*			Critical level 59.26
	No. of errors: 31		T score 74
7. *Spatial Relations:* (Greek Cross) Best: 1 + Worst: 1 = 2			Russell 1

8. *Pegboard:* (Grooved) RH: 75″ T 34　LH: 108″ T 03
9. *Grip Strength:* RH: (1) 48 T55　(2) 40 T52　　LH: (1) 42 T53　(2) 42 T53
　　(Kg)　　　　　　Mean RH: 44 T: 53　　　　　Mean LH: 42 T: 53
10. *IQ Estimate* Kent EGY Scale (similar to WAIS-R Information)
　　　　Raw score: 26　IQ estimate: 97
10a. *IQ Estimate:* Shipley Institute of Living Scale (SILS)
　　　　Vocabulary raw score: 5　Abstraction raw score: 6
11. *Block Design:* Raw score: 20　Scale score: 7
12. *Digit Span:* 4 digits forward, 4 digits backward
13. *Associate Learning:* 4:0; 5:1; 6:3
14. *Fingertip Number Writing:*
　　　　　　　4 6 3 5　3 5 4 6　6 5 4 3　5 4 6 3　6 3 5 4
　　Right　　4 6 3 5　3 5 4 6　0 5 4 3　? 4 6 ?　6 3 5 4　R: 3 errors
　　Left:　　? ? ? 5　3 5 4 6　6 5 4 3　5 4 6 3　6 3 5 4　L: 3 errors
15. *Personality Test:* POMS.
　　BDI = 40

Note: 0–5 severity ratings are from Russell (1975) and Russell, Neuringer and Goldstein (1970) where higher scores indicate greater impairment.

Case notes — long-term consequences of short-term arsenic exposure

The patient is a 31-year-old tractor driver with an 11th grade education. In 1980 he was driving in the field when a crop duster sprayed the field and as a consequence doused the patient with an arsenic-based insecticide. The patient reported no immediate effects, suggesting that he did not inhale the poison. However, the patient began to vomit after an unspecified time, which implies slightly delayed effects of skin absorption. He became unable to retain food and water and began to lose weight. The patient reported losing approximately 40 pounds in the month following his exposure.

The patient initially went to a physician who diagnosed his symptoms as ''heat stroke''. However, since symptoms did not remit, the patient came to the

Occupational Medicine Clinic where he was diagnosed as having arsenic poisoning via an insecticide which contained arsenic acid. The patient denied history of alcohol or drug abuse, head injury, high fever or seizures. Hypertension was controlled with hydrochlorothiazide. Caffeine intake was about five cans of cola per day. He reported periodic (about once a month) attacks of vertigo that began immediately after his arsenic exposure. Other symptoms reported included continuous paresthesias in the hands, lower arms, and the legs, beginning at the knees. The patient described his paresthesias as "tingling" rather than painful.

The patient was cooperative and appeared to try hard during testing; however, he had great difficulty performing tasks which required fine motor coordination and speed. When holding a pencil it was necessary for the patient to grasp it firmly with all of his fingers, in a balled fist instead of a more conventional grip.

In the neuropsychological examination the patient showed sensory changes consistent with peripheral neuropathy, including complete loss of sensation in the palms of his hands and poor ability to perceive numbers written on the fingertips.

The patient's verbal memory and learning was also impaired relative to memory for designs. The discrepancy between recall of the two Wechsler stories in immediate recall was probably due to educational limitations; however, poor recall of the first story after 30 minutes, coupled with slower than usual verbal learning in the Associate Learning Test, suggest encoding difficulties irrespective of premorbid education. The patient's ability to maintain attention and concentration seems likewise impaired, especially on the Trails Tests, where the patient was not hampered by sensorimotor dysfunction, but rather by the ability to correctly scan for numerical and alternating number–letter sequences.

On measures of current affect, the patient admits to severe depression which appeared to be reactive to real losses of function and ability to make a living. He was highly focused on his physical symptoms, exhibited early morning awakening, and mild loss of appetite, in addition to other "cognitive" forms of depression. In addition, the patient described himself as forgetful, grouchy, uncertain, discouraged, exhausted and "extremely bitter".

The patient's current neuropsychological profile suggested a combination of structural and reactive emotional components. PNS damage, loss of attention and concentration, and probable verbal memory deficits may be direct effects of arsenic damage, but also certainly contribute to the patient's sense of a futile future as evidenced by severe depression noted in the Beck Depression Inventory. Recommendations for such a patient would include evaluation for supportive psychotherapy, antidepressant medication and re-entry into the labor force in whatever capacity he is able.

BISMUTH

Bismuth has been used in large quantities by individuals in France and other countries to control chronic colon disorders. In the United States, bismuth drugs are prescribed to decrease odor and increase bulk of bowel movements, and are also used in colostomy patients after colon carcinoma surgery (Goetz, 1985). The phenomenon of bismuth encephalopathy has only been recognized since the early 1970s; however, by 1981 over 1050 cases and 72 deaths have been attributed to this neurotoxic disorder (Buge *et al.*, 1981; Le Quesne, 1982). The syndrome is characterized by a prodrome of several weeks or months of "depression, anxiety, irritability and tremulousness" (Le Quesne, 1982, p. 537). Further deterioration may occur without warning, sometimes after several years of exposure (Kruger, Weinhardt and Hoyer, 1979). Symptoms include confusion, myoclonic jerks, dysarthria and gait apraxia (Goetz, 1985; Nordberg, 1979). Goetz (1985) reports other neurotoxic effects of bismuth when injected intramuscularly as a systemic treatment of syphilis. Sequelae of multiple injections include acute myelopathy, flaccid paraplegia and loss of bladder control (p. 50).

Little is known about the underlying neuropathology of bismuth intoxication although CT scans show hyperdensities in basal ganglia, cerebellum and cerebral cortex. The pattern of gray matter cortical hyperdensities found in bismuth intoxication has not been seen in any other type of heavy metal intoxication (Buge *et al.*, 1981).

CADMIUM

As cadmium dust:

OSHA exposure limit	0.2 mg/m^3 8 hr TWA
	0.6 mg/m^3 ceiling
NIOSH exposure recommendations	reduce exposure to lowest feasible limit
ACGIH	0.05 mg/m^3
IDLH level	40 mg/m^3

As cadmium fume:

OSHA	0.1 mg/m^3
	0.3 mg/m^3 ceiling
NIOSH	reduce exposure to lowest feasible limit
ACGIH	0.05 mg/m^3 ceiling
IDLH	40 mg/m^3

Cadmium's uses include pigments, alloys and electroplating. Principal effects of cadmium intoxication are on the kidney and lungs rather than the brain, although rat studies have shown CNS changes in early development and demyelinating PNS changes in adult rats. Rats also appeared to become irritable and showed lowered motor activity (Katz, 1985). No human neuropsychological studies of cadmium-poisoned individuals are available.

CHROMIUM

Chromium (metal and insoluble salts):
Exposure limits

OSHA	1 mg/m^3
IDLH	500 mg/m^3

soluble:

OSHA	0.5 mg/m^3
IDLH	250 mg/m^3

(NIOSH, 1985)

Not heretofore thought to be neurotoxic, a recent study suggests that chromium can enter the brain under certain unusual conditions. Duckett (1986) describes three cases with unrelated encephalopathic diseases who showed evidence of CNS chromium neurotoxicity at autopsy. Sources of chromium were radiological contrast media, KCl solution, and mylanta, an antacid. Chromium was thought to enter the brain through pathological pallidal blood vessels which showed vascular siderosis and possible breakdown of the blood–brain barrier. This appears to be the only report of pure chromium neurotoxicity in the literature, and thus, the finding must be considered tentative. The results suggest caution in the use of chromium-containing substances in older patients, or those with damaged vasculature.

COPPER

Dust and mist:

OSHA	1.0 mg/m^3

Fumes:

OSHA	0.1 mg/m^3
ACGIH	0.2 mg/m^3

(NIOSH, 1985)

Neurological and neuropsychological symptoms of copper toxicity occur during the development of Wilson's disease, a genetic disorder of abnormal copper metabolism. Copper is found in brain autopsies of patients with Wilson's disease, and it is likely that many neurological manifestations of the disease are caused by toxic accumulation of brain copper. Structural damage from copper toxicity includes "neuronal degeneration, spongy focal change in cortex, corpus striatum and central myelin" (Feldman, 1982a, p. 150). The basal ganglia and cerebellum are said to be particularly affected (Bornstein, McClean and Ho, 1985). Generalized brain atrophy may or may not be present. Cirrhosis of the liver and deposits of excess copper around the cornea (Kayser-Fleischer rings) are also present in some degree.

Neurological symptoms of Wilson's disease include choreic movement,

Parkinsonian-like rigidity and masked facies. Dementia and death within 4–5 years can result if copper is not chelated from the body. Wilson's disease is rare, and its exact pathophysiology remains open to debate, i.e. whether neurological changes are indirectly produced by copper accumulation in the liver or directly within the brain. It is also unclear whether an individual exposed to heavy amounts of copper in the environment can develop copper neurotoxicity without having a selective metabolic vulnerability to copper (Feldman, 1982a).

Individuals with copper toxicity from Wilson's disease exhibit a variety of neuropsychological and emotional symptoms which appear to be a function of disease progression. Initial testing reveals abnormal motor functioning with intact IQ, while more advanced cases exhibit intellectual dysfunction, and the possibility of dementia in the late stage of the illness. Psychological abnormalities may also accompany Wilson's disease, and a recent review of case studies concluded that affective and behavioral or personality changes are the most common sequelae, with two less common profiles showing schizophrenic-like or cognitive deterioration (Dening, 1985).

While the exact etiology of patients' psychological and intellectual deterioration is not known, patients with other types of extrapyramidal disorders (e.g. Parkinson's) have shown similar neuropsychological deficits. In addition, the generalized losses found in some Wilson's disease patients are consistent with a more global form of encephalopathy (Bornstein, McLean and Ho, 1985).

Reitan and Wolfson (1985) report neuropsychological effects in a 48-year-old high school-educated male with "a long history" of Wilson's disease. IQ was still intact, although Digit Symbol and Block Design were abnormally low. Spatial abilities were poor, with the patient showing constructional dyspraxia and markedly deficient left-hand performance on the Tactual Performance Test (TPT). Fine motor speed was also impaired as was cognitive flexibility (Trails B) and abstract reasoning (Category Test). The patient's impairment index on the Halsted–Reitan Battery was 1.0. Emotional complaints included high perceived stress, with a very low threshold of annoyance or irritation, and occasional outbursts of violent rage.

Bornstein, McLean and Ho (1985) report an even more severe case in a 25-year-old college-educated male who, after experiencing what was thought to be mild depression for several months, presented with unsteady gait, dysphagia, slurred speech and intermittent urinary incontinence. A neuropsychological examination was performed 4 months later, using the WAIS-R, Wechsler Memory Scale, Halstead–Reitan Battery, the Wisconsin Card Sorting Test and several other measures. Verbal IQ at that time was 85 and Performance IQ was 70, scores quite inconsistent with the patient's previous position as a budget analyst. The patient's performance on all tests was impaired; the only tasks with scores less than one standard deviation below the mean were immediate verbal recall and a test of verbal concept formation. This patient's course became chronic despite chelation therapy, and at the time of the report he required total supportive care.

Finally, a somewhat more optimistic outcome for Wilson's disease was found in the case examined by Rosselli, Lorenzana, Rosselli, and Vergara (1987). The authors describe a case of Wilson's disease in a 30-year-old female born of consanguineous parents. The patient was neuropsychologically tested before and after penicillamine chelation treatment.

Initial presentation revealed a Performance IQ of 63 and a Verbal IQ of 73. There were marked impairments in memory, constructional abilities, motor speed and slowing of verbal responses. Speech was dysarthric without aphasia. The patient showed tremor, rigidity and bradykinesia.

The authors characterized the patient's improvement after chelation as "dramatic", although some deficits remained. Her Performance IQ increased to 91 while verbal IQ remained constant at 72. Improvements were seen in both verbal and non-verbal memory for immediate and delayed recall. The patient's learning curve also showed significant improvement. The authors suggest the course of recovery is consistent with the reversibility of Wilson's disease dementia, speculating that remaining deficits in their patient were due to a 13-year prodrome. They hypothesize that earlier treatment would have arrested or eliminated expression of the disease in this patient.

GOLD

History

It has been suggested that the first recorded "medicinal" use of gold was recorded in the Old Testament, where Moses "took the calf which they had made and burnt it in the fire and ground it to powder, and strawed it upon the water, and made the children of Israel drink of it" (*Exodus*, cited by Marks and Beatty, 1975, p. 15).

Gold also may have been used as a medicinal preparation by the Chinese as early as 2000 years before Christ. The Taoist philosopher Pao Pu Tzu (253–333?) believed that gold, when taken internally, was second only to cinnabar in producing immortality. The sixteenth-century Swiss physician, Paracelsus, used gold as a blood purifier, poison antidote, miscarriage preventative and as a cardiac medicine (Marks and Beatty, 1975).

Current uses and neurotoxic effects

Organic gold compounds are currently used to treat rheumatoid arthritis, lupus erythematosus and bronchial asthma (Goetz, 1985; Hanakago, 1979), although "potentially severe toxic reactions limit their use" (Schaumberg,

Spencer, and Thomas, 1983, p. 121). Gold neurotoxicity is rare and no neuropsychological studies are available in the gold toxicity literature. Neurological signs of ataxia, blurred vision and tremor have been reported (Hanakago, 1979), although psychiatric symptoms of depression and hallucinations are possible without other CNS signs (Sterman and Schaumberg, 1980). Subcortical infarction and meningeal irritation have been cited in clinical case reports, and ventromedial hypothalamic damage has been produced in animals exposed to gold thioglucose (Sterman and Schaumberg, 1980). Peripheral neuropathy has also been reported in reaction to organic gold ingestion; however, it is unclear whether peripheral nervous system effects are due to actual gold toxicity or a secondary allergic reaction (Schaumberg *et al.*, 1983). Polyneuritis from gold ingestion has also been found to be associated with gold therapy (Hanakago, 1979), as has Guillain Barré syndrome, radiculopathy and myokymia (Goetz, 1985).

IRON

Iron oxide fume:
OSHA 10 mg/m^3
ACGIH 5 mg/m^3

(NIOSH, 1985)

Abnormal brain iron accumulation may cause neurotoxic effects in two medical disorders — hemachromatosis and Hallervorden–Spatz disease. In the former, iron absorption from a normal diet is abnormally high, with neurological and neuropsychological changes noted in adulthood. Accumulation of iron in the globus pallidus and the reticular zone of the substantia nigra, as well as severe degeneration and demyelination of neurons, are believed to induce dementia, ataxia and neuropathy (Feldman, 1982a). The latter (Hallervorden–Spatz) disease is an often familial, probably metabolic disorder which appears in childhood or adolescence. The disorder causes iron accumulation in the globus pallidus and the reticular zone of the substantia nigra, although there is no systemic disorder of iron metabolism. Demyelination may occur in the globus pallidus, and axonal swelling has been noted in the pallidonigral system and the cortex (Feldman, 1982a). The disorder produces choreoathetosis, rigidity, indistinct speech and progressive impairment in intellectual functions. Hallervorden–Spatz disease is eventually fatal, with death occurring approximately 10 years after onset (Richardson and Adams, 1977).

LEAD

Inorganic, fumes and dust: Pb
OSHA 0.5 mg/m^3 (Feb. 1979)

NIOSH < 0.1 mg/m^3 10h TWA
ACGIH   0.15 mg/m^3
Lead arsenate
OSHA   0.05 mg/m^3
NIOSH   2 mg/m^3 (15 min ceiling)
ACGIH   0.15 mg/m^3

Organic lead:
Tetraethyl lead Pb $(C_2H_5)_4$
   OSHA   0.075 mg/m^3
   IDLH level   40 mg/m^3
   ACGIH   0.1 mg/m^3
Tetramethyl lead Pb $(CH_3)_4$
   OSHA   0.075 mg/m^3
   IDLH level   40 mg/m^3
   ACGIH   0.15 mg/m^3
(NIOSH, 1985)

History

Lead was one of the earliest neurotoxins produced by humans. Easily smeltable from galena ore, lead beads have been found in Asia Minor dating back to 6500 B.C. (Wedeen, 1984) The ancient Romans were extensive users of lead, producing an estimated 80,000 tons of lead annually at the peak of the Roman empire, using it in paint pigments, makeup and lead plumbing (Windebank, McCall and Dyck, 1984). Wine was undoubtedly a major cause of lead poisoning to the Romans since their prominent philosophers advocated the boiling of wine in lead containers to increase sweetness and halt fermentation (Wedeen, 1984).

The number of birth defects and developmental abnormalities produced by lead during the Roman era can only be guessed, but may have been substantial, particularly since Roman women reportedly coated their cervixes with lead compounds to prevent conception (Wedeen, 1984). A high rate of sterility in the Roman aristocracy may have been induced by an elevated concentration of lead in wine and cooking utensils as well as by the use of lead compounds as sweetening agents.

Lead has no known biological benefit and, like all non-essential heavy metals, it is hazardous to living matter (Niklowitz, 1980, p. 27). The toxic effects of lead have been known almost as long as it has been mined. The physician Nikander of Colophon wrote of lead's poisonous effects in 200 B.C.:

But may the hateful painful litharge (lead oxide)

be unknown to you,
If oppression rages in your belly,
    and all around your middle,
Pent up in your howling bowels,
    winds roar,
The sort which cause deadly disturbances
    of the bowels, which,
Attacking with pains unexpected,
    overpowering mankind.
The flood of urine does not stop it,
    but all around
The limbs are swollen and inflamed,
And, no less, the skin's color
    is that of lead
(Nikander, cited in Weeden 1984, p.14).

Current uses of lead

Lead in its pure form and its various compounds continues to be utilized in diverse capacities; as a component of ceramic glazes, in batteries and in paint pigments. It had been widely used as an octane-increasing gasoline additive; however, growing knowledge of lead's deleterious health effects, and ensuing legal regulation, have caused this form of lead pollution to diminish.

Current world output of lead exceeds 3.5 million tons per year, an amount greater than any other toxic metal. More than 800,000 American workers are exposed to lead in their jobs and up to 20% have elevated blood lead levels (Schottenfeld and Cullen, 1984). Thus, in terms of quantity produced and number of workplace exposure victims, lead's potential effect on human health is perhaps greater than any other neurotoxin except alcohol. Perhaps because of this ubiquity and serious health risk, there is more information and research about lead than any other neurotoxic metal.

Intake

In humans, lead is accumulated via inhalation and ingestion. It is transported throughout the body by the erythrocytes and is deposited in soft tissue and bone. Precise measurement of body lead is complicated by the variability in storage capacities and biological half-times among tissues. The biological half-time of bone lead "has been estimated at around 10 years while the half-time of blood lead can be as short as 2–3 weeks" (Krigman, Bouldin and Mushak, 1980, p. 492). These authors also estimate that over 90% of the chronic body burden of lead is contained in bone. Thus, blood lead levels may provide only a very preliminary approximation of body and brain lead burden. Recently, it has been suggested that zinc protoporphyrin (ZPP) level, a substance accumulated in the red blood cell when lead inhibits the cell's ability to contain iron, is a more sensitive indicant of biologically active lead on the nervous system than blood lead levels (Lilis *et al.*, 1977).

Neuropathology

Several mechanisms of lead-related neurotoxic damage have been proposed and the subject remains under investigation. Lead may compete with calcium, sodium and/or magnesium in neurotransmission. Direct and indirect effects on nerve cell mitochondria, inhibiting phosphorylation have been suggested (Silbergeld, 1982). In addition "non-neural effects of lead on such processes as membrane transport, oxidative phosphorylation, and heme synthesis may affect neuronal function by depleting supplies of precursors, reducing energy sources or producing neurotoxic intermediates" (Silbergeld, 1982, p. 18).

There is evidence from animal research and some corroboration in human case studies that lead is a demyelinating agent (Fullerton, 1966; Behse and Carlson, 1978; Nicklowitz and Mandybur, 1975). A possible relationship of chronic lead exposure to Alzeheimer-like symptoms has been posited by Niklowitz (1979) who observed neurofibrillary tangles in animals and in the autopsy of a 42-year-old survivor of childhood lead encephalopathy. Two studies suggest that cerebellar capillaries may be particularly susceptible to calcification as a result of lead exposure (Benson and Price, 1985; Tonge, Burry and Saal, 1977). The latter study found 84% of 44 patients who were diagnosed with lead neuropathy at autopsy to show cerebellar calcification. There are, however, few such human case studies in the modern literature, and Wallerian-type axonal degeneration is the most frequently cited neurological change resulting from lead exposure in adult humans (Krigman, Bouldin and Mushak, 1980). Many questions remain unanswered, including whether lead accumulates differentially in different areas of the brain, and how age, metabolism or other individual differences mediate lead toxicity mechanisms.

Lead exposure in adults — occupations at risk

Adult exposure to lead usually occurs in the workplace. Common avenues of exposure include lead smelters, battery manufacturing or recycling plants, auto repair shops and via contaminated bootleg alcohol. Lead shot manufacture and use of lead-containing industrial paint are also suggested to put the worker at risk for toxic lead exposure (Windebank, McCall and Dyck, 1984). It has also been our experience that workers or home remodelers who must remove old paint are at risk; we have seen high blood lead levels in transit workers assigned to burn old paint from elevated railroad track installations. Perhaps the most unusual form of occupational lead poisoning has been documented in Jewish scribes who must prepare and work with a special ink that contains significant amounts of lead (Cohen *et al.*, 1986).

Lead exposure — children

Incidence

The extent of lead exposure in children appears to be almost as great as that in adults. A recent survey suggests that 3.9% or almost 700,000 United States children have blood levels at or above 30 μg/dl (Mahaffey *et al.*, 1982). Racial and socioeconomic factors strongly influence the prevalence of lead elevation, with only 2% of white children showing elevated blood lead, as contrasted with up to 18% of poor, inner-city, black children.

The majority of these cases have been linked to *pica*, the ingesting of non-food substances (Baloh *et al.*, 1975). Dust, dirt and especially old paint chips (some of which have been found to contain up to 50% lead) are common vehicles of exposure (Otto *et al.*, 1982, p. 733). Houses built before the mid-1950s were commonly painted with interior and exterior lead-based paint. It has been estimated that flaking and peeling paint from such housing puts about 2,500,000 children under the age of 5 at risk (Baloh *et al.*, 1975).

Blood lead levels are also higher in children living within 100 feet of a major roadway, and can be positively correlated with the volume of automotive traffic in the vicinity (Caprio *et al.*, 1974), although federally mandated phaseout of leaded gasoline has produced a reduction in the blood lead levels of United States children (Center for Disease Control, 1985). Living in the vicinity of lead-utilizing heavy industry may also be a risk factor (Winneke *et al.*, 1983). Landrigan *et al.* (1975) found children living near a lead-discharging smelter to have significantly decreased IQ and finger tapping scores compared to socioeconomic status (SES) and race-matched controls. A parent working in a lead-utilizing industry may transport lead from the workplace via skin, hair or clothing, thereby contaminating the home and its occupants. One study found almost half of such children showing blood lead elevations at or above the then current clinical threshold of 30 μg/dl (Baker *et al.*, 1977).

Even where lead is not introduced by industry, paint or auto, it may enter the household through the water supply. Although many municipalities have outlawed lead piping in water supplies, older communities may retain such pipe. At least one major city in the United States (Chicago, Illinois) still mandates the use of lead water pipes.

Relative risk

While complete review of lead's effects on pre- and post-natal development is beyond the scope of this chapter, risk is inversely correlated with age of the child (Niklowitz, 1979). Because children absorb more lead per unit of body weight than adults and have higher mineral turnover in bone, allowing more lead to be released, they are considered to be at greater risk for lead poisoning than adults (Center for Disease Control, 1985). Because of such risk, the Center for Disease Control has recently lowered the definition of "elevated" blood lead levels from 30 to 25 μg/dl (CDC, 1985). However, even these lowered limits may not be adequate to prevent behavioral dysfunction.

In a preliminary study, for example, Bellinger *et al.* (1984) classified several thousand 6-month-old infants by umbilical cord lead content into one of three groups: "low" (mean = 1.8 μg/dl), "mid" (mean = 6.5 μg/dl) and "high" (mean = 14.6 μg/dl). There was a difference of approximately 6 points on the Bayley Mental Development Index (BMDI) between the low cord lead group (< 3μg/dl) and high cord lead subjects ($\geqslant$ 10 μg/dl). Results suggested that a cord blood lead level of only 10 μg/dl or greater "was associated with early developmental disadvantage" measured by the Bayley (Bellinger *et al.*, 1984, p. 396). Further, when Bellinger *et al.* (1986) re-assessed their subjects 6 months later, they found that high cord lead subjects continued to maintain about a 7 point deficit on the BMDI compared to low cord lead children. Since blood levels at 6 and 12 months in these two groups no longer differed from each other, pre-natal lead levels were more predictive of BMDI impairment than later lead assays. Skills most strongly affected by lead at this age were "fine motor and interactional/linguistic skills" (Bellinger *et al.*, 1986, p. 159).

Neurophysiological effects

Childhood diagnosis of toxicity is made when elevated blood lead levels are coupled with an erythrocyte protoporphyrin (EP) level of 35 μg/dl or more (Center for Disease Control, 1985). High-level childhood lead poisoning more often presents with CNS neuropsychological symptoms than peripheral neuropathy. Childhood peripheral neuropathies, when they do occur, involve the legs more than the arms, whereas in adults the reverse is true (Windebank, McCall and Dyck, 1984).

Neurophysiological measures have demonstrated the neurotoxicity of lead in children. Otto *et al.* (1982) measured slow wave potentials evoked by sensory conditioning in children with blood levels of 7 to 52 μg/dl and found data to suggest that even the lowest levels of lead were able to alter conditioning.

Neuropsychological effects of childhood lead exposure

There is some controversy concerning confounding influences in studies of lead-exposed children. Several researchers have questioned whether neuropsychological dysfunctions found in lead-exposed children are due to the effects of lead, or the non-specific conditions highly correlated with lead exposure, including poverty, poor nutrition and an understimulating environment (e.g. Baloh, Sturm and Gleser, 1975). Winneke and Kraemer (1984), in particular, argue that these confounding influences do not receive correct methodological treatment in most childhood lead exposure studies.

Another complicating factor in the design of childhood lead studies is the lack of knowledge concerning childhood lead-ingestion patterns. This might cause inappropriate subjects to be grouped together. For example, if only acute blood lead levels are obtained, children with single acute exposures to lead and no body burden may be compared with others whose blood lead levels are equivalent but which reflect the slow release of lead from a large body burden accumulated over several years.

A third difficulty has been the correct selection of testing procedures which are most sensitive to lead effects. Some authors have criticized the use of insensitive testing procedures in the examination of childhood lead exposure (Needleman et al., 1979).

Despite these methodological and practical complications, evidence has steadily accrued that ingestion of lead in childhood produces neurotoxic sequelae at both clinical and subclinical levels. Several studies show neuropsychological impairment to be associated with subclinical blood lead levels in children (e.g. Rutter, 1980). Hunter et al. (1985) found a small but significant slowing in reaction time in children with lead levels of 5–26 μg/dl (mean = 11.85 μg/dl). David et al. (1982) found a significant negative correlation between supposedly "non-toxic" mean blood levels of 25 μg/dl and mental retardation that could not otherwise be explained by other factors. Yule et al. (1981) studied 141 children with blood levels from 7 to 33 μg/dl and found significant impairments in general intelligence and several achievement test scores (reading and spelling) that remained after social class had been partialed out.

Lead assays taken from shed teeth have also correlated with neuropsychological dysfunction. For example, Needleman et al. (1979) found WISC-R Full Scale IQs to be significantly lower by about 4–5 points between high and low lead groups. High tooth lead children also performed significantly more poorly on all subtests of the Seashore Rhythm Test, suggesting auditory processing dysfunction, and on a reaction time measure, suggesting impaired vigilance or attention. Winneke, Hrdina and Brockhaus (1982) found impaired problem-solving and perceptual-motor integration in children with high lead dentine levels, although they also warn against confounding variables of "socio-hereditary background" in these types of studies (Winneke et al., 1983). Association of hyperactivity with lead has been noted (David et al., 1983) and replicated with a non-disadvantaged group of children (Gittelman and Eskenazi, 1983). Another study examined a total of about 1000 children and found that high lead levels were associated with impaired Verbal and Full Scale IQ on the WISC, especially in the Information, Comprehension and Vocabulary subtests in a group of children matched for parent social status, sex, school and neighborhood. The high lead group also made significantly more errors on the Bender Visual Motor Gestalt and had poorer ratings in a behavioral rating scale (Hansen *et al.*, 1985). Deficits in other visuospatial tasks have also been found (Maracek *et al.*, 1983). These dysfunctions may be cumulative, and with repeated exposure the risk of permanent brain damage approaches certainty (Niklowitz, 1979).

In conclusion, there seems to be no evidence disputing the childhood effects of acute high dose lead exposure or of chronic, prolonged toxic doses to the neuropsychological functioning of the child. Disputes center instead on the long-term effects of low level lead intoxication and on the methodology used to control for social and demographic factors that may be potential confounds. The group of studies which support the subclinical neurotoxicity of childhood lead exposure have consistently reported results suggesting the hypothesis that there is effectively no "safe" level of childhood lead exposure. Methodological refutations of such studies must be taken seriously and may be used to guide future research; however, at this time there remains a preponderance of evidence on the side of a positive association between subclinical lead exposure and neuropsychological dysfunction.

In addition, while the controversy over subclinical effects has not been completely resolved, there may be other reasons to assume a positive association between lead and neuropsychological dysfunction in children. The human consequences in making a Type I error (incorrectly rejecting the null hypothesis and viewing this known neurotoxin as a subclinical poison) would be far less damaging in their clinical and social consequences than would be the commission of a Type II error (that of incorrectly *accepting* the null hypothesis and assuming no effect of lead).

Lead exposure — adults

Organic lead

In adults, lead is associated with two spectra of neuropsychological dysfunctions, depending on its composition. Organic (covalently bonded to carbon) lead, contained in leaded gasoline, solvents or cleaning fluids, produces neuropsychological symptoms that include memory dysfunction and loss of ability to concentrate (Grandjean and Nielson, 1979). Emotional symptoms produced by organic lead exposure include psychosis with hallucinations, restlessness, nightmares and impotence. In high concentrations, organic lead can produce delirium, convulsion and coma.

Organic lead exposure exerts these effects by interfering with energy metabolism and possibly damaging the hippocampus, amygdala and pyriform cortex (see Grandjean, 1983, p. 336 for a detailed discussion of these effects). One form of organic lead (tetraethyl lead) is metabolized into triethyl lead which can cross the blood–brain barrier and disrupt cholinergic and adrenergic central pathways (Bolter, Stanczik and Long, 1983).

Most cases of organic lead intoxication are the result of exposure to leaded gasoline. Leaded fuels contain a variety of other neurotoxic substances, including benzene, xylene, triorthocresyl and ethylene dichloride (Poklis and Burkett, 1977). Therefore the neuropsychological results of organic lead exposure may actually be caused by combinations of triethyl lead and solvents, as well as from hypoxia in cases where intoxication has produced unconsciousness.

Case studies of organic lead intoxication are usually reported either as a byproduct of accidental industrial exposure or through voluntary gasoline "sniffing". Such case reports are rare, and even fewer neuropsychological studies of organic lead intoxication have been performed.

Two cases of high level gasoline exposure with hypoxia in a gasoline storage tank were reported by Bolter, Stanczak and Long (1983). One subject, unconscious for 20 minutes, experienced numerous cerebellar and cortical symptoms, including paresthesias, nausea, anxiety and dysarthria. Neuropsychological testing showed intellectual and short-term memory functions to be in the borderline range. Other neuropsychological tests showed impaired motor functioning of the right hand, decreased bilateral tactile sensitivity, and impairment on phoneme and rhythm discrimination, expressive language, sensorimotor functions, and abstract reasoning. Two years later the patient complained of daily headache, numbness and weakness of the right hand, and continued to show lowered language and verbal memory abilities as well as impaired emotional functioning.

A second subject, unconscious for 2 minutes, also showed left hemisphere deficits which remained 3 years post-accident. Possible reactive emotional symptomatology was also seen in the form of phobic reaction to gasoline fumes, and symptoms of suspicion, distrust and withdrawal. Lowered verbal functioning in both subjects was speculatively attributed by the authors to greater relative impairment of left hemisphere functions which show greater specialization for and potential for disruption of cholinergic activity.

Gasoline sniffing

Neuropsychological and neurological effects of gasoline inhalation are also produced when vapors are deliberately inhaled for their intoxicating effect. Gasoline vapors are rapidly absorbed by the lungs and symptoms begin within 3–5 minutes. Voluntary gasoline abusers report that 15–20 breaths of gasoline vapor will cause a 5–6-hour period of euphoric intoxication. Psychotomimetic concomitants can include visual, auditory and tactile hallucinations, sensations of lightness or spinning, and alterations in shapes or colors (Poklis and Burkett, 1977). Rapid or more prolonged inhalation can result in "violent excitement followed by unconsciousness and coma" (Poklis and Burkett, 1977, p.36).

Rajani, Boeckx and Chow (1978) examined 50 native American Indian patients in Winnipeg, Mannitoba, Canada, who had been voluntary abusers of leaded gasoline. The patients had histories of sniffing leaded gasoline from 6 months to 5 years. Forty-six (92%) had abnormal neurological examinations which resolved in all but one case after 8 weeks. All but one had blood lead levels above 40 μg/dl and chelation was instituted in 39 patients. Twenty-seven of the 46 patients tested had abnormal EEGs with very low voltage and an excess of diffuse slow activity. Ten of 15 EEGs given 8–12 weeks later were normal. The most common neurological symptoms noted on initial intake included abnormally brisk deep reflexes (34 patients), intention tremor (29 patients) and abnormally brisk jaw jerk (28 patients). Various cerebellar signs were also observed and many of the abnormal findings correlated with mean blood lead or ALAD levels (Seshia *et al.*, 1978). The authors also note that 17 (34%) of the patients resumed sniffing gasoline upon discharge, a finding which could suggest effects of peer pressure or the addictive potential of gasoline inhalation.

An even more severe form of encephalopathy from organic lead intoxication has been reported by Goldings and Stewart (1982). The subject was a 15-year-old male with a several year "sniffing" history. Serum lead level upon admission was 168 μg/dl. The patient developed a toxic delirium state with buccal and lingual dyskinesias, ataxia, myoclonus and hallucinations of "bugs crawling on my skin". Snout reflexes, bilateral foot grasps, urinary incontinence and a palmomental sign were noted. The patient's premorbid intellectual capacity was probably in the retarded range, limiting speculation about specific intellectual deficits from organic lead. However, symptoms of delirium and encephalopathy were similar to, if more severe than, other reported cases of organic lead intoxication (Goldings and Stewart, 1982).

Inorganic lead

Exposure to pure or "inorganic" lead has been more extensively studied than has organic lead intoxication, probably because more individuals are exposed to inorganic lead. Inorganic lead appears to induce different neuropathological alterations, especially in cerebellar and hippocampal sites. The constellation of neuropsychological symptoms produced by inorganic lead also differs from that of organic lead in both cognitive and emotional spheres.

General symptoms of inorganic lead intoxication

Neurotoxic reactions to inorganic lead usually occur in the context of a systemic illness with classic symptoms. These include "abdominal pain, constipation, anemia and neuropathy". Gout may also be present (Windebank, McCall and Dyck, 1984, pp. 2134–5).

Exposed subjects do not typically complain of these symptoms when blood lead levels are less than 40 μg/dl. However, neurological investigations have found lead-related abnormalities below the level of subjective complaint. Both PNS and CNS effects have been reported. For example, Araki and Honma (1976) found nerve conduction velocities of median and posterior tibial nerves were significantly correlated with blood lead levels in a group of 39 lead workers whose mean blood lead concentration was 29 μg/dl. Another study found a "highly significant decrease in visual sensitivity" (and presumed damage to the optic nerve) in 35 workers with subclinical blood lead levels (Cavalleri *et al.*, 1982, p. 263). This latter result is consistent with Niklowitz's (1979) observation that "Pb is taken up by the brain even when blood-Pb levels are quite low" (p. 28), and suggests that vulnerable brain tissue has no protection against lead damage, even at subclinical exposures.

At higher blood lead levels, "wrist drop", a motor peripheral neuropathy with little sensory involvement, is probably the most frequently cited neurological symptom. However, clinical observations of wrist drop are less common today than in previous years, possibly because exposure levels are more closely monitored in many industries.

Neuropsychological effects of lead

Subjective complaint

As is the case with neurological effects, lead-induced changes in neuropsychological function are not well correlated with subjective complaint. Subclinical blood levels of 40–50 μg/100 ml are the lowest levels where neuropsychological changes have been detected; however, few patient complaints are noted at this value. For example, Hänninen *et al.* (1979) studied a group of 20 workers whose blood lead levels never exceeded 50 μg/dl, and compared them to both a group of 25 workers with blood lead from 50 to 69 μg/dl as well as to a group of controls. Length of exposure in the groups ranged from 2 to 9 years. Subjective complaints were measured using a questionnaire and a Finnish adaptation of the Eysenck Personality Inventory.

Significantly more low lead exposure subjects than controls admitted to fatigue after work, sleepiness, depression and apathy. Cognitive symptoms were reported only in the higher exposure group. The group of subjects with slightly higher lead exposure added forgetfulness and sensorimotor complaints to their subjective list, which also included fatigue, restlessness, apathy, and gastrointestinal complaint (Hänninen *et al.*, 1979).

In patients with lead levels higher than 69 μg/dl, subjective complaints may again be somatic or emotional, rather than cognitive. This could be due to the relative saliency of common accompanying symptoms of gastritis and joint pain compared to more subtle changes in cognition. Alternatively, attention and abstraction deficits characteristic of lead intoxication may so seriously impair introspective abilities as to militate against the patient's realizing the extent of his cognitive losses.

In either event, there is evidence that neuropsychological decrements may precede entry of those complaints into subjective awareness. Neuropsychological evaluation appears to provide an early warning of lead neurotoxicity, and is a more sensitive indicant than subjective complaint alone.

Neuropsychological effects

Neuropsychological functions shown to be deleteriously affected by lead include visual intelligence and visuomotor functions (Hänninen *et al.*, 1978), general intelligence (Grandjean, Arnvig and Beckmann, 1978) and memory, "particularly in learning new material" (Feldman, Ricks and Baker, 1980). Williamson and Teo (1986), using an information processing model of memory, found significant lead-related decrements in sensory storage memory (brief tachistoscopic presentation of letter pairs), Sternberg-type short-term memory scanning and a paired associate learning task. In combination with lowered critical flicker fusion thresholds, the authors interpreted their results as consistent with arousal deficit and/or degradation of retinal or visual pathway input.

Reductions in psychomotor speed and dexterity (e.g. Williamson and Teo, 1986; Repko *et al.*, 1978) have been cited in many studies, perhaps due to either reduced nerve conduction velocities or damage to the motor areas of the cortex (Hänninen, 1982).

When lead levels exceed the subclinical threshold of approximately 30 μg/dl, subjects may develop neuropsychological deficits relatively rapidly. Bleecker *et al.* (1982) examined 13 workers who had been exposed a median of 2.5 months (range of 2 weeks to 8 months). Workers displayed significant deficits on Block Design, Digit Symbol and a decreased rate of learning on the Rey Auditory Verbal Learning Test. Marginally significant impairment of visual memory on the Wechsler Memory Scale was also noted.

The clinical appearance of more severely lead intoxicated patients suggests generalized losses in memory, attention, concentration and abstract thought processing. In severe cases these symptoms can present as globally dementing impairments.

Emotional effects of lead

Lead-induced emotional alterations include depression, confusion, anger, fatigue and tension (Baker *et al.*, 1983a). These symptoms have been observed both in chronically exposed patients, as well as in individuals with lead exposure histories of 2 weeks to 8 months (Bleeker *et al.*, 1982, p. 255). These symptoms may go unrecognized by mental health personnel untrained in neuropsychological effects of neurotoxins (Schottenfeld and Cullen, 1984). Because the emotional concomitants of lead intoxication can resemble major affective disorder, misdiagnosis could potentially occur and delay appropriate administration of chelation therapy (Schottenfeld and Cullen, 1984).

The causes of lead-induced emotional changes are uncertain. Direct organic brain dysfunction may produce depression via cortical and subcortical tissue damage. Hypothalamic alterations and changes in catecholamine metabolism have also been suggested (Schottenfeld and Cullen, 1984). Secondary emotional reactions to diminished cognitive functioning may also contribute to affective changes.

Neuropsychological recovery from lead neurotoxicity

Baker *et al.* (1985d) examined 160 foundry workers during the course of improving hygienic conditions at the plant. Individuals with an initial blood level over 50 μg/dl showed a 20% reduction in tension, 18% reduction in anger, 26% reduction in depression, 27% reduction in fatigue and a 13% reduction in confusion on the Profile of Mood States (POMS). Significant associations between exposure indices and neuropsychological performance were also found on the Santa Ana Dexterity Test (both hands) and a paired associate learning test. Workers failed to show improvement in other lead-impaired tasks.

Case report — Probable lead encephalopathy
The patient is a white male in his late 40s with a 9th grade education. He had worked for 20 years at a steel refinery where his job was to heat-treat steel and quench it in molten lead. He was not issued any protective mask or clothing until OSHA came to the plant in 1979, after the patient had already worked at the plant for about 18 years. The patient reported that he started noticing medical problems around 1976 when he began to feel abnormally fatigued. By 1977–78 he felt ''extreme'' fatigue in his arms. Other symptoms which the patient noted at that time included weight loss, loss of appetite, and poor memory. Although the patient has not worked with lead for approximately 3 years, a blood lead level taken a month before testing indicated 50 μg/dl. The patient's highest measured blood lead while working with lead was over 80 μg/dl.
Current symptoms include constant body aches ''like the flu'', and ''terrible'' hearing in addition to poor memory and fatigue. There is no prior psychiatric history, nor any reported work difficulties prior to the mid-1970s.

Discussion

This patient showed neuropsychological deficits that appear to be fairly

TABLE III.3. Moderate neuropsychological test results in a case of chronic exposure to lead

1. *Finger Tapping:*	RH mean: *46*		Russell 2
(Dom. hand: R)	LH mean: *40*		Russell 2
2. *Wechsler Memory Scale:*			
(a) *Logical*			
Immediate recall:	A: 7.5 B: 6.5	Total: 14	Russell 3
Delayed recall:	A: 1 B: 1.5	Total: 2.5	Russell 5
(b) *Figural*			
Immediate recall:	A: 0 B: 0 C: 2	Total: 2	Russell 4
Delayed recall:	A: 0 B: 0 C: 2	Total: 2	Russell 4
3. *Trail Making Test:*	A: 42 (seconds)		Russell 2
	B: 181 (seconds)		Russell 3
4. *WAIS-R Digit Symbol Test:*		Raw score: 39	Scaled score 2–3
5. *Stroop Test:*			
No. of words: 68 + age corr.: 8		Total: 76	T score 34
No. of colors: 59 + age corr.: 4		Total: 63	T score 39
No. of colored words: 31 + age corr.: 5		Total: 36	T score 41
6. *Luria-Nebraska Pathognomonic Scale:*			
			Critical level 69.21
	No. of errors: 21		T score 58
7. *Spatial Relations:* (Greek Cross) Best: 1 + Worst: 1 = 2			Russell 1
8. *Pegboard:* (Purdue) RH: 12 T 47 LH: 12 T 49 BH: 9			
10. *IQ Estimate:* Kent EGY Scale			
Raw score: 22 IQ estimate: 98			
15. *Personality Tests:* MMPI BDI = 13			

MMPI Scales and T Scores (K corrected where appropriate)

L	53	PD	56	SI	51
F	60	MF	44	A	53
K	48	PA	41	R	51
HS	93	PT	69	ES	40
D	80	SC	65	MAC	67
HY	72	MA	58		

Note: 0–5 Russell ratings are from Russell (1975) and Russell, Neuringer and Goldstein (1970), with higher scores indicating greater impairment.

typical of moderate effects of chronic lead exposure. While his education may limit his abilities somewhat, it seems likely that memory and cognitive efficiency deficits shown here are related to chronic lead exposure and a continuing body burden of lead. Personality evaluation was interpreted as consistent with depression and concern over significant decrements in health and well-being. However, the patient's depression could also be a direct neurological effect of lead intoxication (Schottenfeld and Cullen, 1984). The patient's hearing loss could be due either to factory noise damage to the ear or to lead-related CNS damage.

Case No. 2: Mr. B: severe lead encephalopathy
This patient is a 53-year-old black male who received longitudinal testing to monitor effects of chronic cognitive changes as a result of lead exposure. As

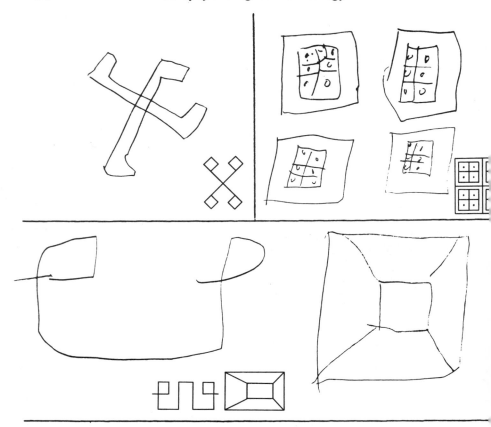

FIGURE III.1. Moderate lead encephalopathy. WMS: Figural memory — immediate recall. For reader comparison, card images were inset subsequent to the evaluation.

can be seen from selected test results, the patient shows global and severe neuropsychological impairment, with marked verbal and non-verbal memory deficit, and poor ability to comprehend instructions and generate internal plans (Fig. III. 4-6, 7-9, 10-12).

Complicating the inference of causality to these data is the fact that the patient was raised in rural surroundings and has had no schooling whatsoever. However, the patient did perform capably in a lead refinery for 20 years, was able to follow directions and showed good work performance before he was finally fired for incompetence. It therefore seems likely that premorbid functioning was substantially less impaired than current data suggest. This patient's current cognitive status was so impaired that he essentially voiced no complaints about cognitive difficulties. In this he was typical of other patients with severe lead encephalopathy/dementia. Like such patients, his lack of complaint probably reflected an inability to observe and reflect upon those difficulties. Further, joint and stomach pain tend to be very salient in patients with severe lead encephalopathy and such symptoms may tend to obscure less noticeable neuropsychological abnormalities.

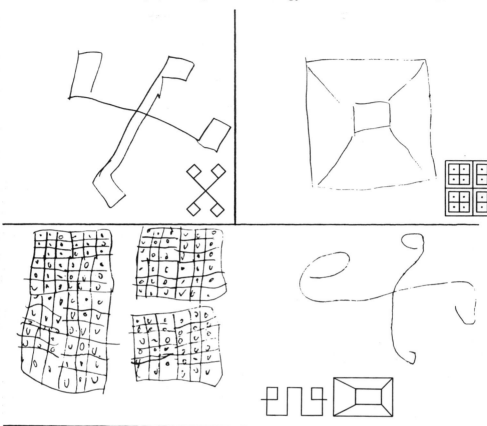

FIGURE III.2. Moderate lead encephalopathy. WMS: Figural memory — 30-minute delayed recall. For reader comparison, card images were inset subsequent to the evaluation.

LITHIUM

See Chapter 6, Neuropsychological Toxicology of Drugs.

MANGANESE

Manganese and compounds (Mn):
OSHA   5 mg/m^3 ceiling (dust)
ACGIH   5 mg/m^3 ceiling (dust)
ACGIH   1 mg/m^3 (fume)
IDLH level   10,000 mg/m^3
(NIOSH, 1985)

The first reported medical use of manganese was as a purgative. Another early observer noted that manganese miners were "uniformly cured of

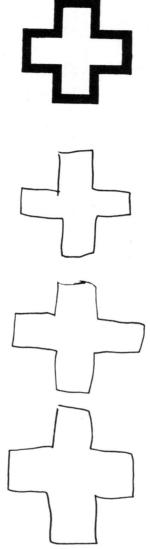

FIGURE III.3. Moderate lead encephalopathy. Spatial Relations Test (direct copy).

scabies and other cutaneous affections during their stay at the works'' which led to the use of manganese to treat these disorders (cited in Marks and Beatty, 1975 p. 128). As early as 1837, however, a Glasgow physician described five workers who inhaled manganese oxide and developed paraparesis, masked facies, drooling, weak voice and propulsion, in the absence of tremor (Cawte, 1985).

Although manganese is not a widely known neurotoxin, intoxication has

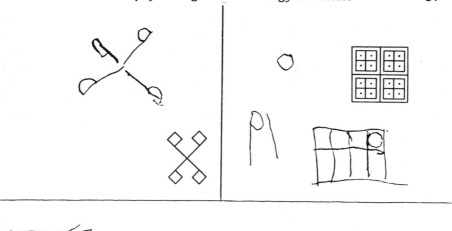

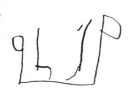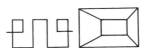

FIGURE III.4. Severe effects of chronic lead intoxication. WMS: Figural memory —
immediate recall, initial testing. For reader comparison, card images were inset
subsequent to the evaluation.

been found to cause serious neurological disturbance, and thousands of
workers are said to have developed manganese neurotoxicity (Politis,
Schaumberg and Spencer, 1980). Manganese miners, welders and workers in
dry-cell battery plants are primary exposure victims (Grandjean, 1983, p.
335). Other occupations where manganese is used include steel alloy plants,
and factories which produce "ceramics, matches, glass, dyes, fertilizers,
welding rods, oxidizing solutions, animal food additives, germicides and
antiseptics" (Katz, 1985, p. 176).

In miners, initial signs of intoxication have been reported in as few as 6
months and as long as 24 years (Politis, Schaumberg and Spencer, 1980).
Symptoms are not inevitably correlated with exposure or high tissue levels,
but appear to depend upon a combination of contributing factors including
"genetic predisposition, age, nutrition, anemia or alcohol" (Cawte, 1985, p.
216.)

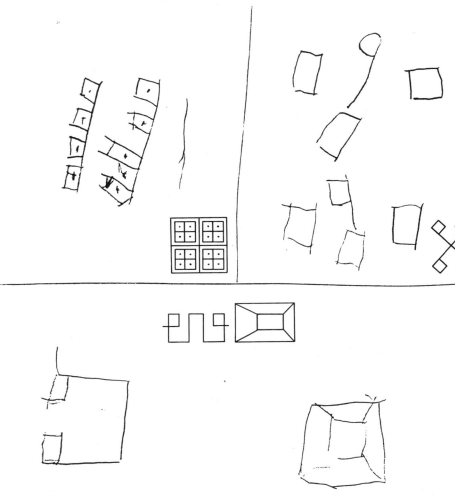

FIGURE III.5. Severe effects of chronic lead intoxication. WMS: Figural memory — 30-minute delayed recall, initial testing. For reader comparison, card images were inset subsequent to the evaluation.

Neurological and neuropsychological aspects of manganese intoxication

Manganese poisoning is said to occur in three stages. The initial manifestations of manganese intoxication, which last approximately 1–3 months, include sleepiness, poor coordination, ataxia and impaired speech (Baker, 1983) as well as other more psychiatric-seeming symptoms, including asthenia, anorexia, insomnia, hallucinations, "mental excitement, aggressive behavior and incoherent talk" (Chandra, 1983; Politis,

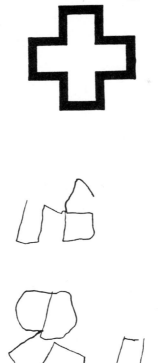

FIGURE III.6. Severe effects of lead intoxication. Spatial Relations Test, first testing (direct copy).

Schaumberg and Spencer 1980; Cawte, 1985. This latter set of early symptoms has led to the disorder's title of "manganese mania". Arousal, judgment and memory deficits have also been reported (Rosenstock, Simons and Meyer, 1971).

The second stage of manganese intoxication is characterized by greater numbers of neurological symptoms, including abnormal gait, expressionless facies, speech disorder, clumsiness and sleepiness. In "third stage" severe cases the syndrome is called "manganism" and presents with "parkinsonian-like" symptoms of "asthenia, staggering gait, muscular hypertonia and hypokinesia, and tremor" (Grandjean, 1983, p. 335). Frontal lobe dysfunction, dementia and emotional lability have also been reported to occur at this final stage (Cawte, 1985).

Neurophysiological aspects of manganese intoxication

While the neurochemical mechanism of manganese-induced aggression remains unknown, Chandra (1983) hypothesizes that increases in activity

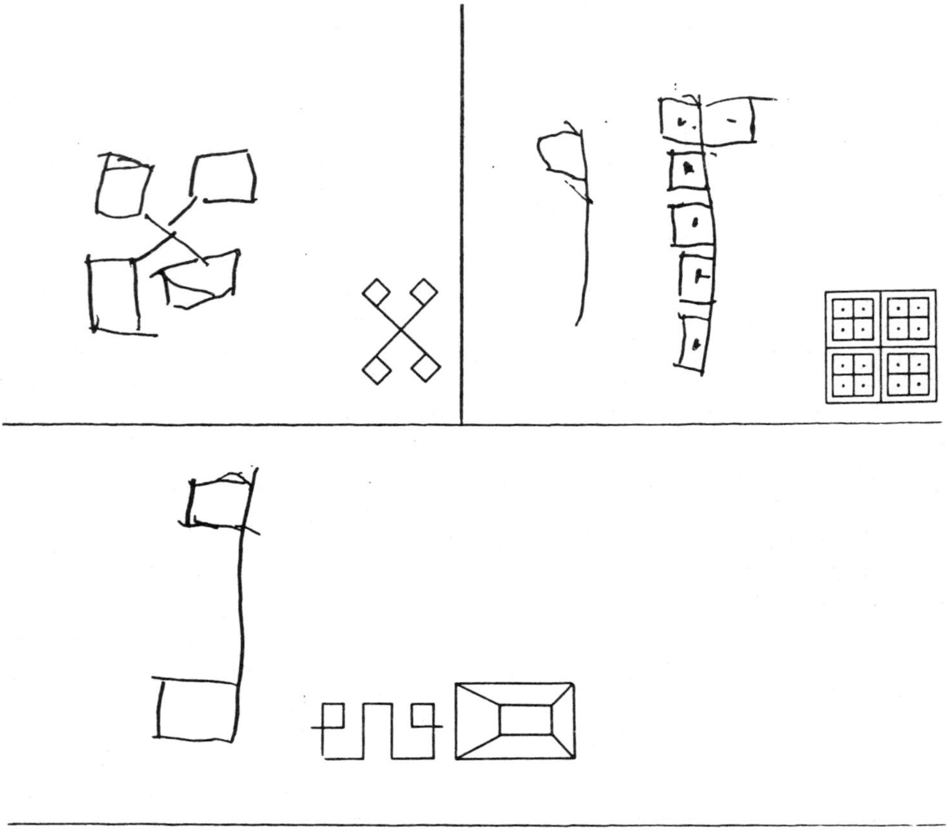

FIGURE III.7. Severe long-term lead exposure. WMS: Figural memory — immediate recall, second testing, 4 months. For reader comparison, card images were inset subsequent to the evaluation.

level characteristic of manganese exposure may be related to elevated striatal catecholamines observed in manganese-intoxicated patients. Cawte (1985) provides a more elaborate hypothesis that catecholamines are first displaced from the ATP complex in the adrenal medulla with consequent "flooding" of the brain by catecholamines, thereby producing the "psychiatric" phase of the disorder. Later, more parkinsonian stages, are byproducts of neurotransmitter depletion. Cawte notes that support for manganese interaction with the dopamine pathway is provided by the observation that L-Dopa "may relieve many of the neurological symptoms in cases of chronic manganism" (Cawte, 1985).

MERCURY

Inorganic (as Hg and compounds) Hg:
OSHA   0.1 mg/m^3 ceiling

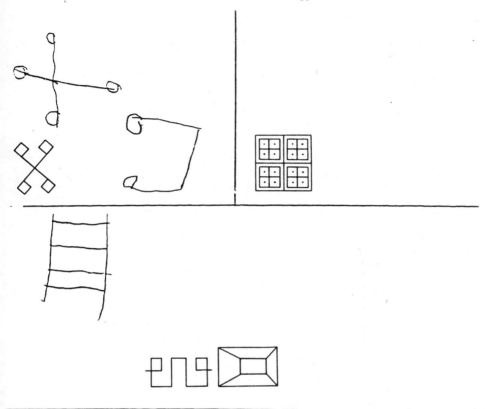

FIGURE III.8. Severe, long-term lead exposure. WMS: Figural memory — 30-minute delayed recall, second testing, 4 months. For reader comparison, card images were inset subsequent to the evaluation.

NIOSH	0.05 mg/m^3 10h TWA
ACGIH	0.05 mg/m^3
IDLH level	28 mg/m^3

Organic and alkyl compounds	0.01 mg/m^3
	0.04 mg/m^3 ceiling
IDLH level	10 mg/m^3
NIOSH, 1985)	

History

Mercury's unusual liquid state at room temperature, coupled with its silvery appearance, have garnered the attention of physicians, philosophers

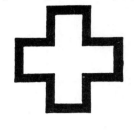

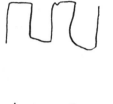

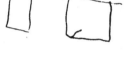

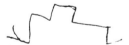

FIGURE III.9. Severe, long-term lead exposure. Spatial Relations Test, second testing, 4 months (direct copy).

and scientists throughout history. In the second and third centuries A.D. the Chinese philosopher Pao Pu Tzu recommended mixing pills of three parts cinnabar (red mercuric sulfide) and one part honey to induce immortality,

Take ten pills the size of a hemp seed every morning. Inside of a year, white hair

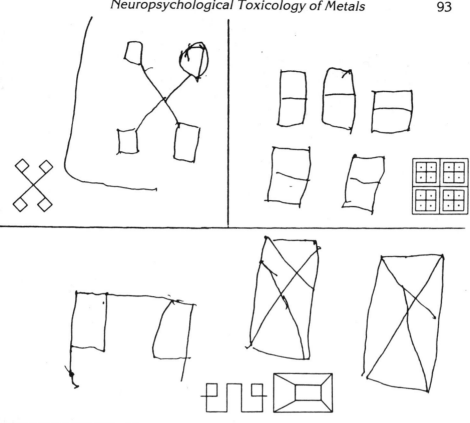

FIGURE III.10. Severe, chronic lead exposure. WMS: Figural memory — immediate recall, third testing, 10 months. For reader comparison, card images were inset subsequent to the evaluation.

will turn black, decayed teeth will grow again . . . . The one who takes [cinnabar] constantly will enjoy eternal life and will not die (cited in Marks and Beatty, 1975, p. 18).

Hippocrates was said to have employed mercuric compounds in his pharmacopoeia around 400 B.C. (Chang, 1980) and Indian physicians of the Brahman period (800 B.C.-A.D. 1000) employed mercury to treat smallpox and syphillis (Marks and Beatty, 1975). Thomas Dover (1660–1742) declared that "To take an ounce of quicksilver every morning . . . [is] the most beneficial thing in the world" (Marks and Beatty, 1975, p. 54).

Children were not spared the "curative" effects of this metal. For example, Antonio Musa Brassavola (1500–55) gave children 2–20 grains of mercury to help them to expel worms. Samuel Bard (1742–1821), a professor of medicine at Kings College, New York, prescribed 30 or 40 grains of

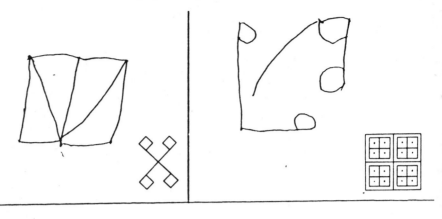

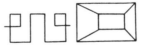

FIGURE III.11. Severe, chronic lead exposure. WMS: Figural memory — 30-minute delayed recall, third testing, 10 months. For reader comparison, card images were inset subsequent to the evaluation.

calomel (mercurous chloride) to children for "sore throat distemper" and proclaimed "the more frequently I have used [mercury compounds], the better effects I have seen from them."

Mercury was cited as a "cure" for syphilis as early as A.D. 1000; one of many metals that have been tried on this disease, including antimony, arsenic bismuth, copper and others (Goldwater, 1972). That mercury cured syphilis "may have been the most colossal hoax ever perpetrated in the history of [medicine]" (Goldwater, 1972, p. 226). As was most likely the case with other metallic cures for syphilis, the belief in mercury's potency may have had more to do with the fact that the early stages of syphilis disappear within a year. If mercury was applied during that time, an association with a remission of symptoms might erroneously be inferred, since visible lesions disappear as the virus enters a second stage.

Like lead, mercury's toxicity has also been recognized for centuries; one of

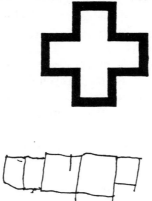

FIGURE III.12. Severe, chronic lead exposure. Spatial Relations Test, third testing, 10 months (direct copy).

the earliest recorded accounts of occupational poisoning is from the supervisor of a mercury mine in 1616:

> sooner or later even the strongest mitayos succumbed to mercury poisoning,/ which entered into the very marrow of their bones/ and made them tremble in every limb (Pereira, cited in Bingham, 1974, p. 199).

Occupational mercury poisoning was noted by Bernardino Ramazzini (1700, cited in Goldwater, 1972) in miners, gilders, those who treated syphilis, chemists, mirror makers, and painters, among others. Hatters were especially at risk because of their exposure to *le secret* or *secretage*, the closely guarded proprietary compound (mercury nitrate) used in the 1600–1800s by members of the hatting guild to cure felt (Hamilton, 1985). Their use of *le secret* caused hatters to develop symptoms of "erethism", a syndrome of irritable and avoidant behavior, in addition to the tremors which became known as "hatter's shakes".

Some authors have understood Lewis Carroll's remarkable "Mad Hatter" to be a caricatured victim of mercury poisoning. Notwithstanding the very real behavioral abnormalities produced by mercury poisoning, it is more likely that Carroll was burlesquing a furniture dealer near Oxford, who was known for his eccentric behavior and inventions; among the latter an "alarm clock bed" which tossed the sleeper on the floor at the predetermined hour (Gardener, cited in Goldwater, 1972, p. 274). Similarly, the phrase "mad as a hatter" may have been a variant on the cockney phrase "mad as an adder" (p. 274).

The history of mercury exposure contains two recent and tragic mass poisonings. The first was at Minamata Bay, off the coast of Japan, where mercuric chloride discharge from an industrial plant was converted to the highly neurotoxic methyl mercury either by microorganisms or from concentration of small amounts of organic mercury along the food chain (Schoenberg, 1982). Whatever the etiology, many individuals died or suffered severe neurological and neuropsychological damage from eating bay shellfish. Many symptoms were noted, including "ataxia, dysarthria and constriction of the visual fields" (Takeuchi, Eto and Eto, 1979, p. 17). In child victims a "decortication" syndrome not found in adult cases was observed, with apraxia, aphasia, agnosia, disorders of consciousness and "loss of all mental activities" (Takeuchi, Eto and Eto, 1979, p. 17). By 1974 over 1200 cases of methyl mercury poisoning had been identified and traced to industrial release of mercury into Minamata Bay (World Health Organization, 1976).

An even larger outbreak of methyl mercury poisoning occurred in Iraq during 1971–72 when grain treated with a mercuric fungicide was taken by peasants and made into bread or cereals rather than kept for seed grain as had been intended. Over 6000 individuals were affected and over 500 deaths were recorded (World Health Organization, 1976).

Industrial risks

The yearly industrial output of mercury is substantial. In the United States alone, more than 11 million pounds of mercury is utilized by various electrical, paint, pharmaceutical and other industries (Chang, 1980). While mercury in its elemental form is poorly absorbed from the gastrointestinal system, it is also quite volatile and may be absorbed from the air in unventilated areas. Because elemental mercury becomes volatile at room temperatures, it may enter the indoor atmosphere from an unsealed container and produce chronic intoxication (Feldman, 1982b). The vapor pressure of pure mercury is also high enough to produce hazardous air concentrations at normal outdoor temperatures (World Health Organization, 1976).

Occupational exposure
Occupations where the volatility of mercury causes risk to workers include those which employ or manufacture barometers or mercury vapor lamps. Also at risk are technicians who prepare dental amalgams, and possibly dentists themselves, since it is reported that 15–20% of United States dental offices exceed OSHA limits for ambient mercury exposure (Uzzell and Oler, 1986). Other occupational groups at risk for mercury exposure include felt-makers, photoengravers and photographers (Feldman, 1982b, p. 147). Industrial workers who manufacture electrical switches and batteries, those using mercuric salts in plating operations, tanners and embalmers are also at

risk. Employees who produce or apply organic mercury compounds as pesticides, fungicides, disinfectants or wood preservatives may also be endangered (Feldman, 1982b; Hamilton, 1985).

Non-occupational exposure

Mercury vapor exposure is not limited to the workplace. The most common non-occupational exposure to mercury occurs via implants of dental amalgam to correct the effects of dental caries. Amalgam is a metallic alloy, usually composed of silver, tin, copper and other metals which are then mixed with between 40% and 54% mercury. Mercury vapor levels three times greater than OSHA safety levels can be produced during initial compression of amalgam in the tooth (Wolff, Osborne and Hanson, 1983). Removing old amalgam, or careless dental techniques, can each expose patients to elevated levels of mercury vapor. The act of chewing with amalgam fillings can release from 4 to 15 times the amount of mercury normally in expired air, even in fillings several years old (Wolff, Osborne and Hanson, 1983).

Wolff, Osborne and Hanson (1983) warn that "patients [with amalgam fillings] could receive a chronic low level exposure to elemental Hg for many years . . . . It is generally agreed that if amalgam was introduced today as a restorative material, they [sic] would never pass F.D.A. approval" (p. 203). While there are no neuropsychological studies on individuals receiving amalgam fillings, such studies would seem strongly indicated to substantiate the allegations of Wolff *et al.*

Mercury exposure has also occurred in home accidents. Windebank, McCall and Dyck (1984) report a case of ataxia, anorexia and lethargy in three members of a family after their 9-year-old son attempted to make "silver bullets" by heating lead shot and thermometer mercury in a frying pan. Air samples in the family's home showed 4 times the maximum industrial limit of mercury.

Neuropathology — methyl mercury

The methylated form of mercury is a far more potent central nervous system poison than mercury in its inorganic state (Weiss, 1978). Methyl mercury is almost completely absorbed from the gastrointestinal tract. By contrast, less than 15% of inorganic mercury is retained (World Health Organization, 1976). Methyl mercury intoxication also produces neurotoxic effects which differ from those of inorganic mercury. Takeuchi, Eto and Eto (1979), reporting on autopsied Minamata victims, found methyl mercury-induced lesions occurred predominantly in the "calcarine cortex, pre- and post-central gyri, superior temporal gyrus and central portion of the cerebellum" (p. 18). The basal ganglia may also show severe destruction (Chaffin and Miller, 1973; Feldman, 1982b). In contrast, elemental mercury lesions have been thought to occur in the occipital cortex and the substantia nigra (Grandjean, 1983).

In addition, chronic exposure to methyl mercury produces systemic central nervous system damage, including constriction of visual fields, ataxia, dysarthria, partial deafness, tremor and intellectual impairment (Windebank, McCall and Dyck, 1984). Feldman (1982b) reports one case of methyl mercury poisoning where members of a family ate pork from animals accidentally fed seed grain treated with methyl mercury fungicide. Several individuals developed initial symptoms of "ataxia, agitation, decreased visual acuity and stupor". Evaluation 10 years later showed blindness, ataxia, retardation, choreoathetosis, myoclonic jerks and abnormal EEGs.

Neuropathology — inorganic mercury

Opinions differ as to the neuropathology of mercury vapor poisoning. Feldman (1982b) suggests that toxic effects are due to mercury-induced enzyme inhibition. Since mercury penetrates and damages the blood–brain barrier (Chang, 1982), and accumulates in the brain, it may also produce direct structural damage. Several authors have speculated about brain localization of inorganic mercury damage. Grandjean (1983) suggests that brain damage from inorganic mercury vapor may be localizable to the occipital cortex and the substantia nigra. Other authors have suggested that inorganic mercury appears to show uniform brain distribution. Conservative estimates of brain mercury able to induce neurotoxic symptoms are 1.2 μg/g, corresponding to a blood level of 200 ng/g (Nordberg, 1976; Williamson, Teo and Sanderson, 1982).

Neurological effects

Neurological sequelae from inorganic mercury exposure begin approximately 24 hours following acute exposure. Levels of mercury in urine greater than 0.5 mg/l have been linked "to the development of mild neurotoxic effects" (Feldman, 1982a, p. 147). Tremor is a common concomitant of urinary excretions above 250 μg/dl of Hg (Grandjean, 1983). Hand and finger tremor, progressing to tremor of the face and eyelid, occurs at a frequency of about 5 Hertz (Grandjean, 1983). Tremor eventually involves the head and trunk (Feldman, 1982a).

These and other changes may be progressive, continuing to worsen after cessation of exposure. Moreover, toxic neurological abnormalities may be permanent.

Neuropsychological effects of mercury

Mercury intoxication may be produced by inhalation, ingestion, or, in the case of one 19 year-old-suicide attempter, injection (Zillmer *et al.*, 1986). Neuropsychological effects are present in all modalities of exposure.

In general, disturbances in behavior and cognition are "the earliest signs of chronic mercury intoxication" (Feldman, 1982b, p. 203), and thus may precede other neurological effects. Intellectual disturbance from mercury intoxication has been found to occur in tests of visuospatial abilities, visual memory, non-verbal abstraction, cognitive efficiency and reaction time (Angotzi *et al.*, 1982, p. 249). Block Design, Digit Symbol and Raven's Progressive Matrices appear to be sensitive indicators of toxic effects, as are Digit Span and tests of visual memory (Hänninen, 1982, p. 169). Lowered eye–hand coordination and decreased finger tapping scores are significantly correlated with urinary mercury levels (Langolf *et al.*, 1978), as are foot tapping scores (Chaffin and Miller, 1974). Mercury exposure increases test fatigue, and decreases initial learning of word associations.

The emotional dysfunction called "erethism" is also thought to be a very common emotional abnormality related to mercury exposure. This syndrome, derived from the French and Greek word "to irritate", denotes an unusual and morbid level of overactivity of the "mental powers or passions" (*Oxford English Dictionary*, 1971, p. 890). In current use the term also connotes symptoms of avoidant, irritable and overly sensitive interpersonal behavior, depression, lassitude and fatigue (Hänninen, 1982, p. 167). Ross and Sholiton (1983) found some evidence of this syndrome when they interviewed nine laboratory technicians exposed to mercury vapor. These authors describe symptoms of irritability in six individuals and "shyness" in three. Two of the nine individuals displayed most of the classical symptoms of erethism; however, three others showed none of the classical symptoms. In another study, Uzzel and Oler (1986) found significant elevations on the SCL-90-R, a psychopathology inventory, in subclinically exposed individuals compared to controls.

For the suicidal adolescent who injected himself with metallic mercury, neuropsychological effects were particularly severe (Zillmer *et al.*, 1986). In the context of a normal neurological examination at 6 weeks post-injection, the patient exhibited a Halstead–Reitan Impairment index of 1.0 and had a Wechsler Memory Scale MQ (memory quotient) of 59, both indicating severe impairment of neuropsychological function. Overall WAIS-R IQ scores, while somewhat depressed, did not appear to particularly sensitive to the patient's neuropsychological abnormalities.

Hänninen's (1982) review concluded that mercury-induced neuropsychological abnormalities fell into three major groups, including 1) motor system abnormalities (e.g. fine motor tremor), 2) intellectual impairment (gradual and progressive deterioration of memory, concentration and logical reasoning), and 3) emotional disability. Occupational studies of mercury exposure have found support for individual symptoms of impairment within these categories. For example, Williamson and Teo (1982) examined 12 mercury-exposed workers who were exposed to the supposedly less toxic organic and inorganic forms of mercury, including mercury-based fungicide, and inorganic mercury amalgam used in gold refining. Exposure length in total time and hours per day was quite variable, from 1 to 8 hours per day and total duration from 3 months to 8 years. Nonexposed controls were age-, sex-, race- and education-matched.

The authors administered an extensive neuropsychological battery to all subjects, including various tests of memory, a paired associate learning test, critical flicker fusion, a pursuit rotor to measure visual pursuit, a Sternberg task, and tests of hand steadiness, reaction time, and vigilance.

No significant differences were found for flicker fusion, or simple reaction time. Speeded tracking of a pursuit rotor was impaired at the higher speed but not at the lower (Williamson, Teo and Sanderson, 1982). Other significant impairments in the mercury group were in the areas of hand steadiness, short-term (but not iconic or long-term) memory, verbal learning and the Sternberg paradigm. The only test which correlated significantly with total duration of mercury exposure was the visual pursuit rotor performance. Only hand steadiness correlated significantly with current urinary mercury levels. The authors explained their results as consistent with mercury-induced effects on "psychomotor coordination and short term memory" (Williamson, Teo and Sanderson, 1982, p. 285).

Treibig and Schaller (1982) also report a significant relationship between mercury exposure duration and short-term memory, but failed to find other signficant neuropsychological deficits. Subjects were exposed a mean of 8 years, and had blood mercury averaging 68 μg/l in one group and 30 μg/l in another. Changes in nerve conduction velocity were not consistently found at this level of exposure.

Uzzel and Oler (1986) used X-ray fluorescence to detect low-level mercury exposure in dental technicians, and compared their performance to dental assistants without detectable mercury levels. Subjects were similar in age, education and years employed in dental work (approximately 15). Tests employed included the WAIS, the Rey Auditory–Verbal Learning Test, Recurrent Figures Test, the PASAT (Paced Auditory Serial Addition Test), Finger Tapping Test, the Bender-Visual Motor Gestalt Test and the SCL-90-R, a symptom checklist.

The subclinically exposed subjects showed deficient performance in the Recurrent Figures Test — an examination of visual recognition memory, as well as significantly elevated SCL-90-R profile compared to controls. The study's small number of subjects in each group (13) may have militated against achieving significance in other neuropsychological measures, since mean subject performance of the experimental group was also worse than the control group's in tests of attention, memory and visual–motor abilities.

Since subjects remained employed and able to perform their work, the authors' neuropsychological results may be indicative of a very early "pre-tremor" phase of mercury intoxication. While elevated levels of psychopathology shown by subjects on the SCL-90-R are suggestive of "erethism", there is no information provided about whether subjects knew their group membership. If subjects had been told of their mercury body burden, the personality results shown could be equally well explained as a reactive consequence of that knowledge.

A fourth study examined subjects with longer exposures, higher average blood mercury levels and a wider range of blood mercury. Piikivi *et al.* (1984) studied the neuropsychological effects of mercury vapor in 36 workers exposed for a mean of 16.9 years. They found significantly lowered Similarities, Digit Span and Visual Reproduction (WMS Figural Memory) in workers with blood Hg levels greater than 75 nmol/l compared to controls with lower blood levels. Individuals with higher blood mercury levels (280 nmol/l) and those exposed to higher peak levels also showed significant deficits in motor coordination on the Santa Ana Dexterity Test. The authors' results are consistent with mercury-induced memory, abstract reasoning and motor coordination deficit. Unfortunately, they did not also test for indications of personality or affective disorder. The authors recommended a maximum metallic mercury exposure limit of 25 $\mu g/m^3$ to avoid neurotoxic effects.

NICKEL

Metal and soluble compounds (Ni):
OSHA   1 mg/m^3
NIOSH   15 μg Ni/m^3 10 h TWA
  ACGIH   1 mg/m^3 metal
              0.1 mg/m^3 (soluble)
Nickel carbonyl [Ni(CO)$_4$]:
OSHA   0.001 ppm (0.007 mg/m^3)
  NIOSH   1 ppb TWA
IDLH level   0.001 ppm
  ACGIH   0.05 ppm
(NIOSH, 1985)

Very little information is available concerning the neuropsychological effects of nickel. Feldman (1982a) describes two cases of toxic nickel encephalopathy after an accident occurred in an electroplating plant where workers were exposed to nickel chloride and nickel sulfate. Symptoms included severe frontal headache, nausea and vomiting. One victim had showed restricted visual fields, and both men's CT scans showed small ventricles, suggesting cerebral edema. With penicillamine chelation complete recovery was reported within 1 month. No neuropsychological testing of nickel-exposed individuals appears to be available.

PLATINUM

Platinum (soluble salts as Pt):
OSHA   0.002 mg/m^3
(NIOSH, 1985)

Platinum is commonly used in the electronics and chemical industries, and is also used in jewelry. Pure platinum has not been linked to neurological symptoms; however, platinum-containing compounds used in cancer treatment are neurotoxic. "Cis-platinum" or cisplatin (cis-diamminedichloroplatinum), is one of the most often used forms of chemotherapy to combat testicular, bladder, and head and neck cancer.

Central and peripheral nervous system damage has been reported as a result of cisplatin use (Walsh *et al.*, 1982). Peripheral nervous system damage takes the form of progressive symmetrical sensory neuropathy (Schaumberg and Spencer, 1983), although intra-arterial injection may induce reversible unilateral cranial nerve palsy. Central nervous system effects may include damage to the optic nerve and spinal cord (Pomes *et al.*, 1986). A postmortem study suggested cisplatin-induced degeneration of the optic disk, optic nerve and long tracts of the spinal cord (Walsh *et al.*, 1982). There are no neuropsychological studies of cis-platinum intoxication.

SELENIUM

Selenium and compounds (as Se):
OSHA   0.2 mg/m^3
IDLH level   100 mg/m^3
(NIOSH, 1985)

Selenium is found in industrial settings as a result of mining or processing selenium-containing minerals including copper, lead, zinc pyrite, roasting lime and cement. Selenium is used commercially in the production of glass and ceramics, and other substances including steel, rubber, brass, paint and ink pigment, and photoelectric materials (Katz, 1985).

In very small doses, selenium is an essential trace element in human diet. In larger amounts from voluntary or industrial exposure, selenium has been associated with neurotoxic effects, including headache, vertigo, convulsions and a motor neuron disease similar to amyotropic lateral sclerosis, a disease reported in four ranchers who grazed their cattle in high selenium soil and ate meat with high selenium content (Goetz, 1985). There are no neuropsychological studies of selenium intoxication.

SILICON

Silicon shares properties of both metal and glass, and therefore can be appropriately included in this section. It is widely used in the glass and electronics industries. Silicon has been controversially linked to dementia in several studies cited by Goetz (1985). However, it is unclear whether elevated silicon levels found in demented patients are causal or secondary to a neuropathological disease process.

TELLURIUM

as Te: OSHA   0.1 mg/m^3

Tellurium exposure occurs in miners; and in the alloy, rubber, glass, stainless steel, copper and lead industries (Katz, 1985). Tellurium exposure in humans has been associated with mild neurological complaints, including headache and sleepiness. Symptoms seem to be the same whether exposure is acute or chronic. Rat studies have suggested that tellurium exposure may produce muscle weakness and behavioral abnormalities. Peripheral nervous system damage is more common than CNS effects in experimentally induced toxicity studies. There are no neuropsychological studies of tellurium exposed individuals.

THALLIUM

Thallium (soluble compounds as Tl):

OSHA   0.1 mg/m^3
IDLH level   20 mg/m^3
(NIOSH, 1985)

Thallium was initially used in the nineteenth century to treat "night sweat" symptoms of tuberculosis. Currently the main uses of this metal are for rodent and pest control, although thallium is also used in tungsten filaments, jewelry, alloys, fireworks and high refractive index glass (Katz, 1985). Thallium poisoning is relatively rare and most case reports consist of homicide attempts or accidental ingestions. Hair loss (alopecia) is a unique identifying sign of thallium poisoning.

Damage to the peripheral nervous system occurs within 24–48 hours of thallium ingestion and may progress for several weeks after ingestion of a single dose (Windebank, McCall and Dyck, 1984). Central nervous system effects may occur with larger doses, and organic psychosis may ensue. Chromolytic changes in the motor cortex, substantia nigra and globus pallidus and third nerve nuclei have been reported (Bank, 1980). Optic neuropathy has been reported in children who have ingested this metal, and a single case report of an exposed worker who also developed optic atrophy has also been cited (Hamilton & Hardy, 1974).

TIN AND ORGANOTINS

Inorganic (compounds except oxides) (as Sn):
OSHA 2 mg/m^3
IDLH level 400 mg/m^3

Organic compounds:
OSHA 0.1 mg/m^3
NIOSH 0.1 mg/m^3 10 TWA
IDLH level 200 mg/m^3
(NIOSH, 1985)

Tin's first recorded medical use was during the Middle Ages as a vermifuge. It was also employed to purge fevers, induce sweat and "cure" venereal disease and hysteria (Marks and Beatty, 1975).

Tin is presently used to plate containers, but is also found in solder and as part of other metal alloys and dental amalgams (World Health Organization, 1980). Organotins are used as polyvinyl chloride (PVC) stabilizers and elsewhere in the plastics industry. Trisubstituted forms of organotin have biocidal properties useful in agriculture and other circumstances where fungicides, miticides, bactericides or similar substances are required (World Health Organization, 1980).

Inorganic tin

Inorganic (elemental) tin is poorly absorbed and rapidly turned over in tissue, hence its toxicity is very low compared with organotin compounds. Although animal studies show inorganic tin can produce "ataxia, muscular weakness and central nervous system depression", no such effects have been cited thus far in human studies (World Health Organization, 1980).

Organotins

In contrast to inorganic tin, organic tin compounds are very neurotoxic; their effects have been documented for over a century (Reuhl and Cranmer, 1984). Of these, trimethyl and triethyl tins are primarily toxic to the nervous system, in contrast to other organotins which target other organ systems.

Triethyltin
Triethyltin exerts its neurotoxic effects by causing "massive" myelin

TABLE III.4. Signs and symptoms of human organotin poisoning. (Reprinted, by permission of the publisher, from Reiter, L. W. and Ruppert, P. H. (1984). Behavioral toxicity of trialkyltin compounds: A review. *NeuroToxicology*, **5**, 197–186.)

TRIETHYLTIN	TRIMETHYLTIN
Headache	Headache
Abdominal pain	Generalized pain
Visual disturbance	Visual disturbance
Vertigo	Disorientation
Weight loss	Appetite loss
Hypothermia	Memory deficit
Paralysis	Sleep disturbances
Papilloedema	Loss of libido
	Depression and rage

edema with consequent raised intracranial pressure (Reuhl and Cranmer, 1984, p.187). The mechanism of edema is not known. In France, during 1954, 200 individuals became intoxicated, and half eventually died from the neurotoxic effects of a compound called "Stalinon", which contained triethyltin impurities and purportedly treated "osteomyelitis, skin infections . . . anthrax" and acne (Hamilton and Hardy, 1974, p.177; Watanabe, 1980). Severe diffuse white matter edema and changes in glial cells were found in four autopsied victims of Stalinon (Watanabe, 1980), and it is probable that most of the Stalinon deaths could be attributed to cerebral edema (World Health Organization, 1980). Clinical symptoms of exposed individuals included "nausea, vertigo, visual disturbances, papilledema and convulsions"; typical symptoms of elevated intracranial pressure (Reuhl and Cranmer, 1984, p. 195).

Trimethyltin

Trimethyltin has different neuropathological properties from triethyltin. Trimethyltin specifically targets the cortex, limbic system and brainstem. Experiments with primates have shown damage to the hippocampus, amygdala, pyriform cortex and neuroretina (Reuhl and Cranmer, 1984). It is capable of also decreasing gamma aminobutyric acid in the hippocampus and dopamine levels in the striatum (Hanin, Krigman and Mailman, 1984). One case study reports two chemists exposed to trimethyltin who subsequently experienced epilepsy, mental confusion, headache and psychomotor dysfunction, but who did not show characteristic manifestations of intracranial pressure common to triethyltin victims (Fortemps *et al.*, 1978).

Reports of neurotoxic exposure to organotins in the workplace are uncommon. One study examined 22 chemical workers who had been exposed to spilled trimethyltin chloride over the period of a month (Ross *et al.*, 1981). Significantly more high-exposure workers reported non-specific symptoms of forgetfulness, fatigue, loss of libido and motivation, and periods of headache and sleep disturbance.

Neuropsychological effects

Neuropsychological tests were also administered in the Ross *et al.* (1981) study, although the authors did not name the tests or report actual scores. Using non-parametric statistics they reported significant decrements in verbal memory, finger tapping, fine motor eye–hand coordination, as well as deficits in "visual-motor integration and learning" (Ross *et al.*, 1981, p. 1093; Ross and Sholiton, 1983).

Personality effects

The authors suggested that a unique pattern of mood disorder was found significantly more often in organotin-exposed workers, which consisted of alternating bouts of rage and deep depression lasting from several hours to several days. Personality deterioration may be long-lasting; when four of the 12 individuals receiving the highest exposure were re-evaluated between 9 and 34 months post-exposure, all were said to suffer long-term deterioration of personality functioning.

As the authors noted, it is not known whether these changes are direct effects of organotin or reactive via post-traumatic stress disorder. It is also unclear whether premorbid personality factors or coping style influenced post-exposure behavior.

ZINC

Zinc chloride (fume): $(ZnCl_2)$
OSHA   1 mg/m^3
IDLH level   2000 mg/m^3

Zinc oxide (fume): (ZnO)
OSHA   5 mg/m^3
NIOSH   5 mg/m^3 10 h TWA
                      15 mg/m^3 15 min ceiling
(NIOSH, 1985)

Zinc is a common metal, found in sheet metal, batteries and various alloys. Two neurological syndromes have been linked to toxic exposure. Oral ingestion of zinc chloride or of acidic foods stored in galvanized containers has been fatal, with survivors showing residual neurological symptoms of dyspnea, weakness, muscle spasm and lethargy (Goetz, 1985). Inhalation of zinc vapor may produce neurological and psychiatric symptomatology, including irritability, "upper extremity coarse intention tremor, incoordination and ataxia" (Brazier's disease) (Goetz, 1985, p. 57). Neuropsychological tests of zinc toxicity have not been performed.

Table III.5. Other metals with neurobehavioral effects

METAL	BEHAVIORAL EFFECT
Barium	Severe neurotoxicity, flaccid paralysis, including respiration
Boron	CNS depression
Vanadium	Tremors, "nervous depression"

OTHER METALS

Metals as a group tend to be neurotoxic. However, there is little or no neuropsychological research on many metals with common industrial applications, e.g. thallium or platinum. There is also no neuropsychological information yet available concerning the neurobehavioral effects of exposure to the substances listed in Table III.5. Further neuropsychological, neurophysiological, and epidemiological studies are clearly needed.

IV
Neuropsychological Toxicology of Solvents

INTRODUCTION

Solvents must be included in any discussion of neuropsychological toxicology, since in the 100 years that organic solvents have been in existence, evidence has slowly accrued to suggest their role in the production of overt and subclinical neurotoxic syndromes.

Definition

The term "organic solvent" is a generic classification for a chemical compound or mixture used by industry to "extract, dissolve or suspend" non-water-soluble materials including fats, oils, resins, lipids, cellulose derivatives, waxes, plastics and polymers (*Organic Solvents*, 1985, p. 3; Arlien-Søborg, 1985). Most solvents are liquids and their chemical composition may be simple, like carbon tetrachloride, or complex, like those solvents derived from petroleum (MacFarland, 1986).

Solvents are also grouped into major classes according to their chemical composition. One major class of solvents is that of the *hydrocarbons* which, in turn, are divided into two subgroups: the aliphatic hydrocarbons that include hexanes, pentanes and octanes, and the aromatic hydrocarbons, including benzene, styrene, toluene and xylene (MacFarland, 1986). Other solvent groups include *halogenated compounds* (also referred to as chlorinated hydrodrocarbons) like carbon tetrachloride, methylene chloride, trichloroethylene and perchloroethylene; *alcohols*, including methanol (wood alcohol) and ethanol (grain alcohol) are also known as *oxygenated solvents*; *glycols*, which include ethylene and propylene glycol; *ketones*, e.g. methyl ethyl ketone, and *complex solvents* (MacFarland, 1986).

Members of the latter group are classified according to their boiling points, on a continuum which includes petroleum ethers, rubber solvent, varnish makers' and painters' naphtha, mineral spirits and Stoddard solvent (also known as "white spirit"). Finally, other classes of materials have solvent properties, including esters, aldehydes and substances like dioxane, isophorone and pyridine (MacFarland, 1986). However, these latter agents have not been subjected to neuropsychological investigation.

Curtis and Keller (1986) state that all solvents share common characteristics including *volatility* (significant vapor pressure) and *solvency* (pass through intact skin). In addition, solvents are *lipophilic* with an affinity for nerve tissue, and are *soluble* in blood and pass rapidly through lung tissue. Further, solvents have relatively *unobjectionable odors* which may not provoke irritation until high concentrations are achieved. Finally, exposure to solvents may cause *chemical dependency* (Curtis and Keller, 1986).

Exposure

Individuals are typically exposed to solvents accidentally and involuntarily in the workplace. However, they may also deliberately expose themselves in the pursuit of an intoxicating solvent "high". Exposure is widespread in each category.

Industrial exposure to solvents began approximately 100 years ago in small cottage industries. Present-day solvent exposure sites include large-scale manufacturing applications involving millions of workers. Workers involved in the manufacture of paints, adhesives, glues, coatings, dyes, polymers, pharmaceuticals and synthetic fabrics are commonly exposed. In addition, workers who directly employ solvents in their trades are also at risk, including painters, varnishers and carpet layers (*Organic Solvents*, 1985).

Solvent abuse is also widespread, with one study estimating that 18.7% of United States high school seniors had tried solvent-based inhalants (Johnson, Bachman and O'Malley, 1979).

Neurophysiological effects

Despite long-standing industrial use and individual abuse, neurophysiological and neuropsychological function changes as a result of solvent exposure did not enter the health literature until 1940, while large-scale investigations were not undertaken until the late 1960s and early 1970s. Current medical and neuropsychological understanding of solvent effects remains far from definitive. Knowledge of peripheral nervous system solvent effects is incomplete, and confined to a small number of solvents. Central nervous system effects are even less well understood and require further research (Cherry and Waldron, 1983).

Intake

One route of solvent exposure is via direct absorption into the skin. The speed of absorption into the skin is related to the solvent's solubility in water.

Solvents as a group are quite volatile so they may just as easily enter the bloodstream via inhalation as from direct absorption through the skin. Solvents entering the bloodstream through the alveoli of the lungs diffuse quite rapidly into the blood. Solvents accidentally ingested (or purposely swallowed in suicide attempts) are easily absorbed from the gastrointestinal tract.

The amount of solvent retained is dependent upon a combination of solvent-related and human-related factors. Some of the former include blood and tissue solubility, and *a priori* toxicity of the solvent (Åstrand, 1975). Solvents may also show great intra-individual variations, and their toxicity may vary according to diurnal metabolic cycles, alcohol use and other individual variations. *Inter*-individual differences may also account for variation in solvent toxicity; for example, solvents are stated to have longer biological half-lives in obese persons than in thin ones (Cohr, 1985). Solvents are excreted unchanged in expired air and their water-soluble metabolites are eliminated in urine.

Physiological measurement of solvent uptake is more usefully obtained with urine sample than with blood concentrations or exhaled air. These latter measures "are usually only of value during the immediate exposure interval in view of the short half-life of these compounds in the blood" (Baker, Smith and Landrigan, 1985, p. 214).

General toxic effects

As a class, solvents produce several types of exposure effects. Some common toxic effects do not involve the nervous system. For example, because of their defatting and corrosive qualities, solvents can irritate the mucosal membranes of the eyes and upper respiratory tract, and cause nausea, loss of appetite, vomiting and diarrhea (Arlien-Søberg, 1985; James, 1985). In addition, solvents can be hepatotoxic, nephrotoxic and can also induce cardiac arrhythmia by sensitizing the heart to catecholamines (James, 1985).

Neurotoxicity

All solvents can depress central nervous system activity via their anesthetic action. Solvent-exposed individuals are rendered progressively less sensitive to stimuli as a function of solvent concentration and/or exposure duration until unconsciousness, coma or death occur. Other acute effects can include light-headedness, feelings of drunkenness and ataxia. Despite these obviously neurological effects, when Spencer and Schaumberg (1985) reviewed the current neurophysiological research, they found lasting neurological sequelae for only five individual solvents, including the hexacarbons *n*– hexane +/–methyl ethyl ketone (MEK), methyl *n*–butyl ketone +/– MEK, carbon disulfide, trichloroethylene and voluntarily abused toluene. The authors also suggest that there is evidence, albeit less definitive, for neurotoxicity of the following solvents: diethyl ether, ethylene chloride, nitrobenzene, pyridine, styrene, tetrachloroethane, trichloroethylene +/– perchloroethylene, xylene, "white spirit", other solvent mixtures, chromogenic aromatic hydrocarbons and methylene chloride (Spencer and Schaumberg, 1985, p. 54).

Neuropsychological symptoms of solvent exposure

While neurological examination is usually normal, except in the most severe cases of solvent exposure, "subclinical" neuropsychological effects tend to be seen much earlier in the subject's history of exposure. Neuropsychological abnormalities include behavioral, cognitive and emotional dysfunction. Commonly reported are complaints of headache, dizziness, fatigue, paresthesias, pain and weakness. Subjective complaints of memory disturbances have been frequently claimed (Edling, 1985).

Symptoms found in solvent-exposed workers tallied by questionnaire and interview by Mikkelson *et al.* (1985) include impairments in memory, concentration, general intellect and problem-solving, speed and initiative. Emotional symptoms which may accompany a solvent dementia can include increased fatigue, depression, anxiety, emotional lability and irritability.

With chronic prolonged solvent exposure there is a consensus (at least in the Scandinavian literature) that symptoms of dementia can result. Dementia is defined by DSM III as

a loss of intellectual abilities of sufficient severity to interfere with social or occupational function. The deficit . . . involves memory, judgment, abstract thought and a variety of other cortical functions. Changes in personality and behavior also occur (American Psychiatric Association, 1980, p. 107).

DIAGNOSTIC PROCEDURES IN SOLVENT EXPOSURE

As is true for metals, the constellation of cognitive and emotional alterations produced by solvent intoxication is "most reliably measured by psychological test methods" (Lindström, 1981, p. 48). However, neuropsychological analyses of solvent effects usually occur in the context of a general medico-diagnostic workup. While neurological examination and other medical procedures tend to be less sensitive to early subclinical solvent effects, they are nevertheless essential for several reasons. First, a complete evaluation is usually needed to rule out alternative diagnoses (e.g. unrelated central or peripheral nervous system lesion). Second, neurological and physical evaluations provide tests for functions not examined by neuropsychologists (e.g. liver function tests, tests of cranial nerve function). Finally, conventional medical examination may complement and further validate neuropsychological findings.

Medical evaluation techniques

Techniques in common use include electroencephalography (EEG) to measure central nervous system effects, and electroneuromyography (ENMG) to detect abnormalities in the electrical activity in nerves and muscles. Tests of regional cerebral blood flow have also been found to be useful. CT scan may be employed to rule out alternative diagnoses, or to expose more serious structural damage found in chronic exposure to certain solvents. However, it is not sensitive to early subclinical effects. There are no data yet available on the utility of MR (magnetic resonance) scans in solvent exposure diagnosis.

International diagnostic criteria for solvent syndromes

Just as there is no single test capable of diagnosing solvent intoxication, there is also no single conceptual system to categorize the effects of solvent exposure. Systems of diagnosis and requirements for impairment both vary somewhat from country to country. Denmark, for example, defines "chronic toxic encephalopathy" in terms of impairment of intellect, memory, affect and personality. Neuropsychological test results are crucial to the diagnosis, and while neurological deficit may occasionally be found, the latter is not esential for diagnostic attribution. In fact, severe neurological deficits may argue for an alternative diagnoses (*Organic Solvents*, 1985, p. 8).

Other Scandinavian countries use criteria similar to Denmark's. Each seeks to verify qualitative and quantitative effects of solvent exposure by clinical history as well as by documenting a symptom picture which may include both objective and subjective data. All seek to rule out other causes of brain dysfunction and all subject the potential exposure victim to a variety of neurological, neuropsychological and neurophysiological tests, including computerized tomography (CT), magnetic resonance (MR) scan, electroencephalography (EEG), electromyography (EMG), evoked potentials (EP), sensory nerve action potentials (SNAP), F-response, muscle biopsy and nerve biopsy. Sweden specifies exposure parameters more than its sister countries, by suggesting that more than 10 years of long and/or intensive exposure is necessary to the diagnosis, which they term "psycho-organic syndrome".

The World Health Organization's (WHO) 1985 Copenhagen conference suggested that solvent intoxication effects should be termed "slight or mild" chronic toxic encephalopathy, depending upon exposure severity. "Slight" encephalopathy was characterized by evidence of subjective complaint and personality impairment without neurological signs or symptoms. As exposure progressed, discernible deficits would be noted in cognition, memory and "neurological deficits, characterized by balance deficits and mild ataxia" (*Neurobehavioral Methods*, p. 31).

There is currently no official medico-diagnostic category in the United States that corresponds with "psycho-organic syndrome" or its equivalents. Baker and Fine (1986) suggest that the DSM-III diagnostic criteria for organic affective syndrome are met for the early, reversible symptoms of fatigue, irritability, depression and apathy encountered in solvent-exposed individuals. Chronic exposure to high concentrations of some solvents (i.e. toluene) may also produce global intellectual deterioration and thereby satisfy the criteria for dementia.

A research conference, held in the United States the same year as the WHO conference, attempted to more completely characterize the progressive nature of solvent neurotoxicity. The panel members at the conference partitioned solvent effects into four separate syndromes, the mildest of which was termed a "Type 1" disorder (Baker and Seppäläinen, 1986). Type 1 solvent intoxication is also equivalent to earlier terminology of "neurasthenic syndrome". This syndrome, consisting of "fatigue, irritability, depression and episodes of anxiety", is not acompanied by deficits on neuropsychological tests, but can be documented on instruments which record subjective complaints, e.g. symptom checklists. A syndrome of this type has been hypothesized to presage neurobehavioral dysfunction (Baker, Smith and Landrigan, 1985, p. 213). Type 1 symptoms are also said to be reversible if exposure is discontinued (Baker and Seppäläinen, 1986).

When exposure continues, neuropsychological methods can identify the next stage which has been variously termed "psycho-organic syndrome" (Flodin, Edling and Axelson, 1984) in the Swedish literature, "mild dementia" in Danish writings and "mild toxic encephalopathy" by the World Health Organization (WHO report No. 6, Copenhagen, 1985).

The 1985 International Workshop on the Neurobehavioral Effects of Solvents held in North Carolina, U.S.A., further divided this middle stage into its emotional and cognitive components. For research purposes, a Type 2A exposure syndrome was said to be characterized by disturbances of mood and personality, fatigue, impulse control and motivation, while Type 2B syndromes would be recognized primarily as intellectual disturbances in memory, learning and concentration, psychomotor difficulties and impairments in other neuropsychological functions (Baker and Seppäläinen, 1986). The relationship between these two intermediate-severity solvent syndromes and their reversibility has yet to be determined.

TABLE IV.1. Categories of solvent-induced CNS disorders*

	CATEGORY OF CNS DISORDER	
Severity of condition	Identified by WHO/Nordic Council of Ministers Working Group, Copenhagen, June 1985[†]	International Solvent Workshop, Raleigh, N.C. October 1985[††]
Minimal	Organic affective syndrome	Type 1
Moderate	Mild chronic toxic encephalopathy	Types 2A or 2B
Pronounced	Severe chronic toxic encephalopathy	Type 3

* In view of the difficulty of categorizing these disorders, correspondence between the two systems of nomenclature is not exact.
† *Source:* WHO, 1985.
†† *Source:* Baker and Seppäläinen, 1986.

The time course for development of a psycho-organic or Type 2B syndrome may be dependent on intensity of solvent exposure. Olson (1982) found that tool cleaners who work with vats of solvent appear to show a more rapid onset of solvent symptoms than did painters. Cleaners who were exposed for a mean of 4.3 years performed significantly more poorly in tasks of reaction time, concentration and memory. Incipient symptoms may begin as early as 3 years with chronic industrial exposure (e.g. Flodin, Edling and Axelson, 1984).

The most severe stage or "Type 3" solvent syndrome is characterized by progressive and global neuropsychological, intellectual and emotional decline which fulfills the medical criteria of dementia and is equivalent to the World Health Organization's "severe toxic encephalopathy" (World Health Organization 1985). This latter stage is rarely seen clinically, and usually only after many years of workplace exposure or severe recreational abuse (e.g. Fornazzari *et al.*, 1983).

It must be emphasized that the tripartite division of solvent effects proposed at the 1985 conference were *working hypotheses* of which not all researchers, even those at the same conference, agreed. For example, Mikkelsen (1986) suggested that solvent effects should instead be classified according to three dimensions: (1) particular combinations of neurotoxic signs and symptoms, (2) severity of effects and (3) reversibility of effects.

Table IV.1 shows the approximate correspondence between proposed categorizations of solvent syndromes.

Diagnostic process

The patient who is under evaluation for solvent intoxication should optimally be evaluated by a team specially trained in the diagnosis of solvent syndromes. The initial evaluation should be sufficiently broad to rule out alternative diagnoses, and sufficiently fine-grained to describe in detail the pattern of the individual's deficits. Thus, a chronic solvent exposure victim might receive neurological, neuropsychological, hematological and neuroradiological evaluations as part of a standard workup. Baker and Seppäläinen (1986) have suggested that data collected from the evaluations can be used to diagnose, control exposure and provide appropriate health-related referrals to patients claiming solvent intoxication.

Conventional medical/neurological techniques are usually employed to obtain objective physiological correlates of behavioral dysfunction. These techniques have included blood, urine and breath assay, EEG, CT, nerve conduction and, more recently, magnetic resonance (MR) scans, as well as several types of evoked potential studies (e.g. Otto, 1983). Regional cerebral blood flow studies may also be of value (Risberg and Hagstadius, 1983).

SOLVENT MIXTURES

Mixtures of solvents are studied for their neurotoxic properties for several reasons. First, industrial personnel are more commonly exposed to mixtures or multiple solvents than to a single solvent (Lindström and Wickstrom, 1983). Painters, for example, have often been exposed to solvent mixtures, including "white spirit", a group of paint solvents with boiling points midway between gasoline and kerosene (World Health Organization, 1982). Although techniques used to study mixtures versus single solvents are similar, one difference seems to be that solvent mixture research proceeds "on the assumption that all organic solvents depress the functions of the central nervous system" and thus tends to look for global rather than solvent-specific effects. (Gregersen *et al*, 1984).

Acute effects of solvent mixtures

Acute solvent mixture effects are prenarcotic, usually reversible and dependent upon dose levels (Winneke, 1982). Symptoms often disappear following an exposure-free interval; workers who have experienced progressive discomfort during the week may experience renewed well-being by Monday (Arlien-Søberg, 1985). Cherry, Venables and Waldron (1983) investigated acute behavioral and mood changes in workers exposed to solvents pre- and post-workshift. Workers rated themselves significantly higher in sleepiness, physical and mental tiredness, and believed themselves to be in poorer health than did controls. Neuropsychological findings were inconsistent, with paint solvents and styrene workers showing somewhat greater effects of exposure than methylene chloride workers.

Impairments in attention and concentration have also been related to acute effects (Gregersen *et al.*, 1984).

TABLE IV.2. Percentages of workers with abnormal EEGs. (Reprinted, by permission of the publisher, from Seppäläinen, A.M. (1985). Neurophysiological aspects of the toxicity of organic solvents. *Scandinavian Journal of Work, Environment and Health*, Suppl. 1, 11, 61–64.)

N	Percentage with abnormal EEG	REFERENCE
72 painters	17%	Seppäläinen and Lindström, 1982
102 car painters	31%	Seppäläinen, 1978
233 workers	40–72%	Seppäläinen, 1973
107 solvent-poisoned patients	65%	Seppäläinen *et al.*, 1980
87 solvent-poisoned patients	67%	Seppäläinen and Antti-Poika, 1983

Chronic effects of solvent mixtures

Chronic effects are much more frequently researched than acute effects (Savolainen, 1982). Chronic neurological and neuropsychological effects have been documented for many solvents and may occur separately from, or in combination with, acute effects.

Physiological

Gross clinical signs of CNS impairment are usually "minor, if any" (Seppäläinen, Husman and Martenson, 1978) and conventional neurological tests "are frequently too imprecise and unchallenging" (Bleecker, 1984). However, chronic central and peripheral nervous system deficits can be found by sensitive tests. Chronic neurological effects include vestibular dysfunction (Arlien-Søberg *et al.*, 1981) and cerebral atrophy (Seppäläinen, Lindström and Martelin, 1980; Arlien-Søberg *et al.*, 1979). Juntunen *et al.* (1980) examined 37 patients with suspected chronic solvent poisoning. Pneumoencephalography (PEG) suggested patterns of "slight asymmetric central atrophy and/or localized cortical atrophy" in 63% of patients. ENMG results suggested peripheral neuropathy in 23 of 28 patients examined.

EEG abnormalities are frequently associated with chronic solvent exposure (Seppäläinen and Antti-Poika, 1983). Physiological changes have been correlated with development of psycho-organic syndrome. Seppäläinen (1985) reviewed EEG changes in chronic solvent-exposed workers and found abnormal EEGs in 17% to 67% of patients. She suggests that EEG results are indicative of an acute loss of neurons or neuronal functions as indicated by increased low-frequency irregular or rhythmic theta or delta activity. This phenomenon is most easily seen in acute solvent-exposed patients, while slowly developing increases in slow wave activity are noted with chronic solvent exposure (Seppäläinen, 1985).

Significant reductions in cerebral blood flow have been observed in painters exposed to solvents for a mean of 22 years (Arlien-Søberg *et al.*, 1982), while Risberg and Hagstadius (1983) observed small but significantly lowered regional cerebral blood flow in workers chronicaly exposed to solvent mixtures for a mean of 18 years. The latter study showed greater differences in bilateral frontotemporal and left parietal regions. Larger differences were also found in those individuals with the highest exposure. Since alcohol intake and other demographic variables were similar for patients and controls, the authors speculate that chronic solvent exposure may cause premature aging of the brain by a process similar to that of chronic alcoholism.

Polyneuropathy is also frequently associated with long-term exposure to solvents (Seppäläinen, 1982; Husman and Karli, 1980). Loss of vibration sense and diminished sensitivity to pain and light touch have been reported (Husman and Karli, 1980), as have lowered sensory and motor nerve conduction velocities and abnormal EMGs (Seppäläinen, 1982). Autonomic nervous system abnormalities have also been found in a group of patients who had been chronically exposed to solvents and subsequently diagnosed as showing features of organic solvent intoxication (Matikainen and Juntunen, 1985).

Significant lowering of regional cerebral blood flow (rCBF) in solvent-exposed workers compared to controls was reported by Arlien-Søberg *et al.*, (1982). Similar results were found by Risberg and Hagstadius (1983), who suggest that solvent-induced lowered rCBF may represent premature brain aging similar to that hypothesized to be present in advanced alcoholism.

Neuropsychological effects of chronic exposure —
workplace

Because painters are more likely to have chronic exposure to solvent mixtures than most other occupational groups, many recent neuropsychological studies have used painters as subjects. Most of these studies have found neuropsychological decrements that seem related to chronic solvent exposure.

Painters exposed for a mean of 6.7 years to approximately "several hundred" ppm of hydrocarbon solvents showed deficits in visuo-spatial functions and psychomotor coordination (Hane *et al.*, 1977). Lindström (1980) studied a population of painters, dry cleaners, degreasers and others exposed for a mean of 9.1 years, and specifically referred for previously diagnosed occupational disease. Relative to controls, subjects performed significantly more poorly on Digit Span, Digit Symbol, Block Design and several visuo-constructive tasks, a pattern characterized by the author as lowered visuo-motor performance and decreased freedom from distractibility (Lindström, 1980).

Eskelinen *et al.* (1986) investigated a group of 21 individuals already diagnosed as being in various stages of an organic solvent syndrome. All but one of these patients had been exposed to solvent mixtures. For the latter patient the mono-exposure solvent was styrene. Comparison groups included 16 patients with vertebrobasilar insufficiency, 16 patients with miscellaneous cerebral traumata and 15 tension headache patients. None of the comparison groups had solvent exposure histories.

The groups were given a neuropsychological battery developed at the Institute for Occupational Health in Helsinki, which consisted of various items from the Wechsler Adult Intelligence Scale (WAIS), the Wechsler Memory Scale (WMS), tests of fine motor speed and coordination and several spatial-constructional tasks (the Mira Test and the Symmetry Drawing Task). A symptom questionnaire was also included.

The results of the study suggest that workers with chronic solvent exposure show a specific pattern of neuropsychological impairment that differs from patients with other forms of peripheral or central nervous system impairment, as well as from tension headache controls who might be expected to show similar emotional symptoms. A discriminant analysis performed by the authors suggested that the best combination of tests to distinguish solvent patients from other groups included Similarities, Block Design Speed and No. of Failures, Digit Span — forward and the Visual Memory subtest of the WMS. Five of the nine subjective symptom scales were included in the model for best power. These included "memory difficulties, fatigue, sleep disturbances, neurovegetative symptoms, and headache" (Eskelinen *et al.*, 1986, p. 249). The study suggests that chronic solvent exposure patients may have a unique diagnostic profile, and that their impairments in intellectual abilities and memory rather than spatial or sensorimotor dysfunction distinguish them from other neurological patients. However, since motor tasks were impaired relative to the only non-neurological group (headache patients), solvent-exposed patients may still be said to be impaired in these functions relative to normals.

The study can be criticized for its use of small numbers of patients, using solvent patients with a slightly lower premorbid educational level and for its failure to include a matched control group of "normals" without medical or psychological symptoms. It is likely, therefore, that future replication studies may observe different discriminative patterns than those found here. Nonetheless, since results found by the authors are consistent with known solvent effects, it is also possible that basic neuropsychological impairments shown here may be real and not artifacts of the study design.

Another study used only a questionnaire to query car painters who had been exposed for a mean of 14.8 years, longer than previously described patients. The workers described themselves as being excessively tired after work, and having difficulty with concentration and memory. They were also significantly more bothered by itching, and admitted to "prenarcotic" acute symptoms during work including nausea, vomiting, feeling drunk and being absentminded (Husman, 1980).

Orbaek *et al.* (1985) investigated workers in a paint production plant exposed to solvents for an even longer period: a mean of 18 years. Compared to controls matched for age and education, solvent workers showed a significant 4% decrease in cerebral blood flow and EEG changes. Neuropsychological tests which measured sustained attention and concentration were impaired in the subgroup with the greatest solvent exposure. Solvent-exposed workers also admitted to significantly more neurological and neuropsychological symptoms on a 60-item rating scale, including inner tension, hostile feelings and short-term memory problems.

Ekberg *et al.* (1986) surveyed general health and neuropsychological performance of solvent-exposed floor layers with age-matched carpenters who had long (> 20 years) or short (5–10 years) of relevant work experience. Floorlayers experienced depressive illness and received antidepressant medication significantly more often than carpenters. The authors also noted small but significant associations between neuropsychological performance on several tests, and exposure to contact adhesives or alcohol-based glues after age effects were controlled. Unfortunately there was no information regarding relative educational attainment between groups. It may also be argued that 5–10 years of exposure to relevant substances may not be an appropriate control, since subclinical solvent effects may have begun to appear by that time.

Painters exposed for a mean of 22 years to white spirit mixtures were compared to matched controls in the construction industry and showed significantly lower performance in reaction time, Block Design, Digit Symbol, Figural Memory (Wechsler Memory Scale) and visuo-constructive tests (Lindström and Wickstrom, 1983). Arlien-Søberg *et al.* (1979) studied a group of painters with 27-year mean exposure selectively referred for evaluation (like Lindström, 1980), because of suspected organic solvent intoxication or dementia. They found 39 out of 50 patients to suffer neuropsychological impairment, after ruling out alternative etiologies. CT or pneumoencephalogram (PEG) showed cerebral atrophy in 31 of these cases with significantly widened sulci in 38 of the 50. Deficits of many neuropsychological functions were found in these individuals, including Visual Memory, Digit Span, Paired Associate learning and Sentence Repetition.

The preceding studies, while using diverse procedures for patient selection and neuropsychological evaluation, nevertheless appear, in aggregate, to support a syndrome of deficits related to solvent exposure. Critics, however, have countered that the Scandinavian literature may not be replicable in American and European settings for a variety of sociocultural reasons. For example, several Scandinavian countries view solvent syndromes as *de facto*

NT—E

grounds for disability pensions, while procedures to prove solvent damage favor the worker. In Denmark, for example, the state must prove that a worker does *not* suffer from solvent poisoning for a disability claim to be denied. In addition, widespread publicity concerning details of solvent intoxication syndromes, as well as the difficulty of *disproving* a syndrome, may serve to encourage claims (A. Gade, personal communcation).

However, given the number of researchers who have found chronic effects of solvent mixtures, it seems equally likely that other countries will eventually corroborate Scandinavian results. Support for this viewpoint is suggested by a recent study by Linz *et al.* (1986), which compared neuropsychological results on 15 industrial painters who worked extensively with solvents to 30 controls, at the Oregon Health Sciences University in the United States. Painters were impaired on a variety of neuropsychological measures, including Trails A, Digit Symbol, Seashore Rhythm and Halstead–Reitan Speech Sounds Perception tests. Tests of memory, learning, construction and abstract reasoning were also impaired relative to controls. Twelve out of 15 painters had HRB impairment indexes > 0.5 with painters also reporting significantly increased numbers of neurological symptoms on a questionnaire, including decreased coordination, personality change and decreased memory. Neurological evaluation showed four of the 15 painters to have mild distal neuropathy, five painters to have sensorimotor peripheral neuropathy measured by EMG and nerve conduction studies, and three to have abnormal EEGs.

Another United States study examined 74 male shipyard painters who were exposed to solvent compounds used in primers, shellac, varnishes and enamels. History included exposure in confined areas to "methyl isobutyl ketone, xylene, perchloroethylene, ethylene glycol and mineral spirits" (Valciukas *et al.*, 1985, p. 48). Compared to a control group carefully matched by age, education, race and sex, the painters performed significantly more poorly on the Block Design Test and an embedded figures test which required subjects to identify superimposed outline drawings of common objects. In addition, painters who admitted to chronic solvent-related symptoms in a questionnaire performed significantly more poorly than asymptomatic individuals on Block Design, Digit Symbol and an overall index of performance (Valciukas *et al.*, 1985).

The following cases are presented as examples of chronic solvent exposure effects. The patients' histories have been changed, and portions of the original reports have been omitted to protect their confidentiality.

Case study A: Chronic solvent exposure and neuropsychological impairment

Reason for referral:
The patient is a white male in his 50s with a history of approximately 13 years

exposure to a mixed group of neurotoxic solvents and chemicals, including toluene, xylene, aromatic hydrocarbons, butyl alcohol, ethylene glycol, monobutyl ether, and methyl ethyl ketone (MEK). Neuropsychological testing was initiated to determine whether current cognitive, affective and behavioral performance patterns can be related to the patient's exposure history.

Tests administered:
Finger Tapping Test
Wechsler Memory Scale with Russell Modification
Trail-making Tests A&B
WAIS-R Subtests:
 Block Design
 Digit Symbol
Stroop Color–Word Test
Luria–Nebraska Neuropsychological Battery:
 Pathognomonic Scale
Spatial Relations Test
Grip Strength Test
Grooved Pegboard Test
Shipley Institute of Living Test (SILS)
Harvard School of Public Health Occupational Health Questionnaire
Minnesota Multiphasic Personality Inventory (MMPI)
Personal Problems Checklist
Profile of Mood States (POMS)
Kent EGY Scale D
Category Test
Clinical Interview

Background information:
The patient is a right-handed white male who reports an exposure history to a mixed group of solvents and chemicals over a 13–14- year period. The patient reports that during this time he was responsible for cleaning a spray paint booth with either methyl ethyl ketone or toluene. MEK was applied by hand, using a brush. In addition, the patient used toluene to clean the paint from his hands. After each application the patient states that he felt intoxicated and that his skin itched. There was no ventilation in the paint booths during cleaning as the ventilating fans were turned off. He also states that he did not have protective gloves during the application of either MEK or toluene.
The patient's current symptoms include weakness, shaking, and pain in his legs accompanied by involuntary muscle contractions (myoclonus). He reports that the pain in his legs is so intense "that it feels like a toe is about to break off", a sensation which can last from 10 to 15 minutes at a time. The patient also reports shoulder and back pain with limitation of movement. Other symptoms include numbness in the arms and shoulders.
The patient has seen many health care professionals for diagnosis and relief from these symptoms, including staff at a nationally known clinic, a chiropractor and a psychiatrist. At the time of testing, the psychiatrist was empirically assessing the effects of Haldol on the patient for "restless leg syndrome", but the psychiatrist reports that the patient's symptoms have not diminished thus far. The patient does report, however, that his sleep has improved somewhat after being given Haldol. Medical reports were not

available as of this writing; however, the patient's psychiatrist reports that the patient does have documented dennervation of the left gastrocnemius, as well as spinal defects of a possibly degenerative nature in L4, L5 and S1.

Neuropsychological symptoms noted by the patient include increased fatigue and memory loss. Appetite is reported to be good with no recent changes in weight. Sleep is poor, with awakening after 2 or 3 hours. The patient reports that he occasionally gets depressed but denies suicidal ideation. There is no history of mental health treatment. There have been occasional episodes of hypertension but blood pressure is currently controlled. Current blood pressure is reported by the patient to be 120/70.

With the exception of hypertension and previously noted symptoms, the patient has no other current medical problems. He denies history of diabetes, arthritis, epilepsy, chronic neurological illness, fracture, frostbite or orthopedic injury. Though he is a pack-per-day smoker, he denies cardiac or pulmonary disease. The patient's medical history includes a car accident where his head struck the windshield and cracked the glass; however, there was no loss of consciousness and the patient reports that he recovered fully within a few hours. The patient's current medications include: Tenormin, 1/ day, Haldol 1mg/day and Hydrochlorothiazide 50 mg. Alcohol use is currently low, approximately 6 beers during the last calendar year. Starting 13 years ago, for about 10 years, the patient had a social drinking history of approximately 2 six-packs of beer per weekend when he played cards with friends. Current coffee intake is 4–6 cups per day.

The patient graduated from the 9th grade and he reports that his favorite subject was arithmetic and his worst was spelling. He does not remember his grades. The patient is currently employed as a store room clerk and has not had any contact with solvents or other chemicals for approximately 2 years.

Behavioral observations:
The patient is a heavyset, white male of shorter than average height. Speech was clear and somewhat laconic, spoken with accentless midwestern pronunciation. Affect appeared to be blunted or depressed and the patient's 'flat' expression appeared similar to that found in patients with Parkinson's disease. The patient's responses to history-taking questions tended to be short and somewhat difficult for this examiner to organize. Many questions had to be asked to determine the relationship between time, chemical exposure and symptoms.

The patient's behavior was appropriate at all times during the testing session. He was cooperative and appeared to try hard during all tests. He was able to maintain attention throughout the examination. The only unusual behavior displayed during the testing session was a convulsive arm twitch, triggered by a light pencil touch to the palm.

The patient denied or minimized cognitive changes during the past decade. His principal cognitive complaint was of increasingly poor memory for day-to-day information. The complaints for which he has received multiple medical consults are somatic and related to limb pain.

General cognitive functioning:
The patient was oriented to time, place, person and situation for the testing session. Speech was unremarkable in volume and timbre, although somewhat slow in rate. There were no indications of aphasia or alexia.

The patient's estimated premorbid intellectual functioning was in the

TABLE IV.3. Neuropsychological test scores in a patient with chronic solvent exposure

1. *Finger Tapping:*	RH mean: 41.5		Russell 3
(Dom. hand: R)	LH mean: 39.2		Russell 2
2. *Wechsler Memory Scale:*			
(a) *Logical*			
Immediate recall:	A: 6.5 B: 4.5	Total: 11	Russell 4
Delayed recall:	A: 5.0 B: 1.5	Total: 6.5	Russell 4
(b) *Figural*			
Immediate recall:	A: 3 B: 3 C: 5	Total: 11	Russell 1
Delayed recall:	A: 0 B: 0 C: 2	Total: 2	Russell 4
3. *Trail Making Test:*	A: 39 (seconds)		Russell 2
	B: 97 (seconds)		Russell 2
4. *WAIS-R Digit Symbol Test:*		Raw score: 41	Scaled score 6
			Age corrected: 8
5. *Stroop Test:*			
No. of Words: 93 + age corr.: 8		Total: 102	T score 47
No. of Colors: 51 + age corr.: 4		Total: 55	T score 33
No. of Colored Words: 25 + age corr.: 5		Total: 30	T score 35

6. *Luria-Nebraska Pathognomonic Scale:*

Critical level 66.27

No. of errors: 23   T score 61

7. *Spatial Relations:* (Greek Cross) Best: 1 + Worst: 2 = 3   Russell 1
8. *Pegboard:* (Grooved) RH: 81″ T 39   LH: 85″ T 42
9. *Grip Strength:* RH: (1) 55   (2) 50   LH: (1) 48   (2) 48
   (Kg)   Mean RH: 52.5   Mean LH: 48
10. *IQ Estimate:* Kent EGY Scale: Raw score: 33   IQ Estimate: 133
    SILS: (V: 29   A: 10)   CQ: 63
11. *Block Design:* Raw score: 28   Scaled score: 9 (age corr. 11)
12. *Category Test:* No. of Errors: 94   Russell 3
13. Associate Learning: 5;0, 5;0, 6;1
14. Digits Forward: 8   Digits Backward 4
15. *Personality Test:* MMPI, POMS
    MMPI Scores (T Scores, K corrected where appropriate):

L 53	PD 64	SI 67
F 55	MF 49	A 49
K 68	PA 50	R 74
HS 88	PT 74	ES 51
D 85	SC 69	MAC 34
HY 71	MA 45	

Note: 0–5 Russell ratings are from Russell (1975) and Russell, Neuringer and Goldstein (1970), where higher scores indicate greater impairment.

Average range or above for most abilities. In contrast, many of the patient's abilities appear to have deteriorated from this level. During testing, the patient displayed several types of general cognitive deficits, most notably in cognitive efficiency/flexibility, and abstract reasoning ability. Each of these was moderately impaired. For example, the patient showed reduced ability to separate essential from distracting stimuli (Stroop Test) and made many errors in a task which required inductive reasoning (Category Test). In the latter test, the patient made almost double the number of errors beyond a pathognomonic cut-off level.

Memory and learning:
The patient showed moderate to severe deficiencies in memory and learning.

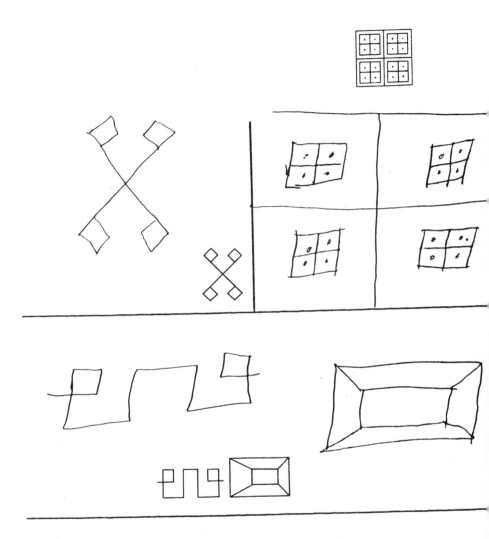

FIGURE IV.1. Chronic exposure to solvent mixtures. WMS: Figural memory — immediate recall. For reader comparison, card images were inset subsequent to the evaluation.

Both verbal and non-verbal encoding was involved. Verbal memory items were poorly encoded and poorly remembered later. Educational limitations may have affected scores somewhat on this particular task. However, non-verbal memory, which is less dependent upon education, was also affected. In a task requiring the memorization of line drawings, the patient was able to perform adequately only when he was asked to recall the drawings

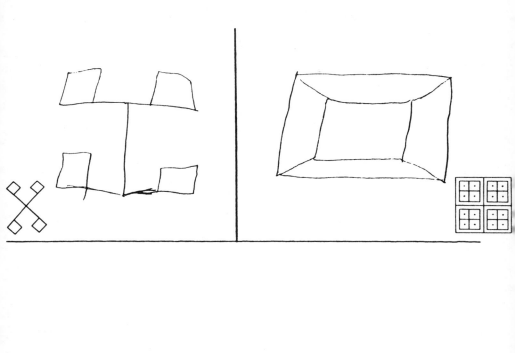

FIGURE IV.2. Chronic exposure to solvent mixtures. WMS. Figural memory — 30-minute delayed recall. For reader comparison, card images were inset subsequent to the evaluation.

immediately (Fig. IV.1). When recall was requested 30 minutes later, the patient scored in the range of severe impairment, recalling almost nothing of the previously presented figures (Fig. IV.2).

When presented with a task requiring the memorization and learning of easy and difficult word associations (e.g. north–south, vs. crush–dark), the

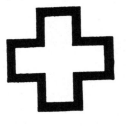

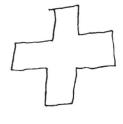

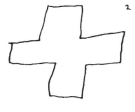

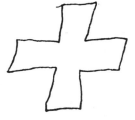

FIGURE IV.3. Chronic exposure to solvent mixtures. Spatial Relations Test (direct copy).

patient was almost completely unable to learn any of the more difficult word pairs, even after three trials.

Sensorimotor functions:

Sensory and motor abilities appear to be mild-to-moderately impaired. Fine motor speed and dexterity were mild-to-moderately impaired in the dominant hand. Left hand performance was closer to normal in fine motor speed, but also shows mild decrements in dexterity. Pencil drawings performed by the patient appeared to suffer from a very fine tremor in their execution (e.g. Fig. IV.3). Gross motor strength was normal bilaterally.

The patient did not show any basic sensory deficits in his hands; however, when his palm was lightly touched with a pencil during a test of body location, his entire arm twitched convulsively. In addition, the patient showed mild-to-moderate deficits in translating proprioceptive cues into verbal descriptions. For example, he could not correctly name letters that were drawn on the back of his wrist. The patient showed no evidence of hearing impairment.

Visuospatial functions:
The patient showed no evidence of constructional apraxia; he was able to correctly draw complex figures, and could correctly name objects placed in his hand. In addition, the patient performed well in a task that required him to assemble blocks in abstract patterns.

Personality functioning:
Personality testing suggests that the patient experiences significant depression and is very concerned with his abnormal physical symptoms. He appears to cope with anxiety and tension by repression and being concerned with details rather than the "big picture". In several inventories of emotional symptomatology, the patient reported extreme inability to concentrate, and forgetfulness, as well as fatigue, uneasiness and exhaustion.

Summary and recommendations:
This is a white male in his 50s referred by his psychiatrist to determine if the patient's symptoms were consistent with a 13-year exposure history to various central and peripheral neurotoxic solvents. Current neuropsychological evaluation suggests that the patient functions significantly below estimates of premorbid abilities in memory, cognitive efficiency and flexibility, and abstract reasoning. The pattern of impairment is consistent with known neurotoxic effects of some of the solvents to which the patient has been exposed. Chronic exposure to toluene, for example, has been linked to both central and peripheral nervous system deficits including depression and flattened affect, memory impairment and other cognitive abnormalities, including dementia. Methyl ethyl ketone is a peripheral neurotoxin, and ethylene glycol may cause sensorimotor neuropathy and central nervous system abnormalities.

Overall, the pattern of impairment in this patient appears to be consistent with chronic exposure to neurotoxic solvents and chemicals. Prognosis for improvement after exposure to mixed neurotoxins is somewhat cautious, although if patients do not show abnormalities in CT or EEG, their prognosis is better than if such tests are positive. The prognosis for recovery of solvent-related peripheral neuropathy is controversial, and while some reviews cite eventual recovery, other authors report continuing symptoms 3 years post-exposure.

Suggestions for the patient's further care include:
(1) Trial of antidepressant medication.
(2) Referral to an occupational medicine clinic where the patient can be further evaluated for solvent exposure effects.
(3) Magnetic resonance (MR) scan, PET scan, or regional cerebral blood flow study may yield further information about the level of activation in various brain areas.

Case study B: Neuropsychological consequences of chronic exposure to a solvent mixture of toluene and methyl ethyl ketone (MEK)

Reason for referral:
The patient is a white male in his 30's with chronic exposure to a mixture of toluene and methyl ethyl ketone (MEK).

Tests administered:
Finger Tapping Test
Grooved Pegboard Test
Grip Strength Test
Fingertip Number Writing Test
Two-Point Discrimination Test
Minnesota Rate of Manipulation Test
    Turning Test
    Displacing Test
    Placing Test
    One Hand Placing and Turning Test
Wechsler Memory Scale:
    Logical and Figural Memory – Immediate & 30 minute delayed recall
    Associate Learning Test
Wechsler Adult Intelligence Scale-Revised:
    Digit Symbol Test
    Block Design Test
    Information Test
    Vocabulary Test
Shipley Institute of Living Test
Stroop Color-Word Test
Luria-Nebraska Pathognomonic Scale
Spatial Relations Test
Minnesota Multiphasic Personality Inventory (MMPI)
Beck Depression Inventory
Personal Problems Checklist – Adult
Harvard Public Health Occupational Health Questionnaire
Psychological/Social History Form
Clinical Interview

Background information:
Prior to obtaining his current job with occasional exposure to solvents, the patient worked inside a warehouse for 7 years and was heavily exposed to solvents, primarily toluene and methyl ethyl ketone (MEK). Further details of his solvent exposure history are contained in his medical records.

During the last 2 or 3 years of exposure, the patient began experiencing concentration difficulties. He believes that a growing inability to pay continuous attention had adversely affected his simultaneous pursuit of a Master's degree in Public Administration and caused him to take a year longer than was usual to complete his degree. Loss of concentration is a continuing problem, "I lose track of my thoughts, I can't seem to keep my mind on things." The patient also reports several "close calls" while driving.

The patient's first symptoms of muscle fatigue were partially relieved with prednisone, which he continued to receive intermittently until recently. Currently the patient states he would "rather work through muscle fatigue by forcing yourself to go on" than worry about side effects from continuing the medication. This year, he has again experienced a recurrence of fatigue symptoms. He reports "waking up tired – as much as when I ended the day." The patient also states that his "forearms get real tired when I use a pipe wrench at work" and that he becomes winded after climbing two flights of stairs. He also reports that he has difficulty keeping his eyelids open and that they have a tendency to droop. Other symptoms include occasionally blurred vision, especially in the right eye, and pain in the left knee the cause of which was reported to the patient as polyneuropathy.

The patient has attempted to build up his endurance with a home exercise program that includes "push-ups, sit-ups, windmills, and 15 minutes on an exercise bike." Despite having exercised in this manner for 3 years, the patient reports little increase in capacity, stating that he "feels tired and dead" on the days that he exercises.

The patient denied any episodes of fatigue prior to working at his company. He reports that he "spent four years in the service and never had a problem with muscle fatigue."

The patient currently receives Synthroid subsequent to diagnosis of hyperthyroidism in 1981 and thyroidectomy. He reported that his thyroid levels were normal at last check.

The patient denied any other ongoing medical problems, and in fact, stated that prior to his employment he "never went to a doctor except once as a kid and once in the service." The patient is a non-drinker with no history of drug abuse. There was no history of head injury, hand injury, psychiatric disorder or any other problems capable of interfering with neuropsychological performance.

The patient is married and lives with his wife and their 2 children. While he reports that his marriage is "fine," the patient also admits that his sex life has deteriorated, not because he is impotent, "but because I'm so tired all the time."

The patient's neuropsychological test results are summarized un Table IV.4.

Neuropsychological test results

Behavioral observations:
The patient is a white male of heavy build and shorter than average height. He was casually but neatly dressed for the testing session in slacks and a blue oxford shirt, giving him a somewhat collegiate appearance. The patient's grooming and hygiene were excellent. The patient was oriented to person, place, time and situation and appeared to cooperative fully with all phases of testing. The patient's display of effort was particularly evident in a sustained performance task (Minnesota Rate of Manipulation Test) which appeared to become unusually tiring over time.

Affect was calm throughout the evaluation, with no evidence of depression or anxiety. In the interview, the patient presented his symptoms in a laconic, straightforward manner that did not suggest exaggeration. In fact, the patient appeared to underestimate the degree of fingertip sensory deficit later elicited in examination.

General cognitive functioning:
The patient's estimated premorbid intellectual abilities were in the Average to High Average Range. There were significant discrepancies between verbal school-learned abilities, and non-verbal skills. The patient's vocabulary and

TABLE IV.4. Neuropsychological test battery – scoring sheet D. Hartman, Ph.D., 1987.

Name _____ Date:___/___/___ ____Testing Age:_____

Address: _____

BD:___/___/___ Education:_____ Tested by: _____

Place of Testing:_____

Reason for Referral: Toluene and MEK exposure   Referral Source:_____

[] 1. Finger tapping: RH mean: 34.2   Russell 3
    (Dom. hand: R)   LH mean: 34.4   Russell 3

[] 2. Wechsler Memory Scale: Logical
    Immediate recall: A: 10 B: 6   Total: 16   Russell 3 AC____
    Delayed recall: A: 7.5 B: 2   Total: 9.5   Russell 3 AC____ %R 59
            Figural
    Immediate recall: A: 3 B: 4 C: 5   Total: 12   Russell 0 AC____
    Delayed recall: A: 1 B: 2 C: 1   Total: 4   Russell 3 AC____ %R 33

[] 3. Trail Making Test: A: 41 (sec.)   Russell 2 AC____
               B: 70 (sec.)   Russell 1 AC____

[] 4. WAIS-R Digit Symbol Test: Raw score: 43   Scaled score: 6 AC____

[] 5. Stroop Test: No. of Words: 74 + age corr.: 0   Total: 74   T score 33
           No. of Colors: 51 + age corr.: 0   Total: 51   T score 30
    No. of Colored Words: 29 + age corr.:___   Total: 29   T score 34

[] 6. Luria-Nebraska Pathognomonic Scale:
    68.8 + Age value:___ – Education value:___ = Critical level 48.97
               # Errors: 13   T score 45

[] 7. Spatial Relations: (Greek Cross) Best: 1 + Worst: 2 = 3 Russell 1
[] 8. Associate Learning: 1) E 5 H 1 2) E 6 H 2 3) E 6 H 3
[] 9. Rey Auditory Verbal Learning Test (ALVT):
    1____ 2____ 3____ 4____ 5____ (IRL)_____ (Recall)_____ (Recog.)_____
[] 10. Block Design: Raw score 22   Scale score 7 AC____
[] 11. Tactual   RH: Time_____ No. of Blocks____   Russell____ Memory____ Russell____
    Performance LH: Time_____ No. of Blocks____   Russell____
    Test   BH: Time_____ No. of Blocks____   Russell____ Location____ Russell____
   12. IQ Estimates:
[]   a) Kent EGY   Raw____   IQ est.:____
[]   b) SILS: V Raw 30 T 50 A Raw 30 T 57 Total 60/54   CQ 97
        Pred. Abs. from, Age. Ed. & Vocab. 28 AQ Conversion   104
        Estimated WAIS-R Full Scale IQ from Total SILS by Age   102
[]   c) WAIS-R: Information   Raw 21   Scale score 10 AC____
            Vocabulary   Raw 52   Scale score 11 AC____
[] 13. Category Test: No. of Errors: 54   Russell 2
[] 14. Grip Strength: RH: 1 48 2 51½   LH: 1 46½ 2 46
    (Lb/Kg)   Mean RH: 49.75 T____   Mean LH: 46.25 T____
[] 15. Pegboard: (Purdue/Grooved) RH: 89 T 19 LH: 100 T 12 BH:___ T____   [] 22.
                                              WAIS-R
[] 16. Minnesota Rate of Manipulation Test: VIQ ____

							1 Hand		2 Hand			
	Placing			Turning	Displacing		Placing & Turning		Placing & Turning		Info	____
											DSp	____
											Voc	____
P	R 77	L 73		81	R 56	L 66	R 89	L 93	____		Arit	____
											Comp	____
1	R 77	L 80		76	R 59	L 66	R 97	L 93	____		Simi	____
											Tot	____
2	R 83	L 79		68	R 59	L 66	R 95	L 105	____			
											PIQ	____
3	R 85	L 90		75	R 65	L 67	R 96	L 103	____			
											PCom	____
4	R 86	L 89		67	R 68	L 70	R 95	L 105	____		PArr	____
											BlkD	____
			2/3/4 Trial total								ObjA	____
											DSym	____
	R 331	L 338			R 251	L 269	R 383	L 406	____		Tot	____
SS	<25	<25	<25	25	<25	<25	<25	<25	____			
%R	<1	<1	<1	2	<1	<1	<1	<1	____		FSIQ	____

2/3/4 Trial mean

R 82.75 L 84.5   71.5   R 62.75 L 67.25   R 97.75 L 101.5   ____

[] 17. Aphasia Screening Test:_____

[] 18. Fingertip Number Writing:

Finger	1	2	3	4	5	
	4 6 3 5	3 5 4 6	6 5 4 3	5 4 6 3	6 3 5 4	
Right	7 6 3 4	2 5 9 0	6 5 4 3	5 7 9 2	6 3 5 4	R 9
Left	9 2 8 4	8 5 4 8	6 5 4 3	8 9 8 2	6 3 5 4	L 11

[] 19. Rhythm errors _____   Russell____
[] 20. Speech errors _____   Russell____
[] 21. PASAT _____
23. Personality Tests:
[] MMPI: (T scores) ?____ L 52 F 66 K 48 Hs 77 D 94 Hy 74 Pd 48 Mf 57 Pa 62
[] BDI:____   Pt 73 Sc 76 Ma 50 Si 78 A 64 R 54 Es 33 MAC 41
[] POMS (T Scores): T____ D____ A____ V____ C____ F____
[] Other Tests: _____

[] Occupational Health Questionnaire
[] Psychological Social History

[] Personal Problems Checklist
[] Other 1–2 point touch discriminations: pt. could not perform accurately, even at 20 mm, compass
point distance

AC = age correction   % R = % recalled (WMS)
ss = scale score   %R = % ile rank (MRMT)

recall of school-related information were in the average range. In contrast, his ability to perform tasks which require nonverbal, spatial or constructional skills was significantly impaired and well below estimates of premorbid function. Verbal and nonverbal abstract reasoning abilities were also significantly impaired considering the patient's level of education.

The patient also performed significantly below expectation on several tests of sustained attention and concentration.

Sensorimotor functions:

The patient showed moderate to very severe bilateral impairments in sensory and motor abilities of the hands. For example, fingertip sensation was severely reduced with the patient being unable to discriminate sharp versus dull stimulation. Nor was he able to reliably differentiate one-versus-two point touch on the middle finger, even when the points were 20 mm apart. Finger-tip number writing also showed severe impairment. The only consistently correct number identifications were on the patient's 5th finger, bilaterally. Identification of numbers traced on all other fingers was severely impaired. Identification of larger objects in the hand was more successful, although the patient performed these identifications at a slower than average rate.

Motor functions were similarly decremented. Fine motor speed was in the range of moderate impairment, with the patient failing to show the expected preference in speed for the dominant hand. Fine motor dexterity was also quite limited; the patient's performance on a pegboard task placed him in the bottom 20% of the population. Motor tasks requiring extended use of the hands and arms showed even poorer performance. On a task requiring approximately 10 minutes of speeded and coordinated hand/arm movement, the patient scored in the lowest 1-2% of the normative population sample.

Gross motor strength was approximately normal.

Memory:
The patient showed mild-to-moderate impairments in short-term memory. Most notable was the loss of nonverbal information over the course of 30 minutes when tested by surprise recall. While immediate recall was quite good, after 30 minutes, the patient was only able to recall about one third of the visual information previously presented. Verbal recall was moderately impaired for both immediate and 30 minute delayed recall.
When verbal material was repeatedly presented, the patient was able to retain information adequately. His learning curve on a verbal paired-associate task was normal.

Visuospatial functions:
The patient showed no significant deficits in simple constructional tasks; however, when spatial tasks included an abstract reasoning component (i.e. assembling abstract block patterns to match a template) the patient's performance was below average.

Personality functioning:
While the patient admitted to several difficulties in social adjustment, most of his current difficulties appeared to be reactive to the stress of ongoing litigation, and concerns about his current and future health. He admitted to anxious and depressed feelings and was very worried about his physical health. Perhaps as a result of these stressors, the patient is introverted and suffers from low self-esteem. The patient appeared to be coping with his difficulties by concentrating on individual details and may not have either the preference or emotional resources to plan a more integrated life strategy at this time.

Summary and conclusions:
This is a white male who has been referred for evaluation of neurobehavioral status secondary to chronic solvent exposure. At the present evaluation, the patient experienced severe sensorimotor deficits that were most apparent when performance had to be sustained over several minutes. The patient also appeared to have significantly impaired sensory thresholds in his fingertips; he was unable to discriminate sharp versus dull, one versus two points, and numbers written on the fingertips. Verbal short-term memory showed moderate impairment for immediate and delayed recall, while non-verbal short-term memory is good initially but shows significant loss over time. Other significant deficits relative to the patient's estimated premorbid abilities included abstract reasoning and the ability to sustain attention and concentration.
The combination of central and peripheral deficits shown here is quite consistent with the effects of chronic exposure to central and peripheral neurotoxic solvents (i.e. toluene and MEK) and the patient's symptoms have been documented in the solvent literature. The patient's deficits do not seem easily explainable by any other mechanism, and they are not consistent with abnormalities related to thyroid hormone level.
The majority of the patient's emotional symptoms are consistent with reaction to sustained stresses of poor health and subsequent litigation, although exacerbation of pre-existing personality traits cannot be ruled out. Supportive counseling may help improve coping and lessen the patient's psychological concomitants of his physical injury.

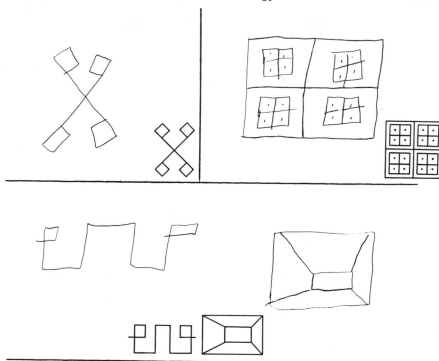

FIGURE IV.4. Chronic exposure to toluene and MEK. WMS: Figural memory — immediate recall. For reader comparison, card images were inset subsequent to evaluation.

Diagnosis:
Sensorimotor, cognitive and memory impairments – probable solvent-related etiology.
Adjustment disorder with mixed emotional features.

SOLVENT ABUSE

Intentional inhalation of substances which alter consciousness may have begun with the Greeks at Delphi where a seer is reported to have foretold the future while inhaling carbon dioxide. Columbus, landing in the Americas, was said to have observed West Indians inhaling various psychotropic substances. Solvents became the inhaled euphoriants of choice during the late 1800s and early 1900s at parties where alcohol, ether, nitrous oxide or chloroform were inhaled (Giovacchini, 1981, p. 18). In the mid-1900s, tons of ether were consumed as a substitute for alcohol in Ireland (Barnes, 1979).

The typical solvent abuser of today is young, male and between the ages of 7 and 17. He tries solvents out of boredom, or to reduce stimulation from an

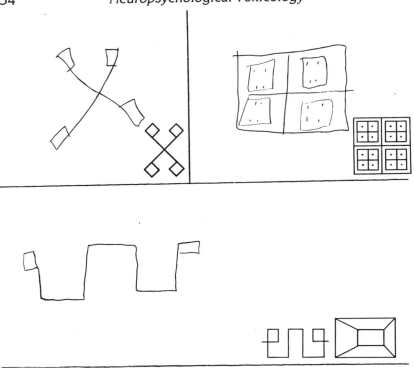

FIGURE IV.5. Chronic exposure to toluene and MEK. WMS. Figural memory, 30-minute delayed recall. For reader comparison, card images were inset subsequent to the evaluation.

environment perceived as hostile. Such abusers are also likely to show delinquency, low self-esteem, poor academic records and social isolation. While many are from low-income minority groups, middle-class abusers have also been reported. Estimates of adolescent abuse rates range from 2.3% to 50% (Giovacchini, 1984). Solvent abuse is more prevalent in some populations than others, e.g. very high use of gasoline-inhalation has been reported in native American populations, and Hispanics tend to be over-represented among solvent sniffers (Barnes, 1979).

Solvents are typically placed in a plaster bag and inhaled; soaked on a piece of cloth which is then sniffed; or inhaled directly from the original container (Barnes, 1979). Unlike other forms of adolescent rebellion or experimentation, solvent inhalation can be fatal. Bass (1970) reports 110 deaths due to inhalation of trichloroethane and fluorinated hydrocarbons, possibly from cardiac toxicity. It has been estimated that solvent abuse currently causes at least 100 deaths per year of young abusers (Cohen, 1978). This has not, unfortunately, diminished its popularity as an intoxicant, and young abusers seek out and experiment with an astonishingly diverse variety

TABLE IV.5. Substances containing abusable solvents. (Reprinted, by permission of Academic Press, from Giovacchini, R. P. (1985). Abusing the volatile organic chemicals. *Regulatory Toxicology and Pharmacology*, **5**, 18–37.)

Aerosol cocktail chillers	Degreasers	Aerosol pain relievers
Nonstick frying pan aerosols	Wax strippers	Aerosol fly sprays
Cold-weather car starters	Lighter fluids	Aerosol antiperspirants
Contact cements	Nail polish removers	Hair sprays
Dry-cleaning fluids	Aerosol shoe polishes	Aerosol paints
Transmission fluids	Refrigerants	Paint lacquers and varnishes
Windshield washer fluids	Sanitizers	Typewriter correction fluids
Brake fluids	Polishes	Anticough aerosols
Fire extinguisher fluids	Disinfectants	Room deodorizers
Liquid waxes	Aerosol deodorants	Gasoline

TABLE IV.6. Constituents of common solvent-containing products. (Reprinted, by permission of PMA Publishing Corp., from Goetz, C.G. (1985). *Neurotoxins in Clinical Practice*. New York.)

PRODUCT	SOLVENT
Aerosols	Dichlorodifluormethane (propellant 12), trichlorofluormethane, isobutane
Fingernail polish	Acetone, aliphatic acetates, benzene, alcohol
Gasoline	Petroleum hydrocarbons, paraffins, olefins, naphthenes, and aromatics (benzene, toluene, xylene)
Household cements	Toluene, acetone, isopropanol, methyl ethyl ketone, methyl isobutyl ketone
Lacquer thinners	Toluene, aliphatic acetates, methyl, ethyl or propyl alcohol
Lighter fluid/cleaning fluid	Naphtha, perchloroethylene, carbon tetrachloride, trichloroethane
Model cements	Acetone, toluene, naphtha
Paint strippers	Methylene chloride
Plastic cements	Toluene, acetone, aliphatic acetates (ethyl acetate, methyl-cellosolve acetate, etc.)
Typewriter correction fluid	Trichlorethane, trichloroethylene

of substances containing solvents. These include substances shown in Tables IV.5 and IV.6.

It would be difficult in some cases, and impossible in others, to substitute non-toxic alternatives for the solvents in these ubiquitous products. Thus the problem of solvent abuse requires more than careful labeling and judicious product development by industry. Professionals in medicine, clinical psychology, law and education will need to work together on the problem of solvent-related chemical dependency. Neuropsychologists may contribute to this effort in both research and clinical capacities; by performing basic neurobehavioral solvent research, and by clinically detecting, monitoring and suggesting rehabilitation strategies for solvent-abusing individuals.

Acute effects of solvent abuse

Symptoms of solvent inhalation abuse have been partitioned into four stages (Wyse, 1973). Initial intoxication is characterized by euphoria, excitation, dizziness, visual and auditory hallucinations. By the second stage, CNS depression has set in and symptoms include "confusion, disorientation, dullness, loss of self-control, tinnitus, blurred vision, diplopia" and other symptoms (Barnes, 1979). By stage 3, increasing CNS depression may produce sleepiness, incoordination, ataxia, dysarthria, diminished reflexes and nystagmus. In the fourth stage, seizures and EEG changes occur (Barnes, 1979).

Chronic effects

Chronic neuropsychological impairments are possible with continued inhalation of at least two types of solvents: methyl butyl ketone and toluene. The former has been linked to the development of peripheral neuropathies while its effects on cortical functioning are unknown. Several studies of toluene abuse suggest that chronic exposure can cause structural brain damage to the cerebellum and cortex (e.g. Fornazzari *et al.*, 1983). Continued toluene inhalation has produced a variety of neurological and neuropsychological toxic effects, including ataxia and dementia.

Allison and Jerrom (1984) used neuropsychological measures to examine a group of 10 subjects, average age $15\frac{1}{2}$, who had 4.6-year mean history of solvent abuse. The type of inhalant used by this group of Scottish adolescents was "EVOSTIK", a combination of toluene and acetone. The neuropsychological battery consisted of the WISC Vocabulary and Block Design tests, the Wechsler Memory Scale (WMS) with immediate and 10-minute delayed recall of the Logical and Figural Memory subtests, and the Paced Auditory Serial Addition Task (PASAT). Compared to a control group matched on age, socioeconomic status and education, the solvent abusers scored significantly more poorly on Block Design, the PASAT and the WMS, the latter test showing impairment on all subtests except Information and Orientation. The PASAT score of the inhalers was 65%, significantly poorer than the 25% error score obtained by controls.

The study has some shortcomings in design, among them lack of verification as to whether subjects continued to use solvents at the time of testing and the fact that the psychologist testing the adolescents was not blind to the purpose of the study, or the group to which each subject belonged. The results are, however, consistent with other studies of solvent abuse.

Another, better controlled, investigation examined the neuropsychological performance of 37 chronic solvent abusers, and did control for acute effects by eliminating any individual with positive urine toxicology screen from the study. Testing was conducted by a technician blind to the group membership of the subjects (Berry, Heaton and Kirby, 1977). Mean exposure duration was 5.5 years, average age was 18.3 and nationality was mixed among Anglo, Hispanic and American Indian. Controls were 11 subjects described as peers or siblings of the experimental subjects, matched on age, ethnicity, education, sex and other sociodemographic variables.

An extensive battery of neuropsychological tests was administered, including the WAIS, the Halstead–Reitan, as well as various memory and motor tests (e.g. Grooved Pegboard). Approximately half of the neuropsychological battery was performed significantly more poorly by the solvent abusers, including Verbal and Full Scale IQ. The Halstead Impairment index was also significantly more impaired in the solvent group, although both groups were under pathognomonic cutoffs established by Reitan. Memory was found to be impaired on the Tactual Performance Test (TPT) and a Story Memory Task. Hand Dynamometer, Maze Coordination Errors and total time per block on the TPT were also impaired.

While not guilty of the same inadequacies as the previous study, the study can be criticized for not specifying the types of solvents under study, and apparent failure to correct for multiple comparisons when using t tests. In addition, verbal, rather than performance, IQ was more impaired in the experimental group, a finding which could suggest lower premorbid functioning in the impaired group relative to controls. Lower premorbid functioning could also have predisposed these individuals to solvent abuse rather than solvents causing current impairment (see also Toluene, covered later in this chapter).

Inhalation abuse of other solvents has not been the subject of neuropsychological studies at this time.

INDIVIDUAL SOLVENTS

While solvent mixture researchers often consider solvent effects as part of a unitary "solvent syndrome", other investigators have attempted to find unique patterns of neurological and neuropsychological damage from individual solvents. Researchers who work with individual solvents state that "exposure data indicate that great differences exist in the neurotoxic potential of even the commonest industrial solvent" (Savolainen, 1982) as evidence that solvent exposure should not be considered a unitary concept. For example, carbon disulfide has long been shown to induce neuropsychological deficit (e.g. Hänninen, 1971) while 1,1,1-trichloroethane researchers have thus far failed to find any evidence of chronic neurophysiological or psychological damage (Maroni, Bulgheroni and Cassitto, 1977).

Several other solvents have been documented to cause direct structural damage to the nervous system, including carbon disulfide, styrene, toluene, trichloroethylene, *n*-hexane, and methyl butyl ketone (MBK). Spencer and Schaumberg (1985) have suggested that several other compounds be considered as putative human neurotoxicants, including diethyl ether, ethylene chloride, nitrobenzene, pyridine, tetrachloroethane, perchloroethylene and xylene, and that further research be performed to determine possible neurotoxicity of the chromogenic aromatic hydrocarbons (e.g. benzene, indane, tetralin, diphenyl) and methylene chloride. The effects of selected solvents entering the neuropsychological and neurobehavioral literature are reviewed below.

CARBON DISULFIDE

Carbon disulfide (CS₂):
OSHA   20 ppm 8 hr TWA, 30 ppm acceptable ceiling
              100 ppm, 30 min maximum ceiling
NIOSH   1 ppm, 10 h TWA
              10 ppm, 15 min ceiling
ACGIH   10 ppm
IDLH level   500 ppm
(NIOSH, 1985)

CS_2 is a sweetish-smelling, clear liquid discovered accidentally by the German chemist Lampodius in 1797. Carbon disulfide was subsequently tried as a narcotic and analgesic agent in the 1800s (Spyker, Gallanosa and Suratt, 1982) and saw its first industrial application in that century when it was used to cure natural rubber.

Psychological symptoms following the use of CS_2 were noted immediately after its industrial debut. The book *Dangerous Trades* (Oliver, 1902) chronicled "the extremely violent maniacal condition" of carbon disulfide workers of that time. "Some of them have become the victims of acute insanity, and in their frenzy have precipitated themselves from the top rooms of the factory to the ground" (Oliver, cited in Wood, 1981, p. 397). Unfortunately, the factories' solution at the time was not better ventilation or otherwise safer working conditions, but rather the placing of bars on the windows to prevent poisoned workers from "precipitating" themselves. Despite the striking observations contained in *Dangerous Trades*, Hamilton (cited in Wood, 1981) noted that no major investigation of carbon disulfide occurred in the United States prior to 1938.

Current uses of carbon disulfide include soil fumigation, perfume production, as a component of lacquers, varnishes, insecticides, and especially as a solvent in the rubber and rayon industries (Spyker, Gallanosa and Suratt, 1982). The World Health Organization suggests that only these latter workers in the rayon or cellophane industries are routinely exposed to CS_2 concentrations high enough to adversely affect health (World Health Organization, 1979a).

Neurotoxicity of CS_2

Carbon disulfide is possibly the most globally neurotoxic of all solvents, and it appears to be the case that virtually all nervous system functions are affected by CS_2. Most clinical cases of CS_2 toxicity are the result of inhalation. Inhalation of "4800 ppm for 30 minutes will usually result in acute poisoning, including narcosis, vomiting, injury to the central nervous system and death" (Spyker, Gallanosa and Suratt, 1982, p. 90). However, doses as low as 20 ppm, the current American "safe exposure" limit, have been shown to produce neurological damage, and workers exposed to a time-weighted average of only 11 ppm have reported headaches (Spyker *et al.*, 1982).

Neuropathology

Very little is known concerning the CNS neuropathology of CS_2, though central and peripheral axon destruction have been observed (Wood, 1981). Toxicological effects are thought to be produced through "alkylation of neural protein by semi-stable epoxide intermediates" (Savolainen, 1982). Other possible, albeit hypothetical mechanisms, suggested to account for CS_2 neuropathological damage include: chelation of essential trace metal metabolites, enzyme inhibition, disturbance of vitamin, catecholamine or lipid metabolism or liver interactions (World Health Organization, 1979). Animal studies have identified severe destruction of the putamen, caudate nucleus, globus pallidus, and substantia nigra (Wood, 1981). Peripheral nerves show neuropathy which may be irreversible even at subclinical exposures (Seppäläinen *et al.*, 1972).

CS_2 has been found to cause general and cerebral atherosclerotic changes in exposed workers (Tolonen, 1975; Key *et al.*, 1977). Thus, secondary neurological and neuropsychological effects of carbon disulfide could occur as a result of CS_2-induced vasculopathy. Workers exposed to levels as low as $30mg/m^3$ for 10 years or more have been suggested to have increased death rates from heart disease (WHO, 1979a). It is not unheard of for rayon workers in their 30s to present for neuropsychological evaluation having already received single and occasionally multiple cardiac bypasses. In a comprehensive review of CS_2's vascular effects, Tolonen (1975) concluded that "disturbed ocular microcirculation" is the first subclinical vascular sign of CS_2 "excessive morbidity" (p. 73) as well as being one of the most common symptoms of CS_2 intoxication (Wood, 1981).

Neuropsychological effects of CS$_2$

Neuropsychological studies of CS$_2$ suggest that symptom questionnaires will be sensitive to very low levels of CS$_2$ exposure (i.e., under 20 ppm). However, few neuropsychological correlates of exposure have been detected at this level. For example, Putz-Anderson *et al.* (1983) examined 131 workers in a rayon plant who had at 1 year or more of CS$_2$ exposure "generally below 20 ppm". These workers, who were also screened for illness with neurological sequelae and substance abuse, were compared with controls having "inconsequential" CS$_2$ exposure.

Exposed subjects reported significantly more symptoms than did controls on a health inventory of CS$_2$ effects. However, when subjects' neuropsychological test results were examined and corrected for multiple comparisons, only an eye-hand coordination task significantly differentiated the two groups.

Another study which examined higher and longer exposures to CS$_2$ in somewhat older subjects, suggested that CS$_2$ is capable of creating more serious forms of neuropsychological impairment. Hänninen *et al.* (1978) studied a group of workers exposed for a mean of 17 years to between 10 and 30 ppm of CS$_2$ (compared to the Putz-Anderson *et al.* (1983) group whose subjects were exposed for a mean of 12 years with only 28% of the workers exposed to levels in excess of 10 ppm). The impairments of the Hänninen *et al.* (1978) subjects were categorized by the authors as occurring in the areas of motor speed, emotionality, energy level and psychomotor performance (Hänninen, *et al.*, 1978).

Findings similar to Hänninen *et al.* (1978) have been generated by a U.S. study conducted by NIOSH (Tuttle, Wood and Grether, 1977). Various reaction time measures, vigilance, visual-motor functions and constructional abilities showed significant correlations with duration of exposure. Partial correlations, with age removed, revealed several neuropsychological tests to be sensitive to duration of CS$_2$ exposure, including simple, choice, and drop reaction time, Santa Ana (right hand), a Neisser vigilance task, Digit Symbol, and to a lesser degree, Block Design.

Neuropsychological measures have also been used to compare the cognitive function of CS$_2$ workers with and without toxic profiles generated by "clinical neurological, otoneurological, and neuro-ophthalmological examination . . ." (Hänninen, 1971). When Hänninen (1971) compared these two groups to a population of non-exposed controls, she discovered that both the "exposed" and the "poisoned" group showed neuropsychological abnormalities with differing discriminent functions for each group. Poisoned workers were characterized by the author as showing "retarded speech, low vigilance, clumsiness . . . inaccuracy of motor functions, diminished intellectual capacity, low level of spontaneous behavior and impoverished capacity of visualization" (p. 376). Workers exposed to CS₂ but not overtly poisoned also displayed neuropsychological deficits compared to controls, albeit with somewhat fewer personality and psychomotor deficits than the clearly poisoned group. Hänninen (1971) characterized these subclinically exposed workers as depressed with mild motor and intellectual impairments. They showed diminished functioning relative to controls in Digit Span, Picture Completion, Block Design and Digit Symbol Tests, as well as on tests of coordination and visual memory.

CS₂-related deterioration of emotional status is a consistent concomitant of other forms of neuropsychological deterioration. Acute manic-depressive psychotic symptoms chronicled in early CS₂ literature are uncommon today because workplace exposures have been regulated to much lower levels than had been the case. However, even these regulated levels of CS₂ appear to be capable of producing a personality syndrome of gradual onset that includes stereotyped behavior, neurasthenic syndrome, depression, irritability and insomnia (Wood, 1981; Hänninen, 1971).

Results from these and other studies, in the absence of consistent neurological test detection of subclinical CS₂ abnormalities have led the World Health Organization to conclude that "psychological test results are almost the only way of assessing involvement of the central nervous system" (World Health Organization, 1979, p. 56).

Testing for CS₂ effects

A battery approach to neuropsychological testing is recommended to quantify CS₂ damage since there is no one pattern of deficit displayed on neuropsychological tests (Wood, 1981, p. 398). Based on the results of the preceding studies, neuropsychological tests sensitive to subclinical CS₂ poisoning include reaction time measures, tests of vigilance and cognitive efficiency like the WAIS-R digit symbol, constructional tests (e.g. Block Design) and tests requiring coordination and manual dexterity (i.e. the Santa Ana Dexterity Test).

CARBON TETRACHLORIDE

Carbon tetrachloride (tetrachlormethane)(CCl₄):

OSHA	10 ppm
	25 ppm ceiling
	200 ppm, 5-min/4-h peak
NIOSH	2 ppm, 60-min ceiling
ACGIH	5 ppm
IDLH level	300 ppm

Once in wide use as a dry-cleaning solvent, carbon tetrachloride has been replaced by less toxic substitutes (e.g. perchloroethylene). Carbon tetrachloride shows initial preference for nervous system toxicity, causing "headache, lethargy, weakness, vertigo, tremor, ataxia and blurred vision (O'Donoughue, 1985, p. 108). These symptoms can be followed by confusional state, coma and convulsion (O'Donoughue, 1985). Central and peripheral neuropathy have been reported including cerebellar signs, blurred vision, constriction of visual fields, optic atrophy and sensorimotor neuropathy. Neuropathological studies suggest pontine, cerebellar and, to a lesser extent, cortical hemorrhage (O'Donoughue, 1985). There do not appear to be any neuropsychological investigations of carbon tetrachloride exposure in the literature.

METHYL CHLORIDE (CHLOROMETHANE)

Methyl chloride CH_3Cl:

OSHA	100 ppm, 200 ppm ceiling
	300 ppm, 5 min/3-h peak
	Lowest feasible limit (occupational carcinogen, no level
	that is risk-free)
ACGIH	50 ppm
IDLH level	10,000 ppm
(NIOSH, 1985)	

Methyl chloride is used as an industrial solvent, a refrigerant and is used in the production of synthetic rubber, methyl cellulose, tetramethyl lead and as a blowing agent for plastic foams (Anger and Johnson, 1985). It is also used as an insecticide propellant. The most common uses of methyl chloride are in the production of methyl silicone compounds and as an antiknock fuel additive. Industrial leaks and defective home refrigerators account for many cases of methyl chloride neurotoxicity (Repko, 1981).

Neurological and neuropsychological effects

The amount of literature on neurotoxic effects of methyl chloride has been described as "meager", even though neurotoxic effects have been stated to resemble encephalitis (Repko, 1981).

Repko (1981) has summarized the neurological effects of methyl chloride exposure as consisting of "profound CNS depression and diffuse toxic damage" (p. 426), with reports of headache, confusion, double vision and damage to the spinal cord and brain. Frontal and parietal atrophy, hyperemia, edema, and various degenerative cortical changes have been reported. Symptoms of neurotoxicity may remain latent for several hours after exposure. Patient symptoms include headache, somnolence, euphoria, visual disturbances and chronic personality changes (Repko, 1981). Ataxia, vertigo, tremor, weakness and loss of coordination have also been reported. There are few data on the long-term neuropathology of methyl chloride exposure, but one case study found EEG evidence of frontal and parietal atrophy in a patient exposed for 10 years (Rodepierre *et al.*, 1955).

Neuropsychological symptoms include depression, emotional lability, psychomotor impairments, ataxia, confusion and incoherent speech (Repko, 1981). Perhaps the most complete neuropsychological investigation of methyl chloride was a NIOSH-sponsored study performed by Repko and his colleagues. They examined 122 workers engaged in the manufacture of foam products and compared them to 49 non-exposed controls (Repko *et al.*, 1976). Mean exposure over all plants tested was 34 ppm, and mean after-work breath concentration of methyl chloride was 13 ppm. Subjects received an extensive neurological evaluation, including EEG, and were also administered eight neuropsychological tests and a personal data questionnaire. Neuropsychological tasks included measures of intellectual abilities, vigilance, visual acuity, equilibrium, strength, tremor, coordination, feeling state and personality.

Test results revealed decrements in vigilance, reaction time and complex parallel processing. Exposed subjects performed significantly more poorly when walking on two different width rails, and did significantly less well on the Michigan Eye–Hand Coordination Test. Neurological examination and EEGs did not differentiate between exposed and control subjects. The authors also failed to find effects of methyl chloride on the Edwards Personal Preference Schedule and the Multiple Affect Adjective Checklist (MAACL).

n-HEXANE AND METHYL BUTYL KETONE (MBK)

n-Hexane $CH_3(CH_2)_4CH_3$:

OSHA	500 ppm (1800 mg/m³)
(NIOSH)	100 ppm, 10 h TWA
	510 ppm, 15-min ceiling
ACGIH	50 ppm
IDLH level	5000 ppm
(NIOSH, 1985)	

These two hexacarbon solvents are classified together because their neurotoxic metabolite 2,5 hexadione (2,5-HD) "is responsible for much, if not all, of the neurological effects" that follow their exposure (Spencer, Couri and Schaumburg, 1980, p. 456; Perbellini, Brugnone and Gaffuri, 1981).

n-Hexane is an inexpensive solvent included in gasoline, glues, lacquers and glue thinners. Its use is as varied as the industries in which it is employed; the food industry uses *n*-hexane to extract vegetable oils, and it is used in the manufacture of perfumes, pharmaceuticals and cleaning agents (Jorgensen and Cohr, 1981). Experimental animal studies have shown *n*-hexane to cause giant axonal degeneration of the central and peripheral nervous system (e.g. Frontali *et al.*, 1981; Spencer, Couri and Schaumburg, 1980). In humans, short-term effects include "narcosis, coma, and eventually, respiratory arrest", possibly caused by infusion of this solvent into CNS cell membranes (Jorgensen and Cohr, 1981). Long-term effects are caused by oxidation to 2,5-hexanedione. In chronic solvent abuse of hexane-containing products, cranial nerve and autonomic function may also be affected (Spencer and Schaumburg, 1985). Clinically, workers exposed to *n*-hexane first report headache, nausea and loss of appetite. Two to six months after initial exposure, exposure victims have shown symptoms of *n*-hexane neuropathy including "symmetrical, predominantly distal, motor deficit, and frequently sensory symptoms" which can progress for up to 3 months post-exposure. Symptoms have been reported to persist on 2–3-year follow-up (Bravaccio *et al.*, 1981, p. 1369) and can accompany positive neurological findings. However, Spencer and Schaumburg (1985) report that "partial or complete recovery (after exposure to *n*-hexane ceases) is the rule" (p. 54). The lowest dose of *n*-hexane that has been reported to cause damage is 194–720 mg/m^3 (54-200 ppm) (Jorgensen and Cohr, 1981).

Although about 200 cases of work-related *n*-hexane neuropathy have been reported in Naples, Italy, alone (Bravaccio *et al.*, 1981), the chief cause of neuropathy is said to be recreational abuse of compounds containing this solvent (Spencer, Couri and Schaumburg, 1980). Recreational abusers have also reported mild euphoria and, in one case, hallucinations (Spencer, Couri and Schaumburg, 1980).

METHYL *N*-BUTYL KETONE (MBK)

OSHA   100 ppm (410 mg/m^3)
NIOSH   1 ppm (4 mg/m^3)
ACGIH   5 ppm (20 mg/m^3)
(NIOSH 1987)

One of the best known epidemics of MBK poisoning occurred in 1973 when 48 workers at a Columbus, Ohio, plastics fabrics plant developed peripheral neuropathy. Their symptoms included mixed motor and sensory findings identified by EMG, and were highly correlated with introduction by the factory of MBK in a print-shop solvent mixture (Landrigan *et al.*, 1980). This episode halted the increasing use of this solvent, which today is recognized for its serious neurotoxic potential (Spencer, Couri and Schaumburg, 1980).

PERCHLOROETHYLENE

Perchloroethylene (tetrachloroethylene) CCl$_2$CCl$_2$:
OSHA   100 ppm, 8 h TWA, 200 ppm ceiling

300 ppm, 5 min/3 h peak
NIOSH   Lowest feasible limit: identified carcinogen, not risk-free
               at any level
ACGIH   50 ppm
IDLH level   500 ppm
(NIOSH, 1985)

Although perchloroethylene (PCE) has widely replaced trichloroethlyene as a dry-cleaning agent, it too has been reported to cause neuropsychological effects similar to those of trichloroethylene, including changes in recent memory and personality (Gold, 1969). There are very few investigations of human PCE neurotoxicity in the literature, and these few studies have suggested that PCE exhibits neurotoxic sequelae similar to, but less severe than, trichloroethylene. Dudek (1985) failed to find effects of acute PCE exposure on reaction time. Similarly, Tuttle, Wood and Grether (1977) tested 18 workers who were occupationally exposed to PCE. Neuropsychological tests were given before and after each work shift over 5 consecutive days. There were no significant findings for any of the tests after a correction for worker fatigue was made. Several problems with the Tuttle *et al.* (1977) study mitigate their conclusions. For example, while the experimental group consisted equally of males and females, the control group contained only females. In addition, exposure was relatively low and the number of subjects was small, suggesting that the definitive study on PCE exposure remains to be performed.

Case study

The following case of chronic PCE exposure is consistent with prior studies in that higher cognitive functions did not appear to be significantly compromised. Instead, results appear to be consistent with central or peripheral neurotoxic "solvent syndrome" as a result of sustained exposure to perchloroethylene.

It is also an example of the need for "flexibility" in conducting such evaluations. Some of the most pathognomonic test results were on examinations decided upon on the basis of history and test results collected *during the evaluation*, and thus usually not typically administered as part of a neurotoxicity screening battery.

Case observations and conclusions:
The patient was a college-educated male in his 30s who had worked with perchloroethylene for five years. He reported constant exposure via ambient air and by direct handling without gloves of perchloroethylene-soaked clothing. The patient's wife corroborated continuous exposure and noted that she continued to smell perchloroethylene on the patient's breath when he

TABLE IV.7. Test scores of a patient with chronic perchloroethylene exposure, with sparing of higher cortical function

1. *Finger Tapping:*	RH mean: 48		Russell 1
(Dom. hand: L)	LH mean: 45.5		Russell 2
2. *Wechsler Memory Scale:*			
(a) *Logical*			
Immediate recall:	A: 9.5 B: 12	Total: 21.5	Russell 2
Delayed recall:	A: 8.0 B: 12	Total: 20	Russell 1
(b) *Figural*			
Immediate recall:	A: 3 B: 4 C: 6	Total: 13	Russell 0
Delayed recall:	A: 3 B: 4 C: 6	Total: 13	Russell 0
3. *Trial Making Test:*	A: 15 (seconds)		Russell 0
	B: 40 (seconds)		Russell 0
4. *WAIS-R Digit Symbol Test:*		Raw score: 55	Scaled score 9
5. *Stroop Test:*			
No. of Words: 100 + age corr.: 0		Total: 100	T score 46
No. of colors: 71 + age corr.: 0		Total: 71	T score 44
No. of colored words: 48 + age corr.: 0		Total: 48	T score 53
6. *Luria-Nebraska Pathognomonic Scale:*			
			Critical level 67.74
	No. of errors: 17		T score 51
7. *Spatial Relations:* (Greek Cross) Best: 1 + Worst: 1 =			Russell 1
8. *Pegboard:* (Grooved) RH: 71″ T 44 LH: 80″ T 29			
9. *Grip Strength:* RH: (1) 47 (2) 49 LH: (1) 45 (2) 58			
(Kg) Mean RH: 48 Mean LH: 51.5			
10. *IQ Estimate:* Shipley Institute of Living Scale			
Raw score: (V: 38 A:40) CQ: 115			
11. Rey Auditory Verbal Learning Test (Rey AVLT)			
12. *Personality Test:* MMPI: BDI: 39			

MMPI T Scores (K Corrected where appropriate)

L 50	PD 80	SI 82
F 68	MF 63	A 77
K 46	PA 65	R 70
HS 65	PT 76	ES 45
D 101	SC 68	MAC 53
HY 67	MA 48	

Note: 0–5 Russell ratings are from Russell (1975) and Russell, Neuringer and Goldstein (1970) with higher scores indicating greater impairment.

fell asleep at night. The patient also admitted to other symptoms which appeared related to chronic solvent exposure, including anosmia, fatigue, dizziness, loss of balance, frequent paresthesias of the face and hands, and a reported history of 4 or 5 brief blackouts.

The patient denied prior head injury or any illness or form of substance abuse which might influence neuropsychological findings. He did report that he had been under acute job-related financial pressure. The patient admitted to increasingly severe feelings of depression, although these symptoms appeared to occur in the context of long-standing dysthymic symptoms. He was prescribed antidepressants and entered psychotherapy.

As can be seen from the summary table (Table IV.7), the patient displayed unimpaired higher cortical functioning. His only neuropsychological deficit in administered tests was significantly decremented fine motor coordination, as shown in Grooved Pegboard scores. Observation of the patient's performance revealed him to be bilaterally clumsy in the Finger Tapping and Grooved Pegboard tasks, missing the tapping paddle and dropping pegs, respectively.

After history-taking and administration of the neuropsychological battery, the patient was further examined with several "cerebellar" tests. He proved unable to sustain a tandem Romberg for more than three seconds and could not sustain his balance when lightly pushed. In addition, the patient displayed mild bilateral dysdiadochokinesia — being unable to perform rapid alternating palm–dorsum slaps on his thigh.

History and neuropsychological test results were interpreted as consistent with possible peripheral or cerebellar neurotoxic effects of perchloroethylene with sparing of higher cortical function. Because the patient was currently experiencing very severe psychosocial stressors, it was not possible to determine if his elevated Beck Depression Inventory and MMPI scores were directly solvent-induced, reactive or unrelated. The patient was diagnosed as experiencing mild neurotoxic effects of solvent exposure, with rule-outs of other cerebellar or peripheral nervous system disorder. He was subsequently referred for further neurological and occupational medical examination.

STYRENE

Styrene $C_6H_5CHCH_2$ (Vinyl benzene):

OSHA	100 ppm, 200 ppm ceiling
	600 ppm, 5 min/3-h peak
NIOSH	50 ppm, 10 h TWA
	100 ppm, 15 min ceiling
ACGIH	50 ppm
IDLH level	5000 ppm
(NIOSH, 1985)	

Styrene (vinyl benzene) is one of the most widely used components in the production of plastics, where the highest levels of industrial exposure occur. (*Styrene*, 1983). It is also a constituent of rubber items, and is widely used in the boat-building industry (Baker, Smith and Landrigan, 1985). Styrene exposure may also occur in the home with the use of styrene-containing materials, including "floor waxes and polishes, paints, adhesives, putty, metal cleaners, autobody fillers, and varnishes" (*Occupational Exposure*, 1983, p. 16). In addition, the general population is exposed to this solvent through tobacco smoke, automobile exhaust and through food wrapped in polystyrene containers (*Styrene*, 1983). In the United States, production of styrene was 6612 million pounds in 1981, and it has been estimated that from 30,000 to 300,000 workers are exposed to compounds containing this solvent.

Styrene is very soluble in blood and tissues. It is detectable in breath samples and in urine metabolites (i.e. mandelic acid) for less than 24 hours after exposure, but has been found in adipose tissue for up to 13 days after experimental exposure to the Swedish threshold limit value of 50 ppm (Engstrom *et al.*, 1978). Chronically exposed workers may show much greater fat storage of this solvent (Engstrom *et al.*, 1978). Rats exposed to 300 ppm have shown "marked styrene accumulation in the brain and perinephric fat" (Savolainen and Pfaffli, 1977, cited in Seppäläinen, 1978, p. 182).

General effects

Common symptoms of styrene exposure include initial irritation of mucous membranes, nausea and dizziness, memory complaints, fatigue, giddiness, headache and paresthesias in fingers and toes (Seppäläinen, 1978; Rosen *et al.*, 1978). Vomiting, vertigo, and anemia have also been reported (*Occupational Exposure*, 1983).

Acute effects

Human experimental study of acute styrene exposure has noted "listlessness, drowsiness and impaired balance" upon initial exposure to 800 ppm, while a 1-hour exposure to 376 ppm produced decrements in "balance, coordination and manual dexterity" (*Occupational Exposure*, 1983, p. 121). O'Donoghue (Table IV.8) summarizes acute effects of styrene exposure.

Chronic effects

Chronic peripheral nervous system changes from styrene exposure have been noted by Rosen *et al.* (1978), who found mild sensory neuropathy in a group of older, more heavily exposed styrene workers. The authors hypothesized that the peripheral nervous system may be synergistically affected by age and chronic exposure, possibly via increased production of intracellular free radicals.

Abnormal EEGs have also been detected in several studies of styrene workers (reviewed in *Occupational Exposure*, 1983, p. 152; Harkönen *et al.*, 1978). In one such investigation, abnormal EEGs were more than twice as likely in a population of styrene workers exposed a mean of 5 years than in the general population (Seppäläinen, 1978).

Anger and Johnson (1985) suggest that chronic styrene exposure produces "EEG abnormalities at 30 ppm, psychomotor impairments at 50–75 ppm and symptoms of fatigue, difficulties in concentration, and headaches at 50 to 100 ppm" (p. 68).

Lowered reaction times related to exposure intensity are the most commonly noted neuropsychological effect of styrene (Mutti *et al.*, 1983; Gamberale and Kjellberg, 1983). Behavioral effects of acute exposure have been suggested to depend upon individual differences in clearing styrene and its metabolites from the body. Subjects who were slow to clear showed longer

TABLE IV.8. Acute effects of styrene inhalation on volunteers. (Reprinted with permission from O'Donoghue, J. L. (1985). *Neurotoxicity of Industrial and Commercial Chemicals*, Volume II, 131. Copyright CRC Press, Inc., Boca Raton, FL.)

STYRENE AIR CONCENTRATION (PPM)	LENGTH OF EXPOSURE	EFFECTS
< 10		Odor not detected (NIOSH, 1973)
50-100	1-6 hours	Styrene odor strong but not objectionable. Transient eye irritation at 100 ppm; tests of coordination and a modified Romberg test were not affected (NIOSH, 1973; Hänninen *et al.*, 1976)
200	—	Strong objectionable styrene odor and nasal irritation occur. (NIOSH, 1973; Hänninen *et al.*, 1976)
350	—	Continuous exposure to 50, 150, 250, and 350 ppm styrene for 30 minutes at each exposure level impaired reaction time only at the 350 ppm level; perceptual speed and manual dexterity were not affected (Cohr and Stockholm, 1979)
376	25 minutes	Unable to perform a modified Romberg test (Hänninen *et al.*, 1978)
	50 minutes	Nausea present; manual dexterity and coordination decreased. (Hänninen et al., 1976)
	60 minutes	Headache and inebriated feeling. (Hänninen *et al.*, 1976)
600	—	Very strong odor; strong eye and nasal irritation (NIOSH, 1973)
800	4 hours	Immediate eye, nose and throat irritation. Pronounced, persistent metallic taste, listlessness, drowsiness and impaired balance; after-effects included slight muscle weakness, unsteadiness, inertia and depression. (Seppäläinen, Husman and Mattenson, 1978)

reaction times (Cherry *et al.*, 1981a). However, this effect was not replicated for workers with an average of 2.5 years of exposure to levels below 110 mg/m³ (Edling and Ekberg, 1985).

Workers with an average of 5 years exposure to styrene showed significant decrements in visuomotor accuracy, psychomotor performance and vigilance as a function of mandelic acid concentration (Härkönen *et al.*, 1978; Lindström, Härkönen and Hernberg, 1976). Lindström *et al.* found one test of visuomotor speed and one of visual memory correlated with exposure duration; however, these effects may have been confounded by significant relationships between age and exposure duration (Lindström *et al.*, 1976).

Workers exposed for an average of 8.6 years showed significant decrements relative to controls in reaction time, Block Design, Rey's embedded figures and Wechsler Memory subtests including Logical Memory (immediate and 30 min delay), and Visual Memory (immediate) (Mutti *et al.*, 1984).

An unpublished study reports chronic central nervous sytem changes in a group of seven patients who were exposed to styrene for a mean of 15 years (range 6–26 years) (Melgaard, Arlien-Søberg and Brulin, cited in *Occupational Exposure*, 1983). "Intellectual impairment" was said to be found in six out of seven patients, with five showing moderate impairment and one severe impairment. Cerebral atrophy was detected in four of these patients by CT scan, and in one patient by pneumoencephalography.

TOLUENE

Toluene $CH_6H_5CH_3$ (Toluol, Methyl Benzene):

OSHA	200 ppm, 300 ppm ceiling
	500 ppm, 10 min peak
NIOSH	100 ppm, 10 h TWA
	200 ppm, 10 min ceiling
ACGIH	100 ppm
IDLH level	2000 ppm
(NIOSH, 1985)	

Introduction

Toluene (methyl benzene) is an aromatic hydrocarbon with primary uses as a cleaner and degreaser, and also as a solvent for paint, varnish and rubber adhesive (Cavanaugh, 1985). Exposure is usually through inhalation. Animal studies imply that toluene's effect is a "U-shaped concentration–response function" (Benignus, 1981) initially excitatory at lower concentrations or shorter exposures but depressant at higher levels/concentrations.

Acute exposure

In humans, depending on the study cited, toluene approaches asymptote in the body between 10 and 80 minutes, with brain asymptote approximately 1.26–2.50 times that of blood (Benignus, 1981, p. 408). Acute effects observable without neuropsychological testing include those listed in Table IV.9, summarized by Von Oettingen *et al.* (1942) and listed by Benignus (1981).

Acute neuropsychological effects of toluene

Several studies have shown decrements in simple and choice reaction time from acute exposure. For example, Gambarale and Hultengren (1972)

TABLE IV.9. Acute behavioral effects of toluene inhalation. (Reprinted, by permission of Pergamon Journals, Ltd., from Benignus, V. A. (1981). Neurobehavioral effects of toluene: A review. *Neurobehavioral Toxicology and Teratology,* **3**, 407–415.)

TOLUENE LEVEL IN AIR (ppm)	BEHAVIOR
0–100	No observable effects
100–200	Variability among subjects including fatigue, headache, paresthesias, slowed pupillary reflex
200–600	All of above plus confusion
600–800	All of above plus "hilarity and exhilaration" and nausea

exposed 12 male subjects to increasing doses of 100–714 ppm of toluene within a single exposure session. They found decreases in concentration which caused reaction time and perceptual speed deficits at concentration levels of 300 ppm and above.

In general, shorter exposures and lower concentrations of toluene do not produce neuropsychological or neurological effects. For example no effects were noted in subjects exposed for 4 hours, either to toluene alone or in combination with xylene (Olson, Gamberale and Ingren, 1985). Benignus (1981) reports no scalp EEG changes during a 6-hour exposure of 200 ppm, and Winneke's (1982) review of the literature finds no effect of acute, short-term exposure at levels below 300 ppm. Somewhat longer exposure intervals may begin to produce observable effects, however, as Andersen *et al.* (1983) report borderline significance levels at a 6-hour 100 ppm exposure levels on three neuropsychological tests (multiplication errors, Landolt's rings and screw plate test).

Laboratory studies which show minimal effects of acute toluene exposure may be misleading, however, because toluene blood levels are cumulative when exposure is extended. Blood toluene levels increase between 10 and 20 times their initial value over the course of 2 weeks exposure to 184–332 ppm (Konietzko, Kailbach and Drysch, 1980). Thus, short-term experimental exposures may not reflect typical workplace blood levels, even if exposure levels are equivalent. Since these high blood levels suggest the possibility of equally high concentrations in sensitive brain tissue, more research on what might be called "intermediate" toluene exposure seems warranted.

Chronic exposure

Chronic exposure to toluene appears to produce general intellectual decrement and increased emotional reactivity, both in the workplace (Hänninen *et al.*, 1976), and as a product of solvent abuse. Toluene is said to be "by far the most widely abused solvent" (King, 1982, p. 76), perhaps because acute subjective effects include exhilaration, euphoria and disinhibition (Cavanaugh, 1985). Toluene abuse shows toxic effects throughout the body — including liver, heart, kidneys and bone marrow — although "the main toxic impact is on the nervous system" (King, 1982, p. 77).

Neurological effects — toluene abuse

As of 1982, the literature on toluene abuse consisted of case studies rather than large-scale group research. In a review of these case reports, King (1982) reported diffuse cerebellar encephalopathy to be a common finding, with or without accompanying cognitive deterioration or dementia. In another case study toluene was apparently able to cross the placenta and create cerebellar damage in an unborn infant (Streicher *et al.*, 1981). Other neurological findings from chronic toluene abuse include optic and peripheral neuropathy. CT scans of toluene abusers have shown widened sulci, enlargement of the subarachnoid cisterns and dilated ventricles (Cavanaugh, 1985). For example, Fornazzari *et al.* (1983) found seven of 14 patients to have abnormal CT scans with significantly more prominent cerebellar sulci, and larger overall ratings of ventricular size. In the same study, 46% of the sample showed cerebellar test abnormalities including gait ataxia and intention tremor. Similar findings have been reported for a group of 20 primarily Hispanic patients who had inhaled solvents (mostly toluene) for at least 2 years (Hormes, Filley and Rosenberg, 1986). The subjects inhaled an average of one $12\frac{3}{4}$ ounce can of toluene-based spray paint per day, and their mean duration of exposure was about 12 years. Neurological dysfunction was found in 65% of these patients, and included pyramidal, cerebellar, cranial nerve or brainstem abnormalities and tremor. Cerebellar signs of gait or leg ataxia or leg spasticity were detected in nine of these patients. Dysarthria, nystagmus and arm incoordination were found in five patients. Miscellaneous other abnormalities were found in several patients, including anosmia, bilateral hearing loss, ocular flutter and opsoclonus.

The underlying neuropathological process induced by toluene is unknown, although volatile hydrocarbons like toluene are all highly lipophilic and are easily absorbed into the lipid-rich nervous system (Hormes, Filley and Rosenberg, 1986).

Neuropsychological effects of toluene abuse

Neuropsychological studies suggest that toluene inhalation may cause more severe neuropsychological consequences than any other form of drug abuse, including polydrug abuse (Korman, Matthews and Lovitt, 1981; Berry, 1976). A representative study found inhalant (toluene) abusers to perform significantly worse than polydrug abusers on 20 of the 67 neuropsychological measures employed (Korman, Matthews and Lovitt, 1981). Fornazzari *et al.* (1983) found 15 out of 24 patients (63%) were classified as impaired on a variety of neurological and neuropsychological measures. Abusers Verbal IQs were less impaired than their Performance IQs, which were in the borderline range. The pattern of impairment led the authors to conclude that toluene abuse causes "profound impairment of motor control . . . intellectual and memory capacity" (Fornazzari *et al.*, 1983, p. 327).

Neuropsychological impairment was also detected in a majority of the Hormes, Filley and Rosenberg (1986) subjects: seven were demented, and another five had mild to moderate degress of impairment, with abnormalities in "attention, memory, visuospatial function, and complex cognition". Personality or emotional dysfunction was noted for all patients who showed characteristically flattened affect and apathy.

Finally, Tsushima and Towne (1977) also investigated combined acute and chronic effects of paint sniffing on neuropsychological performance. While they were unable to specify the precise paint solvent under investigation, it was most probably toluene. Compared to controls matched on age, education, sex and peer group, paint sniffers performed more poorly on 11 of the 13 neuropsychological measures employed. Sensitive tests included Grooved Pegboard, WISC-R Coding B, Stroop Color–Word Interference Test, Memory for Designs and the Peabody Picture Vocabulary Test. Because the latter test is typically seen as tapping premorbid abilities, the study's results could also suggest that paint sniffers may self-select for sniffing because of lower premorbid abilities and intelligence. However, a trend toward significant duration effects suggests that neurotoxic effects may occur over and above self-selection factors (Tsushima and Towne, 1977).

1,1,1-TRICHLOROETHANE

OSHA   350 ppm (1,900 mg/m^3), 8 h TWA.
NIOSH   350 ppm (1,910 mg/m^3), ceiling (15 minutes); action level set at 200 ppm (1,091 mg/m^3) TWA.
(NIOSH, 1987)

Overall, 1,1,1-trichloroethane appears to be one of the more benign solvents with regard to neurotoxic effect. Several days of exposure to 500 ppm of 1,1,1-trichloroethane produced no impairment to psychomotor abilities (Steward *et al.* 1969). Two 4.5-hour exposures of 450 ppm likewise failed to show impaired functioning on neuropsychologial measures (Salvini, Binaschi and Riva, 1971). Alternatively, Gamberale and Kjellberg (1973) found simple and choice reaction time to be impaired as a function of exposure to 350 ppm of 1,1,1-trichloroethane.

Mackay *et al.* (1987) point out that none of the previously cited studies have correlated neuropsychological performance with blood or breath solvent level (a deficiency common to much solvent research). They performed such a study on 12 subjects in a counterbalanced design. Tests included simple and four choice reaction time, Stroop Color–Word Test, as well as tests of verbal reasoning, motor tracking and stress-arousal. Acute exposure to 1,1,1-trichloroethane significantly impaired tracking, Stroop and both reaction time tests. Exposure concentration, duration and the interaction of the two produced different patterns of performance decrement.

There are no neuropsychological studies to indicate whether these patterns of effects are found in workers actually exposed to 1,1,1-trichloroethane, or whether exposure to this solvent can produce "solvent syndrome" as a function of long-term exposure.

TRICHLOROETHYLENE

Trichloroethylene CHClCCl$_2$ (Triclene):

OSHA	100 ppm, 200 ppm ceiling
	300 ppm peak
NIOSH	25 ppm, 10 h TWA
ACGIH	50 ppm
IDLH level	1000 ppm
(NIOSH, 1985)	

Trichloroethylene (TCE) has been recognized as a neurotoxic solvent for over 50 years. Most commonly used to degrease machine parts, TCE is also employed in the dry-cleaning industry, as a household cleaner, and as a constituent of lubricants and adhesives. It has been used as a short-acting anesthetic in dental and obstetric procedures (Annau, 1981). More recently, TCE has become one of the most extensively used solvents in Silicon Valley's (U.S.A.) electronics industry for cleaning, stripping or degreasing (Baker and Woodrow, 1984; Spake, 1986).

Given this variety of applications, it is not surprising that about 3.5 million workers are exposed to TCE, with 100,000 of these exposed on a full-time basis. It has also been estimated that 67% of these workers work with TCE under inadequate safety conditions (National Institute of Occupational Safety and Health, 1978).

Commonly noted neurological effects of TCE exposure include sensory disturbances and trigeminal anesthesia, which can be permanent and spread to other cranial nerves (*Solvent Neurotoxicity*, 1985). The neurotoxic effects of TCE on the trigeminal nerve actually once led to its use as a treatment for tic douloureux. Cranial neuropathies have also occurred as a consequence of TCE's use as a dental and obstetrical anesthetic (Firth and Stuckey, 1945).

While consistent behavioral deficits have not been noted at TCE levels below 300 ppm, "subtle alterations of brain wave-activity" have been observed in subjects exposed to just 50 ppm for 3.5 hours (Winneke, 1982, p. 126).

Neuropathological changes from TCE exposure have been inconsistently reported. Peripheral neuropathy and cranial nerve damage have been found (Cavanaugh, 1982; King, 1982; Annau, 1981), although several autopsy reports of TCE inhalation fatalities fail to cite neurological damage. In at least one subject, however, the brain section showed "striking alterations" in the brainstem, nerve roots and peripheral nerves with "extensive" myelin degeneration (Annau, 1981, p. 418). Case report inconsistencies in both human and animal exposure studies have led to the suggestion that peripheral and central lesions may not be produced from TCE *itself*, but rather by its decomposition product, dichloroacetylene (Annau, 1981). It has also been argued that TCE destroys neural tissue indirectly by acting as a releaser for an otherwise dormant virus (*Solvent Neurotoxicity*, 1985).

Neuropsychological effects

One study of short-term, low-level, experimentally induced exposure to TCE has shown decreases in manual dexterity and visuospatial accuracy (Salvini, Binaschi and Riva, 1971); however, these results have not been replicated and are not consistent with other studies using longer exposures and higher concentrations that failed to find similar effects (Annau, 1981).

Subjects' reports of other non-specific CNS difficulties seem to be more frequent than actual neuropsychological changes. Complaints reported include headache, dizziness, fatigue and diplopia (Steinberg, 1981), as well as tremor, giddiness, increased tear production, decreased skin sensitivity, alcohol intolerance, "neurasthenia and anxiety, brachycardia and insomnia" (Spencer and Schaumberg, 1985).

A 2-year follow-up of a 56-year-old male acutely exposed to TCE showed neuropsychological deficits suggesting posterior cortical lesions. In addition to decreased general intelligence the patient showed losses in efficiency, concentration, dyspraxia, dysgraphia and visual concept formation (Steinberg, 1981).

Field studies of workers exposed to TCE fail to agree on clear patterns of neuropsychological deficit. At least two studies failed to find chronic, low-level neuropsychological effects of TCE. In the first, no effects were found in workers chronically exposed to 50 ppm (Triebig *et al.*, 1977). In the second, female subjects exposed for 6 years to air concentrations ranging from 110 to 345 ppm showed no effects of exposure (Maroni *et al.*, 1977). However, both studies used a small number of subjects, and the absence of vigilance and reaction time tests in the second study mitigates the strength of its conclusions.

In several other studies, TCE-exposed workers did show significant impairment; in choice reaction time (Gun, Grysorewicz and Nettelbeck, 1978), and several types of psychomotor weakness (Konietzko *et al.*, 1975). Grandjean (1950) examined a group of 50 workers exposed to TCE for intervals of 1 month to 15 years. Nine of these workers displayed the "organic psychosyndrome" of "memory disturbances, difficulties in understanding, and changes in affective state" (Lindström, 1982, p. 133).

To summarize, the literature on TCE tends to suggest that short-term acute exposure under the current threshold limit value does not produce neuropsychological deficits. Alternatively, acute exposure to toxic levels of TCE can cause trigeminal anesthesia as well as long-lasting neuropsychological abnormalities.

The effects of chronic exposure to TCE are unclear. Central nervous system dysfunctions and neuropsychological deficits have been inconsistently demonstrated. TCE does not appear to cause overall increases in mortality among exposed workers (Shindell and Ulrich, 1985).

XYLENE

Xylene $C_6H_4(CH_3)_2$:
OSHA   100 ppm (435 mg/m^3)
              100 ppm, 10 h TWA (434 mg/m^3)
NIOSH   200 ppm 10 min ceiling (868 mg/m^3)

IDLH level 10,000 ppm
(NIOSH, 1985)

Xylene is used in paint solvents, varnishes, glues, printing inks, and in the rubber and leather industries (National Institute of Occupational Safety and Health, 1975, cited in Savolainen, Riihimaki and Linnoila, 1979). Histology technicians who prepare tissues for staining and mounting are also exposed through their use of xylene and other solvents to clear fat and paraffin from tissue samples (Kilburn, Seidman and Warshaw, 1985).

In high concentrations, acute exposure to xylene is anesthetic and can be fatal. One report details one fatality among three painters exposed to xylene in a confined space. Xylene concentration was estimated at 10,000 ppm and autopsy revealed petechial brain hemorrhages and anoxic neuronal damage (Morley *et al.*, 1970). Lower concentration acute exposure to xylene was examined by Gamberale, Annwall and Hultengren (1978). In the first experiment, subjects inhaled either ordinary air or xylene at high or low concentration for 70 minutes. No neuropsychological effects were found. Another group first inhaled the higher concentration of xylene (12.3 μmol/l while exercising on a bicycle ergometer to increase uptake of xylene. These subjects did become significantly impaired on three neuropsychological tests: reaction time addition, visually presented Digit Span and choice reaction time. Another study (Savolainen, Riihimaki and Linnoila, 1979) investigated acute effects of xylene on sedentary subjects during more extended inhalation periods (i.e. several successive days for 6 hours each day). Unadapted subjects showed initial problems with equilibrium when exposed to 4.1–8.2µmol/l of xylene in inhaled air, however, they appeared to adapt when tested at double the dose of xylene several days later. The following week, when exposure increased to 16.4 µmol/l, reaction time and equilibrium were both impaired. No effects were found on critical flicker fusion, the Santa Ana Dexterity Test, or the Maddox Wing Test. The study suggests that in acute exposure to xylene, both rapid temporary adaptation and longer-term impairment are possible outcomes of inhalation. Another study suggests that lower doses of xylene (8.2 µmol/l) in short-term exposure may actually improve performance in some neuropsychological tests (Savolainen *et al.*, 1981). Effects of higher doses, consistent with earlier studies, produced impaired functioning.

There are no neuropsychological studies of workers chronically exposed to xylene; however, one study which details subjectively experienced symptoms among chronically exposed laboratory technicians includes reports of impaired work performance and confusion (Hipolito, 1980).

Thus, while there have not been many validating studies, xylene does appear to affect neuropsychological functioning, although at lower, shorter-term exposure, behavior may not be worsened and may even be facilitated. Longer, higher-dose experimental exposures appear to reduce initial adaptive compensation, and produce consistent impairment of reaction time and short-term memory, especially after uptake is increased via exercise.

PROGNOSIS FOR CHRONIC SOLVENT EXPOSURE

Several recent studies address the longevity of neuropsychological impairment secondary to chronic long-term exposure to solvent mixtures. Bruhn *et al.* (1981) followed up their earlier study (Arlien-Søberg *et al.*, 1979) by re-examining 26 of their original 50 painter subjects chronically exposed to solvent mixtures for an average of 28 years. Mild-to-moderate cerebral atrophy was found in two-thirds of these painters during their initial examination (Arlien-Søberg *et al.*, 1979). While subjective complaints of headache and dizziness had declined in most subjects, no subjects showed improvement in neuropsychological, neurological or neuroradiological status after 2 years without solvent exposure. The authors concluded that a syndrome of chronic exposure to solvents does exist, and that once cerebral atrophy or intellectual changes are observed, these symptoms are irreversible.

Another study assessed the recovery of 86 patients exposed to tricholorethylene, perchloroethylene or solvent mixtures (Lindström *et al.*, 1982; Antti-Poika, 1982b). Mean follow-up period was 5.9 years and the patients' average age at the time of the initial diagnosis was 38.6 years. Their mean exposure was 10.7 years. Fifty-three patients stopped working upon initial diagnosis, the remainder continued to work for varying lengths of time after diagnosis.

Group means for Similarities and Picture Completion increased over time, suggesting possible learning effects, but two tests of motor functions showed decline. Prognosis was better among younger patients, those who did not use medicines with neurological effects and those with longer follow-up (Lindström *et al.*, 1982, p. 585). Some relief of subjective symptoms was found in 52% of patients who had no other neurological condition. Symptoms of "abnormal fatigue, headache, dizziness, sleep disturbance, nausea and emotional lability" were reported to be significantly improved, although reports of memory disturbances increased somewhat (Antti-Poika, 1982a, p. 81).

When Seppäläinen and Antti-Poika (1983) examined the EEG recovery of these patients, they found slow recovery of EEG in about 59% of the cases, a finding they equated with the recovery course for closed-head injury. The authors noted, however, that a "substantial" number of patients "still had abnormal EEG's three to nine years after their diagnosis" (Seppäläinen and Antti-Poika, 1983, p. 23).

In a "case-control" or matched subject design study carried out in Denmark, Rasmussen, Olsen and Lauritsen (1985) found a borderline significant difference in risk of development of late-in-life "encephalopathias" as a function of job classifications which involved solvent use. The greatest exposure odds ratios were found for development of psychosis, hypertensive cerebrovascular disease and senile dementia. There was no increased risk of cerebral and cerebellar atrophy or ischemic cerebral atherosclerosis, a finding that is difficult to understand, considering that cerebral atrophy is itself a common concomitant of senile dementia.

Chronically exposed Finnish solvent workers have an increased risk of being "prematurely pensioned due to neuroses" (Lindström, Riihimaki and Hänninen, 1984). Other studies have shown Swedish and Danish solvent workers to have increased risk for neuropsychiatric disability (Axelson, Hane and Hogstedt, 1977; Olsen and Sabroe, 1980) and for "presenile dementia" (used in these countries without the connotation of Alzheimer's disease) (Mikkelsen, 1980).

In conclusion, prognostic studies generally indicate that once chronically solvent-exposed patients have developed cortical atrophy or other brain abnormalities, they recover either very slowly or not at all. Exposed workers who are otherwise healthy and who do not present with actual structural abnormalities appear to be more likely to recover. This conclusion concerns the long-term effects of solvent mixtures or for solvents as a class. Prognostic studies are not available for individual solvents but it may be expected that prognosis will vary, at least, as a function of the solvent's *a priori* toxicity.

NEUROPSYCHOLOGICAL TOXICOLOGY OF SOLVENTS — CONCLUSION

Perhaps the most obvious conclusion that may be drawn from current solvent research is how few definitive answers are available. Very basic questions remain unanswered, including neurophysiological mechanisms of solvent toxicity, the sites of brain effects, the influence of individual physiological differences in metabolism, and the interactive effects of age, medications, alcohol and other toxins. As is true in the field of neurotoxicity generally, current attempts to answer these questions appear to lag far behind the promulgation of new industrial toxins. As solvent effects become more widely known in science and government, perhaps increased multidisciplinary research participation, better governmental funding and enlightened regulatory policies will give researchers a better chance to finally answer these questions.

V
Neuropsychological Toxicology of Alcohol

INTRODUCTION

Alcohol has been described as "the intoxicant of choice in the Judaeo-Christian culture" (Parsons, 1986). Although the average amount of absolute alcohol consumed per person each year in the United States is 2.77 gallons, Parsons (1986) points out that this estimate includes one-third of the population who are abstainers. Thus, the remaining two-thirds of the population must have correspondingly greater per capita consumption rates. Furthermore, 10% of the population is said to consume 50% of the available supply of alcohol (Parsons and Farr, 1981, p. 101). From this subset of the United States population are found an estimated 9 million problem drinkers.

As was seen to be the case for metal and solvent neurotoxicity (Chapters III and IV) neuropsychological evaluation of alcohol-related deficits has been recommended for its "demonstrated efficacy in detection of brain dysfunction" (Eckardt and Martin, 1986, p. 123). Neuropsychological evaluation of alcohol effects is safe, non-invasive, readily administered and normatively based. As neuropsychological abnormalities are said to be found in approximately 50–70% of detoxified alcoholics *without* organic brain syndromes, such an assessment may be particularly useful for evaluating more subtle deficits in cognitive and emotional functioning, especially as those deficits may influence social and vocational plans (Eckardt and Martin, 1986; Wilkinson and Carlen, 1980).

Alcohol is the only neurotoxin whose properties have been extensively debated within the neuropsychological community. In contrast to the dearth of neuropsychological information available about other neurotoxins, the utility of neuropsychological methods in the evaluation of alcoholism has been widely recognized. There are hundreds of research studies extant investigating the neuropsychological concomitants of alcohol. This abundance of alcohol-related neuropsychological research may be related to the availability of specialized federal funding (Grant and Reed, 1985) or may simply be a reflection of alcohol's popularity and visibility as an intoxicant. In either case the volume of available literature precludes an exhaustive survey in the context of a single book chapter. This chapter will instead attempt a general update of neurological and neuropsychological information related to this ubiquitous neurotoxin.

Acute effects

Alcohol produces obvious cognitive and behavioral effects upon human behavior that have been chronicled by saint and scientist alike. As far back as the third century A.D., St. Basil observed that "Drunkenness is the ruin of reason . . . . It is premature old age . . . . It is temporary death" (Byrne, 1982). Modern research investigations of alcohol's acute effects have generally validated such impressionistic observations of impairment by finding decrements in a range of psychological functions. Impairments in these basic functions, in turn, produce the real-world impairments in driving or performance of any occupation requiring these functions (Mitchell, 1980).

Acute neuropsychological dysfunction is demonstrable when blood alcohol levels (BAL) exceed 50 mg/dl. BAL levels above 100 mg/dl elicit marked impairments in almost all behavioral skills (Mitchell, 1985). For any given blood level, neurobehavioral deficits are more serious when alcohol is being initially absorbed into the body (the ascending limb of the blood alcohol curve) than after blood alcohol levels have peaked and begun to decline (the descending limb) (Jones and Vega, 1971).

Acute ingestion of ethanol has been linked to reductions in ability across a range of neuropsychological functions; a typical constellation of impairments in a recent study included losses in attention, concentration, auditory–verbal and visuospatial areas. Fine motor coordination was impaired at low and high doses, although motor speed was impaired at high doses only (Minocha *et al.*, 1985).

Tarter *et al.* (1971) tested medical student volunteers when their blood alcohol level achieved 1.1 mg/kg of body weight on a neuropsychological battery that included the Stroop Test, Purdue Pegboard, Digit Span, a Dichotic Listening task, Critical Flicker Fusion, simple and choice reaction time, and the Shipley Institute of Living Scale. All tests except the Stroop were affected by alcohol ingestion, although only the abstract reasoning portion of the Shipley was worsened by alcohol. Interestingly, test practice eliminated all neuropsychological differences by the second testing session. This suggests the possibility of acute neuropsychological adaptation to alcohol, at least with bright, presumably non-alcoholic subjects.

Acute effects on perception, balance and attention were found by Baker *et al.* (1986). The authors tested 21 non-alcoholic adult males on several measures, including Critical Flicker Fusion, Tachistiscopic Perception, visual after-images, Digit Span and standing stability. Besides applying relatively uncommon psychophysical measures to the study of alcohol intake, the study is notable for its careful methodology, including the use of a breathalyzer to measure alcohol levels, a MANOVA analysis and the selection of a double-blind, crossover design where subjects served as their own controls. Participants received either 0 or 1.4 ml/kg body weight of vodka to produce breathalyzer readings of 0.004% or 0.054% (pre-behavioral testing). Subjects performed significantly more poorly in the intoxicated condition. Significant decrements were found in patients' tachistiscopic perception and one of the stabilometry measures. Trends toward significance were found in Critical Flicker Fusion and cerebellar tests.

Chronic effects

Acute intoxication effects have typically been of less interest to neuropsychological researchers than the chronic effects of alcohol on brain and behavior. These effects could be conceptually divided into at least three areas of research interest: 1) the analysis of long-term "social" use of alcohol, 2) the severe neuropathological and neuropsychological effects produced by Wernicke–Korsakoff syndrome, and 3) the long-term consequences of alcohol abuse uncomplicated by Wernicke–Korsakoff syndrome.

Social Drinking

There has been considerable controversy about the effects of moderate, "social" non-alcoholic drinking on neuropsychological performance. The controversy is probably consistent with the potential impact of a finding that drinkers who average one or two drinks or more each day could suffer impairment; Parsons (1986) estimated that there are millions of such social drinkers in the United States alone.

In an extensive review of the subject, Parsons (1986) concluded that current understanding of the relationship between social drinking and neuropsychological performance is inconclusive, and that the investigation is still in its infancy. Existing studies have suffered from a variety of methodological deficiences, including failing to match for education in alcohol and control groups; failure to measure or control for acute versus chronic alcohol effects; and not including the influence of relevant historical, medical, educational or sociodemographic variables. Considering the potential magnitude of the problem, Parsons (1986) recommends large random sample prospective studies with long-term recording of drinking practices.

In Parsons's (1986) review of several possible relationships between social drinking and neuropsychological function (Table V.1), he found little

TABLE V.1. Possible relationships between social drinking and neuropsychological performance (adapted from Parsons, 1986).

1. Alcohol–causal	Alcohol directly produces brain dysfunction as a consequence of amount of alcohol drunk per occasion
2. Cognitive–causal	Those with poorer intellect drink more than individuals with better cognitive abilities
3. Stress emotional–causal	Subjective stress or emotional problems lead to higher alcohol intake and poorer neuropsychological functioning
4. Genetic–causal	Genetic heritage leads to increased drinking and poorer neuropsychological performance
5. Alcohol–causal–threshold	Same as alcohol–causal but damage occurs only after a threshold has been achieved
6. Alcohol–causal–transient	Alcohol ingestion causes "limited" changes accompanied by neuropsychological and emotional disturbances

support for hypothesis 1, and suggested that hypothesis 2 is worthy of further exploration. There appears to be a small but growing amount of evidence that links genetic make-up with poorer neuropsychological performance in the families of alcoholics (e.g. Schaeffer, Parsons and Yohman, 1984; Diejer, Theilgaard, Teasdale, Schulsinger and Goodwin, 1985). The "alcohol threshold" hypothesis is potentially interesting, since variation in individual thresholds could account for differences among research findings. However, there has been no method identified for establishment of such thresholds in the existing literature. Finally, this hypothesis does not have any direct evidence which would prove that amount consumed per occasion rather than frequency of drinking is related to brain impairment.

CHRONIC ABUSE

Neuropathology

The nervous system is one of the main targets of this well-known neurotoxin (Juntunen, 1982a) with neurochemical, behavioral and neuropathological changes reported as consequences of chronic exposure. Much information remains to be discovered since, except for Wernicke–Korsakoff syndrome, detailed neuroanatomical studies of alcohol's long-term effects have not been performed (Shoemaker, 1980). Animal studies suggest that alcohol decreases the viscosity of biological membranes, which in turn causes neurotransmission abnormalities (Shoemaker, 1980). Neurochemical correlates of acute alcohol administration also include changes in acetylcholine (ACh) release, as well as norepinephrine and other neurotransmitter turnover (Hoffman and Tabakoff, 1979). Neuropathological changes include alterations in neuronal cell membrane structure with chronic use (Hoffman and Tabakoff, 1979).

Similarities and interaction with solvent exposure

Since alcohol is itself a solvent, it would not be surprising if the neurological and neuropsychological features of chronic alcohol exposure resembled those resulting from chronic solvent intoxication. There would appear to be many similarities in symptom development. For example, both disorders have insidious onset and are difficult to diagnose in the early stages. Second, each syndrome is usually caused by repeated intoxicating exposures over a long period of time. Finally, chronic exposure to either toxin may produce deteriorations in occupational and interpersonal coping (Juntunen, 1982a).

Despite such similarities, there has been a notable lack of research concerning the ways in which alcohol and solvents might interact. The topic is more complex than might first be assumed. Questions that would need to be addressed include analyzing how drinking habits effect or potentiate solvent symptoms, whether tolerance to alcohol changes after solvent exposure, and even how prior alcohol intake influences choice of a solvent-related occupation (Baker and Seppäläinen, 1986). Unfortunately, these questions have not been the subjects of investigation at the present time. It remains for alcohol or solvent researchers to extend their investigations to these effects.

Disease pathology

While comparative and interactive effects of alcohol with solvents have yet to be studied in detail, the neurological and neuropsychological effects of alcohol by itself have been widely studied. Alcohol has been linked to an extensive list of disease pathology, and is toxic across the entire human life cycle. For example, alcohol is neurotoxic to the developing fetus and can produce "fetal alcohol syndrome", a constellation of biochemical, behavioral and psychological abnormalities that includes "tremulousness, fine-motor dysfunction, (and) poor sucking behavior" (Rawat, 1979). At the other end of the age spectrum, alcohol appears to produce a wide variety of cognitive deficits in the adult which become increasingly intransigent to recovery with advancing age. Juntunen's (1982a) list (Table V.2) provides the reader with a sense of the pathologic diversity of alcohol. Diseases like those delimited by Juntunen (1985) can be grouped into three etiological categories (Schaumberg and Sterman, 1980):
1. Neurotoxicity occurring from direct toxic effects on the nervous system;
2. Neurotoxic effects as a result of indirect effects, i.e. malnutrition in chronic alcoholism;
3. Effects related to withdrawal from alcohol.

Direct toxic effects
There is growing evidence that the action of alcohol is neurotoxic in itself,

TABLE V.2. Primary or secondary neurological disorders of alcoholism. (Reprinted, by permission of the publisher, from Juntunen, J. (1982a). Alcoholism in occupational neurology: Diagnostic difficulties with special reference to the neurological syndromes caused by exposure to organic solvents. *Acta Neurologica Scandinavica*, **66**: 89–108.)

Alcohol intoxication	Dementia associated with alcoholism
Alcohol idiosyncratic intoxication	Wernicke–Korsakoff syndrome
Alcohol withdrawal	Alcoholic polyneuropathy
Alcohol withdrawal delirium	Alcoholic cerebellar degeneration
Alcohol epilepsy	Retrobulbar neuropathy
Alcohol hallucinosis	Alcohol myopathy
Alcohol amnestic disorder	Hepatic encephalopathy and hepatocerebral
Central pontine myelinolysis	degeneration
	Fetal alcohol syndrome

without accompanying avitaminosis. Recent animal studies have found a variety of alcohol-induced neuropathological changes in animals maintained on a nutritionally complete ethanol diet. For example. Rosengren *et al.* (1985) sought to investigate cortical changes in gerbils fed alcohol for 3 months in an otherwise balanced liquid diet. Neuropathological studies were conducted after 4 additional months when the animals were placed on an ethanol-free diet to allow recovery from acute toxic effects. The authors found results suggesting permanent changes in the composition and volume of brain cells which varied according to the cortical areas studied. They viewed such changes as consistent with gliosis found in the cerebral frontal and temporal cortex and the cerebellar vermis of human alcoholics (Rosengren *et al.*, 1985). Two other studies suggest that mice maintained on a nutritionally complete ethanol diet for 4 months show losses of hippocampal neurons, hippocampal pyramidal cell dendritic spines and dentate granule cells (Walker, Hunter and Abraham, 1981; Riley and Walker, 1978).

Neurotransmitters and receptor sites have also been shown to be affected by chronic ethanol consumption. For example, Pelham *et al.* (1980), found that chronic alcohol use alters brain cholinergic neurons. They suggest such effects may be permanent, or at least persistent. Such findings may help explain the genesis of some alcohol-related forms of memory disorder.

Finally, two autopsy studies suggest chronic effects of alcohol on brain weight (and presumably on cell mass). Harper and Blumbergs (1982) found alcoholics to have brain weights below age-matched controls. In a later study, Harper and Kril (1985) studied the autopsied brains of controls, alcoholics, alcoholics with Wernicke's encephalopathy and alcoholics with liver disease. The authors estimated brain tissue loss to occur for all alcoholic groups, with progressively greater losses in the Wernicke's and liver disease groups.

Indirect toxic effects

The gradual supplanting of nutritive calories for ethanol may produce avitaminosis, and therefore the elimination of thiamine (B_1) from the diet. A completely thiamine-deficient diet, whether from alcoholism or other factors can, in a matter of weeks, precipitate permanent structural damage to the central nervous system in the form of Wernicke's encephalopathy (Hartman, Sweet and Elvart, 1985). If uncorrected, the syndrome can be fatal. Neuropsychological dysfunction resulting from this indirect effect of alcoholism is discussed later in the chapter.

Alcohol may also indirectly damage the central nervous system by producing cerebrovascular spasm and contraction of cerebral microvessels. Altura and Altura (1984) demonstrated that blood alcohol concentrations as small as may result from a single drink are capable of producing significant contractions of blood vessels. With alcohol blood levels high enough to produce stupor or coma, "intense spasm . . . and often rupture" of cerebral microvessels can occur (Altura and Altura, 1984, p. 328). This phenomenon may partially acount for the findings of Hillbom and Kaste (1983), who found that 40% of 100 patients presenting with ischemic brain infarction had used alcohol heavily within the previous 72 hours. A possible relationship of ethanol-induced vascular spasms and hypertension has also been postulated (Altura and Altura, 1984).

Finally, alcohol may be indirectly toxic to the brain via hepatic damage. Various aspects of liver dysfunction have been shown to be highly correlated with neurological and neuropsychological impairment (e.g. Tarter *et al.*, 1986).

Even this catalogue of direct and indirect toxic abnormalities must be considered a subset of the potential physiological, neurological, neuropsychological and psychiatric expressions of this intoxicant on human function. While the many impairments of social and occupational performance found in alcoholics are beyond the scope of this chapter, there are secondary neurological impairments from alcohol not included in Juntunen's list (Table V.2). For example, alcoholism-mediated behavior makes impairment more likely. Alcoholics have a relatively high incidence of closed-head injuries (Tarter and Edwards, 1986). Family violence, criminal behavior and auto accidents leading to head injury have all been associated with alcohol intoxication.

Effects of withdrawal

Neurological and neuropsychological effects of alcohol during withdrawal *per se* are a less salient issue for neuropsychologists than the recovery of neuropsychological function after acute withdrawal. These issues are discussed later in the section on recovery of function.

Locus of damage — hypotheses

The three main hypotheses advanced to explain the neuropathological effects of alcoholism are diffuse injury, lateralized damage to the right hemisphere, or injury to the frontal–limbic–diencephalic area (Loberg, 1986). A brief summary of each is presented below.

Diffuse injury

The diffuse injury hypothesis is controversial. Loberg (1986) considers the evidence for diffuse injury to be the weakest of the three hypotheses and criticizes the ambiguity of the concept; "diffuse" could mean either distributed focal lesions or global, overall damage. In addition, neuropsychological tests which have shown consistent deterioration as a result of alcoholism (e.g. constructional tasks, Performance IQ subtests) have typically been thought of as "right hemisphere" rather than diffuse injury tasks. Verbal abilities that are strongly localized to the left hemisphere do not typically evidence alcoholic impairment.

Alternatively, Goldman (1983) suggests that neuroradiological evidence *favors* the diffuse injury hypothesis, including studies of chronic alcoholics which show bilateral enlargement of the lateral ventricles, the third ventricle and cerebral sulci. Altura and Altura's (1984) theory that heavy alcohol use may cause constriction and rupture of cerebral microvessels, along with hypertension, could also be construed as support for a form of diffuse alcohol-related injury. Goldstein and Shelly (1980) suggest that generalized central nervous system damage would explain why their alcoholics' performance did not resemble either anterior- or posterior-brain-injured controls.

Right hemisphere injury

Alcoholic neuropsychological deficit patterns, including intact Verbal IQ, impaired Performance IQ, visuospatial difficulties and constructional deficits are commonly thought to represent right hemisphere injury (e.g. Jones, 1971; Parsons, Tarter and Edelberg, 1972; Jones and Parsons, 1972). There are several reasons why these data may not provide as strong support for right hemisphere localization as has been thought. First, many of these tasks may not localize as clearly to one hemisphere as has been previously assumed (Loberg, 1986). Second, since such tasks, unlike linguistic abilities, are not practiced day-to-day, the failure to perform well could also reflect the novelty or difficulty of that task (Loberg, 1986). Finally, since most of these tests are timed, any affective or neuropsychological impairment interfering with arousal or cognitive efficiency may cause deficit patterns looking much like right hemisphere injury.

Frontal–limbic–diencephalic injury

This hypothesis predicts alcohol damage to the anterior and basal areas of the brain. This theory is consistent with studies that show frontal lobe and memory deficit. For example, deficits in abstract reasoning as exemplified by poor performance on the Halstead Category Test are prototypical of alcoholism (e.g. Fitzhugh, Fitzhugh and Reitan, 1960, 1965; Smith, Burt and Chapman, 1973; Long and McLachlan, 1974). Alcoholic deficits on the Finger Tapping Test (Long and McLachlan, 1974) and motor impersistence on a Knob Turning Task (Parsons, Tarter and Edelberg, 1972) support localizing impairment to the frontal lobe, while commonly reported deficits on tests like the Wechsler Memory Scale's Russell-modified delayed recall tasks (Russell, 1975) also support this axis of injury. PET scans have identified diminished glucose metabolism in the frontal lobes as a function of alcoholism (Kessler *et al.*, 1984).

However, the frontal–limbic–diencephalic hypothesis does not receive uniform support. Goldstein and Shelly (1980) suggested their alcoholic subjects' pattern of performance on neuropsychological tests was different from either anterior-injury or posterior-injury comparison groups.

While the chronic effects of alcohol on the brain have not been definitively localized, radiological and neurobehavioral investigations continue to discover the structural, metabolic and neuropsychological correlates of this form of chronic substance abuse. Each method has contributed unique information to the overall understanding of chronic alcoholism.

Evidence of chronic effects — imaging studies

CT scan

CT (computerized tomography) scan has been shown to be a reliable and valid method of measuring brain changes of alcoholic etiology. Depending upon the study, the criteria, and the location of atrophy, from 33% to 95% of alcoholics show some form of atrophy on CT scan (Begleiter, Porjesz and Tenner, 1980). There is general accord that CT scan is able to discriminate alcoholics from non-alcoholic controls (e.g. Bergman *et al.*, 1980b). For example, Bergman *et al.* (1980a) examined 130 alcoholics with CT and neuropsychological tests. Diagnosed alcoholics and heavy drinkers from the control group showed greater widening of cortical sulci, larger ventricles and cerebellar atrophy. While these abnormalities also correlated with aging, sulcal widening was common in alcoholics below age 40. Similar results have been found by Ron (1983).

CT also appears to be useful in differentiating alcoholics with Wernicke's encephalopathy from non-amnesic alcoholics. Wilkinson and Carlen (1980c), for example, compared these two groups who were diagnosed by Wechsler Memory Scale performance and neurological evaluation. Alcoholics with amnesic memory and positive neurological examination had significantly larger sulcal width and ventricle and sulcal scores on CT scan.

In contrast, CT alone may be less able to discriminate among non-Korsakoff alcoholics with different drinking histories. Ron (1983) surveyed

100 alcoholics using CT, and collected information on alcohol intake in terms of peak daily amount (g/day) and duration (number of years during which the patient had drunk more than 150 g of alcohol per day, "several" times per week. Measures of drinking pattern and abstinence duration were also collected (Ron, 1983, p. 12). CT measures included ventricle size, and width of sulci, Sylvian and interhemispheric fissures. Within older and younger age groups, alcoholics showed significantly greater structural abnormalities on all four variables. However, when Ron divided her groups into patients of similar age, but different drinking histories (mean = 10 versus 26 years), no significant CT differences were observed between the two groups.

While a majority of CT studies appear to demonstrate some form of cortical atrophy in chronic alcoholic patients, the lack of well-controlled studies, and continuing development of more accurate machines, make definitive conclusions impossible at this time. There are also several problems common to CT research design, including possible selection bias in referral of alcoholics for CT; it may be that only more visibly impaired patients are labeled as alcoholic and referred for CT. Second, many CT studies have not required or controlled for abstinence periods prior to CT, potentially confounding acute and chronic effects. Third, some studies have used mixed populations of alcoholics who have other forms of neurological or physical illness, or have not controlled for the effects of cirrhosis. Fourth, the mere presence of CT deficits in alcoholics does not necessarily suggest a causal relationship between alcohol and atrophy. The study by Bergman, Borg, Hindmarsh, Ideström, and Mützell (1980) found significant CT abnormalities in *all* age groups of alcoholics compared to non-alcoholic controls. This may indicate global, acute toxic influence of alcohol across all age groups, but may also suggest pre-existing neuropathological abnormalities among these subjects. Support for the latter hypothesis can be extrapolated from studies of alcoholic families (e.g. Alterman *et. al.*, 1984; Alterman and Tarter, 1983). Finally, age and population differences may account for CT effects (Ron, 1983).

CT relation to neuropsychological test results

The relationship between CT scan results and neuropsychological tests has been examined in several studies. Wilkinson and Carlen (1980a) found that Wernicke's alcoholics had both poorer CTs and greater impairment on the WAIS Digit Symbol Test and the memory subtest of the Tactual Performance Test. Gebhart, Naeser and Butters (1984) analyzed the relationship of CT scans to neuropsychological performance in 24 chronic alcoholics who were administered a verbal Paired Associate Learning Test a four-word short-term memory test, the Digit Symbol Substitution Test and the Symbol Digit Paired Associate Learning Test. CT density in the thalamic dorsomedial nucleus correlated with verbal paired associate learning scores and with Symbol Digit performance. Third ventricle intracranial width also correlated with verbal paired associate learning scores. The authors suggested a relationship between the integrity of mid-line thalamic structures and the ability to form new associations in long-term verbal memory. Alcoholics who showed the lowest mean CT density numbers were also the most impaired on a verbal paired associate learning task. In contrast, tests of short-term memory or their corresponding brain structures did not show impairment. In another study, Hill (1980) found the ventricle/brain index correlated with Category Test errors in a sample of 42 subjects using alcohol and/or heroin.

Finally, Bergman *et al.* (1980a) surveyed a mixed group of binge and daily drinkers on CT with a median 11.7 years of alcohol abuse. The Halstead–Reitan Impairment Index, Block Design, Category Test and TPT-location correlated significantly with an index of sulcal width. Verbal reasoning, Synonyms, Block Design, the Category Test, Trails A and B, as well as several tests of memory correlated with indices of ventricular size. The authors suggested that the Halstead–Reitan Impairment Index is sensitive to cortical changes on CT, while neuropsychological tests of learning and memory reflect subcortical integrity.

Not all studies have confirmed the relationship between CT and neuropsychological impairment. For example, Ron (1983) examined 100 male alcoholics and compared them to 50 volunteers on CT and neuropsychological tests. Ventricles, sulci and interhemisphere fissures were wider in alcoholics, and cerebellar sulci were "visible only in the alcoholic group" (Ron, 1983, p. 13). However, other significant correlations between CT scan results and neuropsychological measures went in the opposite direction; some measures of atrophy correlated with *better* performance on a visuoperceptual task as well as measures of immediate recall and partial cued recall. The lack of correlations between CT results and psychometric data in the direction of impairment was termed "disappointing" by the author, who hypothesized that the discrepancy between immediate and delayed recall of verbal material may have been better correlated to ventricular abnormalities than sulcal or sylvian fissure width (p. 26).

However, Wilkinson and Carlen (1980b) found no significant relationship between the Halstead Reitan impairment index and ventricle size or sulcal width. CT results were unrelated to impairment index scores, whether or not alcoholics had neurological abnormalities. A wide variation (between 2 and 20 weeks) in abstinence among patients before receiving CT scan may have obscured a relationship between neurological and neuropsychological results in this study.

Lusins *et al.* (1980) studied 50 alcoholic patients with CT and a battery consisting of the WAIS and Trail Making Tests A and B. Duration of drinking, rather than neuropsychological test results, was the only factor that correlated with cerebral atrophy as imaged by CT. However, this study can be faulted for its use of the WAIS, a relatively insensitive measure to chronic alcohol intoxication. The authors correctly pointed out the need for a more comprehensive neuropsychological battery in future studies. Melgaard *et al.* (1986) examined the CT scans of 46 male, chronic alcoholics and compared CT abnormalities to neuropsychological test performance. They were also unable to show alcoholism history (as sampled by the Modified Missouri Alcohol Severity Scale) to be significantly correlated with CT or neuropsychological data. It may be, however, that questionnaire surveys of alcohol history were not valid for the particular populations surveyed, particularly since several neuropsychological tests also failed to correlate with the two indices of alcohol exposure. Cala *et al.* (1980) were also unable to confirm a general relationship between neuropsychological performance and CT results. The disparity among various studies remains unresolved, although variations in test sensitivities, population differences, willingness to disclose drinking histories and the multifactorial nature of chronic alcohol damage each undoubtedly contributes to the disparity among results.

PET scans

Positron emission tomography, or PET scan measures local tissue concentrations of positron-emitting radioactive isotopes. Unlike more conventional computerized tomography (CT) scans, PET scans can image active regional brain metabolism. PET apparatus is expensive and relatively uncommon; thus, few investigations of alcoholic patients using this methodology have thus far been conducted. Some preliminary PET research has detected lower glucose metabolism in the medial prefrontal and temporal cortex, the thalamus and basal ganglia of Korsakoff syndrome alcoholics (Kessley *et al.*, 1984).

Regional cerebral blood flow

Cerebral blood flow (CBF) and regional cerebral blood flow (rCBF) studies directly measure cerebral activity and show high correlation with brain oxygen consumption (Berglund, 1981). The utility of CBF and rCBF to localize the effects of alcoholism has been reviewed by Berglund (1981), who notes the effects of ethanol toxicity (Table V.3).

Wernicke–Korsakoff syndrome

Wernicke–Korsakoff syndrome is a brain disorder produced by a thiamine-deficient diet, a condition which produces destruction of brain tissue in the midbrain surrounding the third ventricle. The syndrome is believed to result from the alcoholic's increasing reliance on ethanol as a primary, non-nutritive calorie source. While only a small percentage (under 10%) of hospitalized alcoholics will present with neurological and

TABLE V.3. Review of CBF and rCBF effects of alcoholism.

1. CBF decreased in Wernicke's encephalopathy
2. CBF shows large variability of flow in Korsakoff's psychosis
3. Normal CBF in "average alcoholic" but alcholics with DTs and physical illness may have lowered CBF
4. Possible accelerated reduction in CBF as a function of aging in alcoholics over 50 years old
5. Reduced mean hemispheric blood flow does not improve after the first week of abstinence in most alcoholics; after 3 weeks of abstinence "there are hardly any changes"
6. Regional CBF has also been found to positively correlate with neuropsychological test scores.

Source: Berglund (1981).

neuropsychological symptoms of Wernicke–Korsakoff syndrome, the syndrome is of theoretical interest because it is one of the few consequences of alcoholism that is well understood; extensive neuropsychological and neuropathological investigations have been performed on victims of this syndrome.

Wernicke–Korsakoff syndrome is also almost certainly more common than hospital statistics would suggest. Harper (1983) found that 80% of patients with features of Wernicke–Korsakoff syndrome were diagnosed during autopsy rather than during life. Harper, Giles and Finlay-Jones (1986) argue that many cases are missed because conventional diagnostic criteria for this disorder are too strict, and would identify only 30 out of 200 potentially diagnosable cases in their city each year.

Wernicke's encephalopathy

The clinical course of Wernicke–Korsakoff syndrome occurs in two stages, the initial acute phase of which is called ''Wernicke's encephalopathy'', a disorder that can be fatal if left untreated. Carl Wernicke first observed this neurological syndrome in 1881. Diagnosis, then as now, is made by history and clinical observation of pathognomonic symptoms, the most common of which are related to impairments in higher mental functions and consciousness (Harper, Giles and Finlay-Jones, 1986). The classic ''Wernicke's triad'' of ataxia, ophthalmoplegia and memory deficit has been cited as diagnostic by Victor, Adams and Collins (1971), although Harper, Giles and Finlay-Jones (1986) suggest that all three signs are ''by no means invariably present'' in these patients (p. 344). Other common peripheral and central nervous system abnormalities have been reported, including polyneuropathy of the arms and legs (Victor, Adams and Collin, 1971), a confusional and/or obtunded state, apathy and an inability to maintain spontaneous conversation. If treated with large doses of thiamine at this point, the patient may show some evidence of improvement after several weeks, although only about 25% of Wernicke's patients are said eventually to recover to premorbid levels of cognitive functioning (Victor, Adams and Collins, 1971). Wernicke's encephalopathy has been induced by other thiamine-deficient etiologies, including hyperemesis gravidarum (prolonged vomiting during pregnancy), anorexia nervosa and gastrointestinal disorders that interfere with vitamin absorption. Alcoholics, however, are by far the group most at risk for developing the syndrome (Hartman, Sweet and Elvart, 1985).

Wernicke's encephalopathy is probably more common among alcoholics than diagnostic statistics would indicate. Torvik and Lindboe (1982) found that only three of 68 cases of Wernicke's encephalopathy diagnosed at autopsy had been suspected prior to death. The neuropathology of Harper's (1979) patient group was similarly underestimated. Only 17 out of 51 cases of Wernicke's encephalopathy were diagnosed before autopsy.

Korsakoff's syndrome

About 6 years after Carl Wernicke's research had been published, S. S. Korsakoff published a number of papers that detailed amnesic and confabulatory symptoms of the disease which came to bear his name. In current use, a "Korsakoff syndrome" denotes the chronic residual symptoms of Wernicke's encephalopathy, most commonly confabulation and a severe anterograde amnesia, or the inability to learn new information, dating from the time of illness.

Neuropsychological investigations of Wernicke–Korsakoff syndrome

Severe anterograde amnesia has also been extensively documented in neuropsychological research. Reviewing the research of his colleagues, Butters (1985) finds that Korsakoff patients are virtually unable to learn short lists of paired associates, or retain even three words in memory for 9 seconds if a distractor task intervenes. He notes that susceptibility to distractors during rehearsal is particularly characteristic of Korsakoff patients.

The extensive neuropsychological investigations that have been performed on Wernicke-Korsakoff patients have been reviewed by Brandt and Butters (1986). These authors note characteristic patterns of neuropsychological functioning in Korsakoff alcoholics. For example, overall IQ scores of these patients are stated to be "indistinguishable" from education, age and socioeconomic class-matched controls (Brandt and Butters, 1986, p. 456). While the WAIS-R Digit Symbol subtest score is low, Digit Span is normal.

Other neuropsychological tests detect the patterns of neuropsychological dysfunction in Korsakoff's syndrome far more sensitively than IQ tests. For example, Wechsler Memory Scale (WMS) scores are severely depressed and may be 20–30 points below IQ score (Butters and Cermak, 1976). Logical

Memory, Figural Memory and Associate Learning are the most sensitive measures, within the WMS, to Korsakoff syndrome. Further, given Korsakoff syndrome patients' susceptibility to distractors, Russell's (1975) modification of the WMS to include incidental delayed $\frac{1}{2}$-hour recall of the Logical and Figural Memory subtests would make the WMS even more sensitive to Korsakoff syndrome memory deficit.

Other neuropsychological impairments of Korsakoff patients may be found on tests having constructional or visuospatial components, including the Tactual Performance Test, and tests containing embedded figures. Tests of planning, categorization and rule learning (e.g. the Wisconsin Card Sorting Test and the Category Test) are also impaired.

Wernicke–Korsakoff patients compared to chronic alcoholics without Wernicke–Korsakoff syndrome

What is the relationship between chronic alcoholism with and without Wernicke-Korsakoff syndrome? Butters (1985) outlines the similarities and differences. Both groups are poor performers in problem-solving tasks and tests involving abstract reasoning. Visuoperceptual deficits are also common to both types of patients.

However, Korsakoff patients show much more severe anterograde amnesia than chronic alcoholics without this syndrome. The quality of recall in experimental tests is also different between the two groups. While Korsakoff patients tend to produce intra-list intrusions of words (proactive interference) from previous lists, chronic alcoholics without Korsakoff's make errors of omission.

Wilkinson and Carlen (1980c) compared the neuropsychological performance of Wernicke's alcoholics with other, non-amnesic alcoholics on the Wechsler Memory Scale (WMS), the WAIS (IQ) and a modified Halstead Reitan battery. The two groups were most consistently differentiated by the WMS, all of whose subtests except Mental Control were significantly different between groups. Digit Symbol from the WAIS and TPT-Memory were the only other tests significantly different between groups, although several other scores, including Category Test and Trails B were above standard impairment cutoffs.

Such results cast doubt on the validity of the "continuity hypothesis" originally proposed by Ryback (1971), which implied that Korsakoff syndrome could be the end-product of chronic alcoholism. The continuity hypothesis suggests that neuropsychological deficits shown by Korsakoff patients are part of a continuum of cognitive decline as a function of alcohol quantity, frequency of use and years of intoxication. Thus, for the continuity hypothesis to be supported, a similar, though less severe, pattern of "pre-Korsakoff" deficits should be seen earlier in chronic alcoholics' drinking histories.

Butters (1985) argues that such pre-Korsakoff patterns have *not* been found in alcoholics without Korsakoff's syndrome. While certain cognitive abilities do show continual decline during the course of chronic alcoholism, these functions have been localized to the *association cortex* rather than to the *subcortical* areas involved in memory and learning. Neuropsychological studies do not indicate that subcortical structures gradually decline to the degree of Korsakoff impairments; chronic alcoholics without Korsakoff's syndrome are not nearly as severely impaired in memory functions as Korsakoff patients. The impairments of these latter patients may best be understood as to consequence of acute trauma (vitamin B_1 deficiency) superimposed on the chronic traumata of long-term alcohol abuse. Thus, available evidence does not support the continuity hypothesis. Instead, separate but possibly additive effects of chronic alcoholism with and without Wernicke–Korsakoff syndrome have been found.

CHRONIC ALCOHOLISM WITHOUT WERNICKE–KORSAKOFF SYNDROME

Alcohol exerts direct toxic effects on the brain beyond those caused by vitamin depletion. These effects have been shown on autopsy, CT scans, cerebral blood flow studies and neuropsychological test results. For example, Harper and Kril (1985) autopsied the brains of controls, alcoholics, alcoholics with Wernicke's encephalopathy and alcoholics with liver disease. Using an index of cerebral atrophy the authors estimated a mean loss of 41 g brain tissue in the alcoholic group, 89 g in the Wernicke's sample and 109 g in the group with both alcoholism and liver disease. Alcoholics who show loss of cerebral tissue may do so in the absence of other alcohol-related organ pathology. A CT examination of alcoholics with no clinical evidence of liver disease revealed significantly greater cerebral atrophy than was present in an age-matched control group (Carlen *et al.*, 1981). However, neuropsychological performance is not simply an additive combination of cerebral atrophy and liver disease. There are many other variables that also appear to influence the neuropsychological performance of alcoholics.

Factors influencing the neuropsychological performance of alcoholics

Recent neuropsychological investigations have strongly emphasized the multifactorial nature of alcohol-related neuropsychological impairments (Tarter and Edwards, 1986; Eckardt and Martin, 1986; Alterman and Tarter, 1985). Many previously unidentified subject variables have been found to influence neuropsychological performance of alcoholic individuals;

variables which strongly suggest that familial, genetic and indirect environmental and physical concomitants of alcohol abuse may be as likely to be associated with neuropsychological impairments as is actual alcohol-caused brain damage. Grant's (1987, p. 320) flow chart captures the complex interplay of influences related to the neuropsychology of alcoholism (Fig. V.1).

For the neuropsychological researcher, the knowledge that alcohol effects are multifactorial may cause re-evaluation of existing research; many early studies which equated impaired neuropsychological performance with alcohol use may have been influenced by one or more of these pre-existing or concomitant variables, and not necessarily by the direct toxic effects of alcohol on the nervous system. For the clinician involved in the assessment of alcoholism, the many new variables found to be related to neuro-psychological performance should spur an increase in data collection of these variables, and at the same time should temper any tendencies to make direct causative inferences about any single influence of alcohol upon observed neuropsychological performance.

Age

'Premature aging' versus independent decrement

The effects of age upon neuropsychological performance are inherently complex, and made more so by the chronic assault on the nervous system by alcohol. Several studies have noted that chronic alcoholics tend to perform neuropsychological tasks at a level more appropriate to the norms of older intact subjects. The basic theory, called "premature aging", makes ambiguous performance predictions and other authors (i.e. Noonberg, Goldstein and Page, 1985) have suggested alternatives. The following alternatives have been proposed.

1. *Premature aging.* The basic theory proposed by Ryan and Butters (1980), which suggests that the neuropsychological performance of chronic alcoholics will resemble older non-alcoholic controls.
2. *Accelerated aging.* A variant of the premature aging hypothesis which hypothesizes that alcoholic performance and underlying neuropathology may occur at any age following an appropriately long and intensive drinking history. Thus, alcoholics will perform more poorly compared to controls at any point across the life span.
3. *Increased vulnerability.* A second variant of the premature aging hypothesis which predicts younger alcoholics are less vulnerable or temporarily protected from the neuropsychological dysfunctions of alcoholism. Deficits may occur in these subjects with increasing age and consequent neuronal depletion (Noonberg, Goldstein and Page, 1985). This hypothesis would predict a fan-shaped interaction between aging and

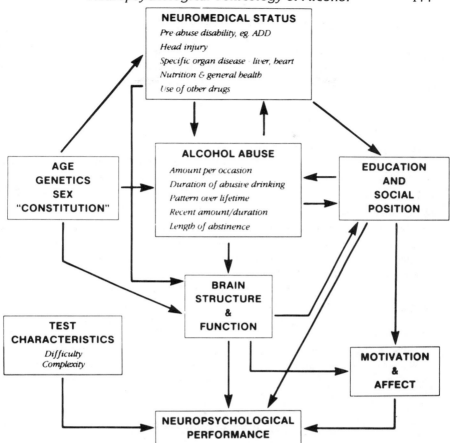

FIGURE V.1. Variables to consider in any causal model of alcohol-associated neuro-psychological deficit. ADD = attention deficit disorder. (Reprinted, by permission of the author, from Grant, I. Alcohol and the Brain: Neuropsychological correlates. *Journal of Consulting and Clinical Psychology,* **55:** 310–324. Copyright 1987 by The American Psychological Association.)

alcoholism. "Novice" alcoholics would initially look like their neuropsychological controls, but the two groups would gradually diverge, with alcoholics becoming increasingly poorer performers compared to controls as a function of age and drinking history.

4. *Independent decrement.* Alcohol and age affect cognitive functioning differently. These effects may or may not overlap.

Support for "accelerated aging" or independent decrements in alcoholics could be extrapolated from several studies, including the original study performed by Ryan and Butters (1980). The authors administered a battery of neuropsychological tests to detoxified younger (34–49) and older (50–59) alcoholics and controls. In several learning and memory tests, including the Symbol Digit Test, a four-word short-term memory test and a paired associate learning test, the younger alcoholics performed more like the older controls than their age-matched non-alcoholic peers. No interactions were observed between age and alcohol impairments. A study by Brandt *et al.* (1983) also found effects of alcohol and of age, but no interaction, suggesting independent decrements from each variable.

Independent decrement effects could be differentiated from premature aging if there was evidence of different patterns of functioning in old alcoholics compared with old controls. One study found such differences in behavior between normal old adults and alcoholics; the former but not the latter showed psychomotor and attentional difficulties (Grant, Adams and Reed, 1984). Reige *et al.* (1984) also found results consistent with independent effects of age and alcoholism. In tests of verbal and nonverbal memory, older alcoholics did not perform to the same pattern as controls, but were distinguished by deficits in auditorily presented memory stimuli. Younger alcoholics were statistically indistinguishable from their non-alcoholic "social-drinking" controls.

Finally, other types of evidence suggests the independence of aging and alcoholism effects. First, severe memory deficits of alcoholic etiology (e.g. Wernicke–Korsakoff syndrome) do not have any equivalent in the normal aging brain. Second, alcoholics make more frequent self-reports of cognitive errors than do non-alcoholics, suggesting potentially different introspective capacities in the two groups. Finally, Brandt *et al.* (1983) suggest that older non-alcoholic patients show naming difficulties not found in middle-aged alcoholics, while older alcoholics have much more pronounced nonverbal learning impairments than elderly control subjects.

To summarize, most current evidence appears to favor the effects of alcohol and age as independent decrements upon neuropsychological performance. That these factors separately impair behavior does not, however, obviate the possibility of additive or synergistic effects.

Onset of impairment

The age at which neuropsychological deficits begin to appear is an issue with serious social, political and clinical implications. For example, when Grant, Adams and Reed (1978) investigated alcoholics in their 30s with a 6-year drinking history, and found no deficits compared to controls, their results were criticized for minimizing the serious effects of alcohol abuse and other concerns (Eckardt, Ryback and Pautler, 1980). In addition the study has been criticized for its overly strict selection criteria, since subjects with mild residual organic brain syndrome were eliminated (Parsons and Farr, 1981).

Other investigations of alcoholics in their 30s have found results contrary to Grant, Adams and Reed (1978). Noonberg, Goldstein and Page (1985) evaluated alcoholics in their mid-30s, with the Brain Age Quotient (BAQ) battery, a collection of neuropsychological tests which included the Category Test, Tactual Performance Test and Trails B from the Halstead-Reitan Battery, and Block Design and Digit Symbol Tests from the WAIS. Even the youngest group of alcoholics performed more poorly on the BAQ than did their age-matched peers. Eckardt, Ryback and Pautler (1980) also compared neuropsychological performance of alcoholic males in their mid-30s on 24 neuropsychological measures. Subjects' primary diagnosis was alcoholism with no secondary psychiatric disorder. Those who were tested from 2 to 6 days after their last drink showed impaired levels of functioning on 13 of the 24 tests administered. A second group examined after 14–31 days of abstinence were impaired on 11 of the 24 tests. An all-possible-subsets regression analysis on the first (acute) group showed, when drinking variables were removed, that amount of alcohol consumption was related to 70% of the variance. Age contributed an additional 20% and education another 10%. Patients in this study had significantly longer drinking histories with significantly greater alcohol intake than those in the Grant, Adams and Reed (1978) study, which may account for the differences between the two studies.

Drinking pattern

There are conflicting findings about the influence of drinking pattern on neuropsychological performance. Specifically, the debate revolves around whether neuropsychological decrements are a function of amount consumed per sitting, recent drinking pattern or lifetime alcohol consumption. Svanum and Schladenhauffen (1986) examined 40 inpatient detoxified alcoholics to determine whether recent drinking pattern or lifetime consumption accounted for Halstead–Reitan testing scores. Drinking pattern proved to be as important as duration in accounting for neuropsychological deficits. Tarbox, Connors and McLaughlin (1986) compared daily drinkers (5 or more days a week) to "bout" drinkers (drinking for days, weeks or months with intervening abstinence). Bout drinkers scored significantly higher on age-corrected performance IQ measures as well as Wechsler Memory Scale Mental Control and Digit Span tests. Post hoc comparisons also found older bout drinkers performed better than older daily drinkers across neuropsychological tests.

Drinking history

Early drinking onset has been associated with greater social maladjustment (Lee and DiClimente, 1985) as well as neuropsychological impairment.

Pishkin, Lovallo and Bourne (1985) investigated the influence of both age of onset and years of drinking. Older controls and late-onset alcoholics performed significantly better than younger, early-onset alcoholics on the Shipley–Hartford test. The authors concluded that early-onset alcoholism is particularly likely to result in eventual cognitive impairment. It is equally likely, however, that younger alcoholics may be more predisposed to neuropsychological deficits because of the same premorbid factors which elicited early use of alcohol.

Familial factors

Several current studies suggest that non-alcoholic relatives or family members of alcoholics may themselves have neuropsychological deficits. Schaeffer, Parsons and Yohman (1984) found males with an alcoholic close relative to perform significantly less well on verbal and nonverbal abstraction and perceptual-motor tasks than did the matched controls without an alcoholic relative. Another group of papers by Alterman and his colleagues suggest that other familial factors should be considered. For example, Alterman and Tarter (1983) reviewed possible genetic factors related to alcoholism and concluded that histories of childhood hyperactivity (with presumed attentional deficits and low impulse control) may be a factor in poorer neuropsychological performance among alcoholics. Another study presents data which suggest that children of alcoholic fathers exhibit learning and neuropsychological difficulties compared to children of non-alcoholic parents (Tarter *et al.*, 1984). Finally, studies which find impairments among young alcoholics may be consistent with either pre-existing cognitive deficit or subtle neuropsychological insult. The study of Alterman *et al.* (1984), which examined 30-year-old male alcoholics, would fall into this category. Subjects showed significantly impaired performance on tasks which required organization, sequencing and sustained goal-directed behavior (Alterman *et al.* 1984).

Handedness

Handedness is another variable which has been suggested to correlate with alcoholism. Studies by London (1985) suggest that larger percentages of alcoholics are left-handed than is true for the general population (17–39% versus 10%). In addition, significantly fewer left-handed alcoholics were classified as "improved" after 1 year (29% versus 56%). While other factors, such as small sample size or having an alcoholic father, may equally explain London's results, other studies not specifically investigating the effects of alcoholism have linked certain kinds of left-handedness to minimal brain dysfunction or subtle neurological disability (e.g. Geschwind and Behan,

1982). It is possible that whatever mediating variables create this form of pathological left-handedness may also increase the likelihood of developing alcoholism.

Hepatic dysfunction

Several studies suggest that alcoholic liver disease may be related to brain damage and neuropsychological dysfunction. Acker *et al.* (1982) found that cerebral atrophy covaried with liver disease. Two studies suggest that EEG abnormalities are worse in cirrhotic alcoholics than those without liver disease (Kardel and Stigsby, 1975; Kardel *et al.*, 1972). Cirrhosis without alcoholism may cause neuropsychological difficulties that are similar to those of alcoholics (Tarter *et al.*, 1983).

In what may eventually prove to be a landmark study in the neuropsychology of alcoholism, Tarter *et al.* (1986) examined the neuropsychological performance of 15 subjects whose alcoholism was confirmed by the most direct evidence possible; all subjects received a diagnosis of Laennec's cirrhosis after liver biopsy. Subjects had been detoxified before their most recent hospital admission and all had been abstinent for 2 months or more.

The authors found that abnormalities of hepatic biochemistry in a large neuropsychological battery accounted for between 23% and 56% of the variance depending on the particular combination of biochemical measure and neuropsychological test score (Tarter *et al.*, 1986; Table V.4). Without longitudinal data and corresponding neurological test results (e.g. CT, MR scan), it is not possible to determine whether liver and other biochemical abnormalities *cause* neuropsychological impairment, or whether abnormal liver enzymes simply correlate well with concurrent neuropathology. Until definitive research answers the question, neuropsychologists may wish to be more cautious in their attempts to attribute the neuropsychological effects of alcoholism to brain abnormalities on the basis of psychometric test data alone. This area of study also awaits larger replications and follow-up research designs to examine subjects over time and determine reversibility.

Psychopathology

Neuropsychological deficits shown by alcoholics are often clinically paired with emotional disturbance and serious psychosocial problems. The relation between this toxic brain disturbance and emotional functioning remains obscure. Løberg's (1986) review of the literature concluded there is "no uniform alcoholic personality" (p. 431), although it suggests the possibility that demographically similar groups of alcoholics may also have consistent profiles and that these profiles, in turn, may be related to neuropsychological

TABLE V.4. Correlation between liver function variables and neuropsychological test performance.

Neuropsychological test	LIVER/FUNCTION								
	Alanine transaminase	Aspartate transaminase	Alkaline phosphatase	Bilirubin direct	Albumin	Globulin	Prothrombin time	Indocyanine green serum (level at 20 min)	Fasting plasma ammonia level
Digit Span Plus One					-0.51*			0.62*	0.66*
Fluency		-0.55*	0.48*				-0.49*		
Confrontation Naming	-0.50*								
TPT-Memory	-0.72**					-0.74*			-0.84**
TPT-Location	-0.54*							-0.71*	
Raven's Matrices IQ		-0.53*							
Visual Memory							-0.71**		
Logical Memory — Delayed				-0.49*					
Trail Making Test	0.57*						0.51*		
Star Drawing Test — Errors									0.59*
Purdue Pegboard			0.62**						

*p < 0.05; **p. < 0.01

Source: Tarter et al. (1986) p. 76.

measures. Future research may also extend the investigations of depression and neuropsychological deficit (e.g. Fisher, Sweet and Pfaelzer-Smith, 1986; Newman and Sweet, 1986) to alcoholic populations. It is unclear how other forms of affect alter neuropsychological performance; for example, the anxiety states so commonly noted in alcoholics. There is very little research that addresses these potential sources of variance in neuropsychological performance (Alterman and Tarter, 1985).

Head trauma

Recent studies suggest that alcoholic individuals with a family history of alcoholism are twice as likely to have a history of significant head trauma than non-familial alcoholics (Tarter and Edwards, 1986). Moreover, in general, the social and environmental context of alcoholism leads to increased risk of head injury. Thus, some observed neuropsychological deficits may be in part or whole the effect of exogenous brain injury rather than endogenous toxic assault.

Gender

Acker (1986) compared male and female alcoholics' performance on a variety of neuropsychological tests including Logical Memory, Benton Visual Retention, Trails, Digit Span and an automated battery of neuropsychological tests. She found female alcoholics to show greater impairment than males, on immediate recall, psychomotor speed, abstract reasoning and visuoperceptual tasks. Acker suggests that females may be more sensitive than males to neuropsychological effects of alcohol for an equivalent amount of drinking; however, since her study lacks statistical comparison with female non-alcoholic controls, her findings cannot discriminate between alcohol-based and premorbid sex differences in the abilities she suggested were impaired.

Support for a non-alcoholic explanation of Acker's results could be extrapolated from the results of Fabian, Jenkins and Parsons (1981), who administered the Tactual Performance Test (TPT) to four groups of subjects; male and female alcoholics were compared to male and female non-alcoholic controls matched for age and education. There were main effects for both gender and memory, as women remembered more shapes but localized fewer of them than men. There was a main effect for alcoholism but not for gender in TPT completion time, with the alcoholic group performing more slowly than controls. Thus, the study indicates effects of alcoholism and effects of gender, but no interaction between the two. The lack of interaction supports the existence of premorbid processing differences.

One recent study does provide some support for differential vulnerability to alcohol in women. Hannon *et al.* (1985) found that amount of alcohol consumed was significantly related to an increased number of total errors on the Category Test, an effect not found for men. The Hannon *et al.* (1985) study awaits replication.

Finally, results suggesting an opposite conclusion were obtained by Silberstein and Parson (1979), who found that alcoholic women were *less* impaired on visuoconstructive tasks than were men.

In summary, theoretical arguments for differential vulnerability of women to alcohol can be made, including differing degrees of cerebral lateralization, lower body mass (and hence higher blood alcohol levels for a given number of drinks) or otherwise unspecified sex-related differences in processing alcohol. However, available studies on gender differences have thus far failed to verify any of these hypotheses. Currently there is no consistent evidence for differential vulnerability to alcohol or a unique pattern of neuropsychological effects due to gender.

WHICH TESTS SHOW IMPAIRMENT?

The neuropsychological complexities of alcoholism make it understandable that testing methods be similarly multifactorial. Almost every neuropsychological test or test battery has at one time been investigated for its sensitivity to the effects of alcoholism. As is the case with other neurotoxins, not all neuropsychological tests are equally sensitive to the effects of alcohol. Those which have been found to be impaired typically assess a common set of functions. These include abstract reasoning, visuospatial abilities, memory and cognitive flexibility. Not surprisingly, test batteries which load heavily on these abilities have also been shown to be sensitive indicators of alcoholic effects.

Individual tests

Abstract reasoning

Loss of ability to form hypotheses and reason abstractly has been a frequent finding among alcoholic subjects. Tests of abstract reasoning shown to be consistently impaired have included the Category Test. For example, Jones and Parsons (1971) found alcoholics to perform significantly more poorly on the Category Test but not on the Shipley–Hartford test of verbal abstraction. Alcoholics had "normal and surprisingly good performance" on the Purdue Pegboard, Finger Tapping and Grip Strength, leading the authors to speculate about a prefrontal cortical or subcortical locus. An elaboration of this study published a year later successfully replicated Jones and Parsons' (1971) findings on the Category and Shipley–Hartford (Jones and Parsons, 1972). Alcoholics also performed more poorly than controls on the Raven's Progressive Matrices, but not on the Embedded Figures Test. The authors suggest their results are interpretable as a deficit in visuospatial concept formation, possibly coupled with defective visual scanning. In a later study another test of abstract reasoning, the Wisconsin Card Sorting Test, was also found to be impaired (Klisz and Parsons, 1979).

Visuospatial tests

There is ample evidence that alcoholics, with and without Wernicke–Korsakoff syndrome, are impaired in tests of spatial abilities. Block Design, Object Assembly and Picture Arrangement subtests of the Wechsler Adult Intelligence Scale (WAIS) were impaired in 70% of the studies reviewed by Parsons and Farr (1981).

Tests of general intelligence (IQ)

IQ test results of alcoholic subjects typically suggest that overall Verbal and Full Scale IQ scores are insensitive to alcohol effects. Performance IQ is much more frequently shown to be impaired, because that section of the WAIS or WAIS-R loads on subtests requiring spatial and constructional functions, nonverbal reasoning, cognitive efficiency and flexibility. Similarity in the pattern of impairments between WAIS subtests and parts of the Halstead–Reitan Neuropsychological Battery have also been noted by Parsons and Farr (1981).

Test batteries

The Halstead-Reitan Neuropsychological Battery

A great number of neuropsychological investigations with alcoholics have used the Halstead–Reitan Neuropsychological Battery (HRB) (Løberg, 1986). Deterioration of Halstead–Reitan performance with respect to controls or to relevant age norms is a usual finding. Parsons and Farr (1981) observed that chronic alcoholics share a pattern on the WAIS and the Halstead–Reitan Neuropsychological Battery that is similar to, albeit not as great as, that of brain-damaged and aged non-alcoholics. Parsons and Farr (1981) concluded that alcoholics exhibit consistently poor performance on three HRB subtests. Impairment reached 87% on the Category Test, 73% on Trails B and 62% on Tactual Performance Test—Localization in the studies they reviewed. Fabian, Jenkins and Parsons (1981) further elaborated a specific pattern of performance on the Tactual Performance Test that appears to be specific to alcoholics. Unlike controls, alcoholic subjects failed to improve their performance times on the second trial using the non-dominant hand. In addition, alcoholic subjects improved more than controls from the second to the third trial (both hands). The authors hypothesize that right hemisphere dysfunction, or perhaps disruption of less well-established behaviors, may explain this pattern of TPT performance (Fabian, Jenkins and Parsons, 1981).

The Luria-Nebraska Neuropsychological Battery

Only a few studies have used the more recently developed Luria–Nebraska Neuropsychological Battery (LNNB) (Golden, Hammeke and Purisch, 1980) to investigate the effects of alcoholism. One such study was performed by Obaldia, Leber and Parsons (1981), who examined 30 male alcoholics. Half were in the acute phase of detoxification between 2 and 3 weeks after hospital admission, the other half between 10 to 12 weeks post-admission. The alcoholic groups were compared against a group of age-and education-matched controls recruited from the community. Controls were significantly superior to both alcoholic groups on every LNNB scale except reading. Only the Rhythm scale (Scale 2) differentiated the alcoholics in the acute phase of detoxification from those 8–10 weeks later.

Despite the ability of the LNNB to differentiate the two groups statistically, it was apparently not an especially sensitive clinical measure. For example, the mean T-score of the *alcoholics* on the Luria–Nebraska was about T50. Using Golden's cutoffs for "brain damage" only 50% of the alcoholics were identified, suggesting either that the alcoholic groups employed by De Obaldia, Leber and Parsons (1981), were not especially impaired, or that the LNNB may not be as sensitive as the Halstead–Reitan in detecting alcohol-related impairment.

Results from the few other studies using the LNNB on an alcoholic population suggest the latter possibility. For example, Chmielewski and Golden (1980) found six impaired scales in alcoholics relative to controls: Visual, Receptive Speech, Arithmetic, Memory, Intelligence and the Pathognomonic Scale. However, just as in the De Obaldia, Leber and Parsons (1981) study, Chmielewski and Golden (1980) differentiated controls from alcoholics on several scales, but failed to show significant clinical elevations in themselves; with the exception of one scale (Pathognomonic) all scales were below T60. Also, as in De Obaldia, Leber and Parsons (1981), Chmielewski and Golden (1980) were led to conclude that "the brain is fairly resilient to the effects of alcohol" (p. 103), a supposition that does not seem to be supported by the more extensive Halstead–Reitan alcoholism literature.

Finally, a third research report (Rebeta *et al.*, 1986) described testing of 100 male V.A. alcoholics using the LNNB and finding no association between drinking variables and LNNB scale scores when age, education and SES effects were factored out.

Thus, available studies do not support the clinical use of the LNNB to test for impairment of alcoholic etiology. The Halstead–Reitan battery appears to have a clear advantage over the LNNB for testing alcoholics for several reasons. First, the few available studies using the LNNB have reported inconsistent results and pattern elevations (e.g. Rhythm scale in one study, six scales but *not* including Rhythm on another and no elevations on a third). In contrast, the extensive HRB literature shows fairly consistent impairments on the Category, TPT and Trails tests. Second, while alcoholics may be clinically differentiated from controls on the LNNB, their actual level of performance is not generally in the range of clinically meaningful impairment using Golden's cutoffs. HRB-tested alcoholics more often fall into a range of clinical impairment using widely accepted cutoffs, both for specific tests and for the battery as a whole (i.e. Impairment Index).

In conclusion, although hit rates for detecting structural brain abnormalities have been suggested to be comparable between the Luria–Nebraska and the Halstead–Reitan, the two batteries nevertheless appear to show differential sensitivity to alcoholism. The Halstead–Reitan loads more heavily on neuropsychological functions that are difficult for alcoholics, including sustained attention, abstraction and complex perceptual processes. By contrast, the Luria–Nebraska emphasizes discrete simple tasks which are heavily mediated by verbal functions that have been shown to be resistant to alcohol effects.

RECOVERY OF FUNCTION

Tracking recovery of neuropsychological functions is difficult, not only because improvement is not uniform across abilities, but for the same reasons that determining precise etiology of neuropsychological impairments in alcoholics is difficult. Alcoholism, in its etiology as well as its pattern of recovery, is a multifactorial syndrome (Goldman, 1986). Drinking pattern and severity, degree of abstinence, age, education, emotional status and drug use are just a few of the factors capable of influencing recovery. Other variables related to alcoholic recovery include one's particular definition of "recovery" and the time at which recovery is assessed.

Neurological recovery

Carlen and Wilkinson (1980) studied the recovery of 122 chronic alcoholics with at least a 10-year history who were admitted to an inpatient treatment center. Over the course of a 6-week study, the authors found continuing neurological improvement on "simple standardized neurological testing" with a "rapid drop during the first 5 weeks" (p. 109). The authors note that practice may have improved performance somewhat, but cite other studies which controlled for practice that have also shown significant improvement. Carlen and Wilkinson's results may not apply to the most severely impaired alcoholics since these patients were excluded from the study.

CT scan

Initial assessment of recently abstinent alcoholics reveals cortical atrophy (Wilkinson and Carlen, 1980a,b). Carlen *et al.* (1978) demonstrated some reversal of atrophy in four of eight patients examined with CT. A later extension of the study, using more patients, did not confirm results of the initial study. However, alcoholics who claimed abstinence during the inter-test interval had a significant negative correlation between age and sulcal measurements, while non-abstinent alcoholics showed no correlation between age and sulci, suggesting the possibility that younger abstinent alcoholics show acute recovery while older alcoholics do not.

Ron (1983) performed follow-up CTs on 56 of her original 100 alcoholic patients at periods ranging from 30 to 152 weeks. Patients were divided according to their drinking history into abstinent and non-abstinent groups. Initial CT examination showed no significant radiological differences between these subgroups. On follow-up no significant CT differences were found between these groups, although "trends toward lessened sulcal and Sylvian fissure widths" were found in the abstinent group (Ron, 1983, p. 20). In addition, the alcoholics rated as abstinent showed significantly smaller ventricles at follow-up, in contrast to the non-abstinent group who failed to improve. The meaning of this finding is obscured by the fact that the abstinent group showed a trend toward larger ventricles upon initial testing. Thus, the "improvement" may be artifactual. When Ron analyzed the results of individual patients, five of the seven rated to be improved at follow-up were abstainers, while only one of five in the deteriorated-at-follow-up group claimed abstinence.

The evidence for alcoholic recovery on CT is complicated by questionable alcohol history self-reports, inability to exactly reproduce prior head positions in follow-up CT evaluation, sample attrition, and an unknown proportion of variance contributed by other factors correlated with alcoholism. Perhaps the best conclusion that can be made about CT data at this time is that while abstinence will not *necessarily* produce structural recovery that is viewable on CT, such recovery is far more likely to be observed during abstinence than if drinking continues. There is no evidence to suggest that CT scans of non-abstinent alcoholics improve with time.

Regional cerebral blood flow

Berglund *et al.* (1980) studied recovery during the first 7 weeks of alcoholism using measurements of global and regional cerebral blood flow. Mean cerebral blood flow remained stable after the first week of abstinence. Within the first 2 days of abstinence an average 20% decrease in cerebral blood flow was found, a result Goldman (1983) associates with ionic imbalance. Significant increases in regional blood flow subsequently occurred in the upper frontal and parieto-occipital regions of the right hemisphere. The right temporal region showed significantly decreased blood flow compared to the left. The authors found recovery of rCBF in the frontal and anterior temporal cortex to be associated with improved performance on the Koh's block and Trails B neuropsychological tests.

Berglund (1981) summarizes rCBF relationships to recovery as follows:

1. Mean hemispheric blood flow in most patients is not reversible after one abstinent week, although a minority of patients will show partial recovery during the first few weeks.
2. Relative reductions of blood flow in lower frontal regions without changes in mean hemispheric flow may be "related to reversibility of impaired spatial ability" (p. 298).
3. Older alcoholics show larger reductions of blood flow in lower frontal regions compared to younger alcoholics.
4. Wernicke–Korsakoff alcoholics may also show recovery of cerebral blood flow "but . . . the flow normalization probably takes more than a few weeks in many patients" (p. 298).

Neuropsychological recovery

There are many types of neuropsychological deficits identified in alcoholics, including impairments in motor abilities, perception, verbal and nonverbal abstract reasoning, conceptual shifting and memory. Recovery from such impairments is dependent upon many factors. First, the pattern of neuropsychological recovery is not uniform; some abilities return completely while others may fail to improve significantly above initial levels of impairment. Second, recovery of neuropsychological functions appears to depend upon remaining abstinent; neuropsychological improvements noted in alcoholics who have maintained sobriety do not occur in alcoholics who continue to drink (Guthrie, 1980).

Acute neuropsychological recovery

Short-term (under 6-month) recovery has been summarized by Goldman (1986), who finds that while alcoholics continue to show impairments on the Halstead-Reitan neuropsychological battery during their first week of treatment they show some improvement over the next 2–3 weeks and then remain at that level. They do not become "fully normal" even at 6 months after the last drink (Goldman, 1986, p. 137).

Interaction of recovery with age

There are several reasons to believe that alcoholics' neuropsychological recovery may interact with age. First, older drinkers may simply have a longer history of alcoholism. Second, aging alcoholics may have developed other direct and indirect consequences of alcohol abuse, including

TABLE V.5. Time course of neuropsychological test recovery for selected tests during the first 6 months of recovery.

TEST OR NEUROPSYCHOLOGICAL FUNCTION	TIME TO RECOVERY AFTER DRINKING CEASES
Halstead–Reitan Battery	Impaired first week; considerable recovery in next 1–2 weeks. Normal levels *not* seen in 6 months.
Vocabulary	Existing vocabulary not affected at any point. Learning new vocabulary severely impaired during first week of abstinence; recovers thereafter.
Verbal Learning	Impaired first week of abstinence, improves thereafter.
Nonverbal (Visuospatial) Learning	Impairment first 2 weeks after drinking cessation, improvement in *younger* alcoholics. Older alcoholics do not improve during first abstinent week.
Cutaneous Pressure Threshold	Significantly impaired during early abstinence. No recovery after 1 month.
Form Discrimination	Impaired during early abstinence. Recovery after 2 weeks.
Bilateral transfer of motor skills (from one hand to the other)	Impaired first week, full recovery 2 weeks after last drink.
Short-term memory	Differential recovery as a function of age. All ages impaired first week after drinking and all ages show improvement after 4 weeks. No further recovery next 4 weeks. Longer studies suggest alcoholics under 40 show full recovery; alcoholics over 40 continue to be impaired regardless of how long they had been drinking previously.
Learning the content of an alcohol treatment program	Little improvement in learning during first month after detoxification.

Source: Summarized from Goldman (1983, 1986).

malnutrition effects, head injuries and hypertension or related vascular injuries (e.g. Altura and Altura, 1984). Finally, loss of brain mass from chronic alcoholism may limit the adaptive capacity of the aging brain to recover completely from chronic toxic assault.

Several studies have suggested that alcoholics over 40 recover neuropsychological function more slowly and less completely than younger alcoholics. For example, in alcoholics with a mean age of 37, Grant, Adams and Reed (1979) showed that those abstinent a minimum of 18 months scored equivalently to matched controls on the Halstead–Reitan battery. Normal performance was maintained upon follow-up 1 year later (Adams, Grant and Reed, 1980). In contrast, Yohman, Parsons and Leber (1985) studied alcoholics with a mean age approximately 11 years older (48) than the Grant, Adams and Reed study. Yohman, Parsons and Leber (1985) found neuropsychological differences in abstracting, perceptual-motor and learning-memory tests to persist 13 months after detoxification.

Goldman, Williams and Klisz (1983) monitored the visuospatial recovery of alcoholics over the course of 3 months. Alcoholics over age 40, while demonstrating some recovery over repeated testings, remained significantly impaired relative to controls or younger alcoholics on Digit Symbol Substitution, Trails B and Grooved Pegboard—dominant hand. Three months of 14 test sessions "were not sufficient to permit full recovery" (p. 373) in the older group. Age, and not years of drinking, was the predominant predictor of neuropsychological test scores for alcoholics. However, as the authors point out, since older controls failed to show impairment, chronic alcoholism must be added to normal aging to account for studies results.

Other factors

Alcoholic recovery interacts not only with age, but with abstinence or other factors. This question was addressed by Grant, Adams and Reed (1984), who compared 4-week abstinent alcoholics with 4-year abstainers and non-alcoholic controls. Results of their factor analysis suggested the existence of independent, non-interactive factors consisting of recency of active drinking and aging. Regression analysis further suggested that age, education and head injury scores contributed to the variance in several factors, although the "number of weeks since the last drink" predictor contributed only about 3–6% of the variance in the various factors. Multivariate analysis of factor scores suggested that recently detoxified alcoholics had significant difficulty in problem-solving and learning new material. Their findings led Grant, Adams and Reed (1984) to suggest that, while alcoholics continue to show neuropsychological impairments at approximately 1 month of abstinence, somewhere between 18 and 48 months, many seem to recover neuropsychological functions.

Long-term recovery

Obvious practical difficulties in maintaining contact with an experimental population and verifying their drinking histories make studies of long-term recovery from alcoholism quite difficult. One of the longest periods to have been investigated was 5 years, in a study by Brandt *et al.* (1983). They compared three groups of alcoholics with progressively longer periods of abstinence, including a "short-term abstinence" group (sober between 1 and 2 months), a "long-term abstinence group" (abstinent from 1 to 3 years) and a "prolonged abstinence" group (who remained alcohol-free for 5 years or more) (p. 439). Age, years of drinking and WAIS vocabulary score were covariates in the analysis.

Time of abstinence had an effect on some neuropsychological measures but not on others. Recovery of function in the prolonged abstinence group equal to the performance level of matched non-alcoholic controls was demonstrated in verbal and visual short-term memory tasks (Four Word STM and Benton Visual Retention Test), and one test of cognitive efficiency and flexibility (Digit Symbol). Another test of efficiency (Symbol Digit Substitution Test) improved over time but failed to return to the controls level, and no recovery was observed in the Symbol Digit Paired Associate Learning Test or the Embedded Figures Test (Brandt *et al.*, 1983). The authors concluded that, while psychomotor and short-term memory may recover with prolonged abstinence, certain neuropsychological functions in the realm of long-term memory may be refractory to recovery.

CONCLUSIONS

Parsons and Farr (1981) concluded in an earlier review of alcohol's neuropsychological effects that it was "impossible to escape" the many variables that can influence the neuropsychological performance of alcoholics. Recent alcoholism research has borne out the validity of that observation. The days are long gone when a direct causal relationship could be assumed between the intake of alcohol and neuropsychological impairment. That simplistic relationship has been replaced by the concept of multiple causation in alcohol-related neuropsychological impairment. Familial, genetic, sociodemographic and biochemical factors have been shown to contribute, sometimes substantially, to the variance tapped by neuropsychological tests. Direct toxicity to the brain, indirect hepatic and circulatory abnormalities, thiamine deficiency, genetic predisposition and even an injury-prone alcoholic lifestyle, have all been shown to affect neuropsychological functioning. Such diverse etiologies await re-synthesis in future models of neuropsychological function in alcoholism.

The individual clinician must, by extension, also be aware of this diversity of factors when evaluating single cases. Detailed clinical history of alcoholic patients may benefit from inclusion of these new factors. These include information on developmental history (e.g. hyperactivity history or family alcoholism), demographic factors, pre-existing or concurrent psychopathology, age, physical disorders (e.g. liver disease), history of head injuries and nutritional status (Alterman and Tarter, 1985).

Future neuropsychological research on alcoholism will undoubtedly become more multidisciplinary as psychologists utilize increasingly accurate brain-imaging and metabolic scans to better validate patterns of impairment shown on neuropsychological tests. The interaction of alcohol with drugs and other toxic substances (e.g. solvents) on neuropsychological performance is another area which deserves increased research attention.

The goal of understanding each and every interaction between alcohol and all of its co-factors is an idealistic one, to say the least. However, the extensive existing corpus of neuropsychological data and ongoing research in these areas can be viewed as paradigmatic of the way in which neuropsychology can contribute to toxicology. Neuropsychologists who wish to become neuropsychological toxicologists need look no further than alcoholism research to appreciate the very real current and potential contributions of neuropsychological methods to the understanding of neurotoxic effects.

VI
Neuropsychological Toxicology of Drugs

PRESCRIPTION DRUGS
ANTIDEPRESSANTS

Antidepressants, especially the tricyclics (e.g. amitriptyline, imipramine, desipramine and doxepin) have several side-effects capable of affecting neuropsychological performance, including tremor and blurred vision. Postural hypotension may also interfere with performance on some neuropsychological tasks.

Several neuropsychological examinations of subjects receiving tricyclics have failed to find significant neuropsychological impairments, either after a single dose (Heimann, Reed and Witt 1968) or extended (6 and 12 weeks) therapy (Kendrick and Post, 1967). In studies finding deviations from baseline performance there appear to be an approximately equal number showing positive and negative effects. For example, Liljequist, Linniola and Mattila (1974) found that nortriptyline slightly worsened Paired-Associate and Digits Backward scores. Legg and Stiff (1976) examined subjects given clinical trials of imipramine for 3 weeks and found significant impairments relative to controls on the Benton Visual Retention Test, the Wechsler Memory Scale—Logical Memory subtest, the WAIS Digit Symbol and prorated Performance IQ. In contrast to Liljequist, Linnoila and Mattila (1974), however, Paired-Associate Test performance was *not* impaired.

Alternatively, Sternberg and Jarvik (1976) found that tricyclics actually *improved* performance of depressed patients on a battery or memory and learning tests.

As can be seen from available results, there is little consistency among neuropsychological researchers as to the effects of antidepressant medications. Possibly, individual differences in cholinergic response to antidepressant medications may prove related to neuropsychological effects. Future investigation may benefit from combined input of neurochemical and neuropsychological data.

194

ANTICHOLINERGICS

Many types of drugs and neurotoxins have anticholinergic properties. Anticholinergic drugs have been used to control tremor in Parkinson's disease, and today are common adjuncts to neuroleptic therapy. Neuroleptic medications, without adjunctive antiparkinsonian agents, have anticholinergic effects. Finally, pesticides have potent anticholinergic properties.

Neuropsychological symptoms of anticholinergic substances can include amnesia and short-term memory deficit. High doses induce toxic states of delirium, agitation, confusional state and hallucinations. Dysarthria and ataxia may also be present (Goetz, 1985). Chronic use of multiple anticholinergic drugs may induce dementia that could be incorrectly ascribed to psychiatric disorder (Moreau, Jones and Banno, 1986).

Neuropsychological reactions to anticholinergic substances receive additional discussion in the sections on neuroleptic medications and pesticides.

ANTICONVULSANTS

Drugs which are administered as antiepileptic agents are commonly prescribed for long periods, if not permanently. Neuropsychological studies of anticonvulsant effects may be difficult to interpret, since they are, *a priori*, administered to patients exhibiting or at risk for significant brain dysfunction. A selected sample of neuropsychological and neuropsychiatric effects of anticonvulsants are described below:

Carbamazepine (Tegretol)

Carbamazepine is commonly prescribed for childhood seizure disorders. Carbamazepine has also been found to have several applications in psychiatry and may prove useful in treating depression, bipolar disorder and as treatment for chronic schizophrenia that has been refractive to neuroleptics. Other possible, although not yet approved, indications for carbamazepine include episodic dyscontrol syndrome and miscellaneous behavioral disorders (Evans and Gualtieri, 1985).

Neurological side-effects of carbamazepine can include mild "drowsiness, vertigo, ataxia, blurred vision and diplopia" which occur in about one-third of patients on this medication (Evans and Gualtieri, 1985, p. 223). Less common effects can include nystagmus, tics and various forms of dyskinesias (Evans and Gualtieri, 1985), or reversible dystonias (Reynolds and Trimble, 1985). Diplopia, an early sign of toxicity, occurs when carbamazepine blood levels exceed the normal range of $5-9\mu g/cc$ (Goetz, 1985). Overdose may cause ataxia, nystagmus, seizures and myoclonus with asterixis.

Reviewing the neuropsychological effects of carbamazepine, Evans and Gualtieri (1985) suggest that both children and adults show higher levels of alertness with carbamazepine compared to other anticonvulsants (i.e. phenytoin or phenobarbital). One study tested patients on a single medication, in a cross-over design, and found that patients performed significantly better on the Stroop Color–Word Test and the Trail-Making Test during a Tegretol trial than during a period of Dilantin (phenytoin) use (Thompson and Trimble, 1982). Patients also performed more efficiently on a digit cancellation task when taking Tegretol, a finding the authors attribute to increased ability to sustain attention. The same study found significantly improved recall for pictures and words in both immediate and delayed recall conditions (Thompson and Trimble, 1982). Evans and Gualtieri (1985) failed to find any well-documented neuropsychological studies of carbamazepine influence on psychomotor performance.

Phenytoin (Dilantin)

Phenytoin has been employed for over 50 years in the treatment of seizure disorder and its efficacy in that regard is undisputed. Phenytoin has also been associated with a variety of neurological abnormalities and neuropsychological deficits.

Neurological effects

Reynolds and Trimble (1985) reviewed evidence for long-term phenytoin toxicity and described both peripheral and central nervous system effects. Phenytoin has been linked to peripheral neuropathy, or at least electrophysiological abnormalities, in about 18% of seizure patients, a clinical result not found in other anticonvulsants (e.g. carbamazepine or sodium valproate). Permanent cerebellar syndrome has been noted in several case studies of phenytoin intoxication, although this outcome appears to be rare. Other less common neurological sequelae of phenytoin include various kinds of dystonia, reversible involuntary movement disorders and asterixis (Reynolds and Trimble, 1985).

Neuropsychological effects

Toxic blood levels of phenytoin have produced encephalopathy, along with common concomitants of nystagmus and ataxia. More recently, researchers have become aware of neuropsychological deficits produced by therapeutic or even subtherapeutic blood levels of phenytoin. One study investigated the effects of phenytoin on normal, non-epileptic volunteers who received either placebo or phenytoin 200 mg. T.I.D. for 2 weeks, in a double-blind, crossover design. Subjects receiving phenytoin showed significantly poorer delayed recall of pictures, made more errors on the

Stroop Color–Word Test and showed impaired ability to decide color or category membership in a choice reaction time task (Thompson, Huppert and Trimble, 1981). In addition, the authors report significant correlations of serum phenytoin level with scores on five neuropsychological tests: immediate and delayed picture recall, reaction times to correctly identify words and pictures and decision-making about color categories. In all cases, performance deteriorated as a function of increasing serum phenytoin level (Thompson, Huppert and Trimble, 1981). The authors rightly caution that results may not necessarily be applicable to chronic users of Dilantin, since short-term administration precludes the investigation of possible tolerance or adaptation. Results are, however, consistent with a later study by some of the same authors. They investigated a group of 28 patients who had been prescribed a variety of anticonvulsants, including phenytoin. All patients except one had subtoxic blood levels of anticonvulsant. Significant decrements were noted in measures of immediate recall of words and pictures, although no differences were found in delayed recall or recognition. Other neuropsychological functions found to be affected included concentration in a visual scanning task under auditory distraction, and category decision-making. Similar results were found when the authors re-analyzed their data and included only the 16 patients who did not have toxic or near-toxic levels of anticonvulsant. These patients also showed poorer immediate and delayed word recall, poorer visual scanning under distraction and poorer category membership decision-making. Unfortunately, the results of phenytoin users were not analyzed separately, since some of the patients in the study received phenytoin, while others received carbamazepine, an anticonvulsant with fewer neuropsychological side effects (Reynolds and Trimble, 1985; Evans and Gualtieri, 1985; Thompson and Trimble, 1982).

Other anticonvulsants

Sodium valproate (Depakote) was compared with phenobarbital for neuropsychological effects in children by Vining *et al.* (1983). Using a double-blind, crossover design, the authors examined the effects of both medicines on 21 children. While seizure control did not differ between drugs, significant neuropsychological differences were noted between valproate and phenobarbital. When children received phenobarbital they performed significantly more poorly in Full Scale IQ on an (unspecified) Wechsler Intelligence Scale. Phenobarbital subjects also showed decreased performance on Block Design, Picture Completion and Vocabulary subtests. Two tests of attention span were also impaired, and every item but one on a behavioral questionnaire filled out by parents showed less dysfunction with sodium valproate. Sodium valproate use is not, however, completely free of neuropsychologically related side-effects. Valproate use has been linked to symptoms of mild sedation, ataxia, dysarthria and nightmares (Goetz, 1985).

Another anti-seizure drug, *ethosuximide*, does not appear to have been the subject of neuropsychological study as of this writing. Psychosis has been reported as an effect of ethosuximide use, but many of the reported patients have a prior psychiatric history (Reynolds and Trimble, 1985).

Phenobarbital, a barbiturate used in childhood febrile convulsions, has been shown to produce a reversible behavior disorder in children, characterized by hyperactivity. Irritability, lethargy, insomnia and oppositional behaviors are also sometimes seen (Reynolds and Trimble, 1985). Phenobarbital for childhood febrile seizures has shown unfavorable neuropsychological side effects compared to other anticonvulsants (e.g. carbamazepine). Byrne *et al.* (1987) conducted intellectual and behavioral assessments on a monozygotic twin pair, one of whom had developed febrile seizures treated with phenobarbital from 17-30 months of age. While normal intelligence for both twins was found on the Bayley and McCarthy scales, the twin receiving phenobarbital performed consistently less well than the unmedicated twin. Post-treatment evaluation suggested that the medicated twin had improved in endurance and showed a better emotional tone, although he remained less cooperative than his brother. The originally medicated twin also remained significantly lower in the McCarthy's Quantitative and Memory subtests. The authors discount the possibility that febrile seizure and not phenobarbital may have been responsible for the medicated twin's lasting impairments, citing research to the contrary. They suggest that administration of phenobarbital "during infancy may have mildly attenuated general as well as specific intellectual ability, with such attenuation more evident later in the preschool period" (Byrne, Camfield, Clark-Touesnard and Hondas, 1987, p. 397).

Neuropsychological effects in relation to anticonvulsant serum levels

Thompson and Trimble (1983) examined the effects of anticonvulsant serum levels on memory, concentration, perceptual and motor speed and mood in 28 seizure patients who used a variety of single and dual anticonvulsant medications. While mean serum levels were characterized as subtoxic, 12 patients did have toxic serum levels. Relative to their own low serum level performance, high-level anticonvulsant patients were impaired on immediate recall for pictures, concentration under a distracting stimulus, speeded decision on a color and category membership task, and a related motor latency measure when no decision was required. No differences were found in motor speed, mood or delayed memory recall. The authors then removed date culled from the 12 patients with serum levels above the therapeutic range, leaving 16 patients. Fewer neuropsychological tests were found to be impaired at therapeutically high but non-toxic serum levels. These included immediate word recall, visual scanning, decision-making on categories (the more difficult task) but not color membership.

In conclusion, anticonvulsants have a variety of neurotoxic and neuropsychological effects which vary according to dosage and drug type. Neuropsychological function decrements may be observed even when serum levels of anticonvulsant are subtoxic. Certain common medications like phenytoin have been linked to a variety of neuropsychological deficits including sustained attention, perceptual and motor performance and speeded decision-making tasks. Other anticonvulsants appear to produce fewer neuropsychological deficits compared to phenytoin, especially carbamazepine (Tegretol) and sodium valproate. Administration of single anticonvulsants is associated with better neuropsychological performance than polydrug administration.

Future neuropsychological research is needed to continue investigation into the newer anticonvulsants like valproate and carbamazepine, and it is hoped that researchers will utilize the cross-over, double-blind design favored by Trimble and associates. Such a design would obviate many of the difficulties inherent in performing neuropsychological tests upon populations with pre-existing brain dysfunction.

Norms for individuals using anticonvulsants would also be of use to clinicians and neuropsychological researchers. In the meantime, neuropsychologists engaged in testing individual patients need to take into account alterations in behavioral and cognitive functions produced by these drugs.

ANTIHYPERTENSIVES

There have been several anecdotal accounts of "forgetfulness" attributed to medications that lower and stabilize blood pressure (e.g. Ghosh, 1976; Fernandez, 1976). These observations received preliminary validation in a recent study which used Russell's (1975) modification of the Wechsler Memory Scale (Solomon *et al.*, 1983). Their study compared hypertensives on propranolol or methyldopa with hypertensive subjects on diuretic alone, as well as normotensive subjects prescribed propranolol. Subjects receiving either propranolol or methyldopa displayed significant impairment on the Logical (Verbal) Memory subtest of the Wechsler Memory Scale, both in immediate and 20-minute recall. No other deficits were found, and results could not be explained by variations in patient blood pressure. Because the mean age of normotensive subjects (60.5) differed by about 8 years from other subjects (early 50s), the conclusion of a main effect of propranolol on verbal memory is weakened somewhat because age-related changes in normotensives' memory may have contributed some of the variance the authors attributed to propranolol. Nonetheless, the study presents a potentially significant neuropsychological side-effect of antihypertensive agents, and is deserving of replication.

BENZODIAZEPINES

Benzodiazepines are a group of medications commonly prescribed for their anti-anxiety, hypnotic and muscle-relaxing effects. Prescription use of these products is truly extensive, with recent estimates of over $400,000,000 spent annually on these drugs. A survey taken in the Boston area during the 1970s found that 30% of all hospitalized patients were prescribed diazepam and 32% received flurazepam (Greenblatt and Shader, 1974; Hall and Zisook, 1981). Benzodiazepine neurochemistry involves the stimulation of GABA receptors in the ascending reticular activating system, which inhibits cortical and limbic system arousal. Limbic system discharges are also suppressed (Hall and Zisook, 1981). Benzodiazepine can also decrease catecholamine uptake in parts of the brain, and increase acetylcholine concentrations (Hall and Zisook, 1981).

Valium (diazepam) is the most well known of the benzodiazepine derivatives, a group of minor tranquilizers of varying half-lives and potency. Other benzodiazepines include chlordiazepoxide (Librium), alprazolam (Xanax), lorazepam (Ativan), oxazepam (Serax), flurazepam and clobazam.

Acute effects

The most commonly reported acute neuropsychological effect of benzodiazepine has been memory dysfunction. Acute amnestic reactions have been produced in subjects receiving these drugs immediately prior to surgery. Several studies suggest that benzodiazepines may impair recall of words presented after drug administration, but not influence prior word learning, a finding interpreted as consistent with impairment in encoding but not of retrieval (Lister, 1985).

A recent study by Block and Berchou (1984) used the Buschke Selective Reminding test to examine the acute effects of lorazepam and alprazolam. Both drugs impaired total recall compared to placebo. Impairment in total recall was greater over successive trials. Both drugs also significantly reduced the imagery advantage inherent in remembering high-imagery words. In the same study, benzodiazepine administration also impaired performance in a discriminative reaction time task and reduced the frequency for which Critical Flicker Fusion could be perceived. Main effects of impaired learning and retrieval found in this study are consistent with reductions in memory and/or motivation to encode information seen in other studies. However, the authors' use of multiple ANOVAs over the same data makes it difficult to vouch for their many significant findings.

Lucki, Rickels and Geller (1986) examined acute benzodiazepine effects on 22 chronic users of these medications. Subjects received a fixed dose of their usual benzodiazepine and were tested 60–90 minutes later. Compared to their pre-drug status, subjects showed significantly reduced Flicker Fusion but improved their performance on the Digit Symbol substitution test. Memory was tested for immediate and 20-minute recall using a 16-item word list of noncategorized nouns. While immediate recall was not affected, delayed recall was significantly reduced.

Bornstein, Watson and Kaplan (1985) failed to find neuropsychological effects of triazolam on normal university volunteers given single doses of flurazepam or triazolam. Other studies which used higher doses of benzodiazepines and more complex tasks found significant impairments. For example, Hindmarch and Gudgeon (1980) found that lorazepam impaired a four-letter cancellation task in doses of 1 mg.

Finally, a recent study examined memory decrements as a function of increasing doses of diazepam (Wolkowitz *et al.*, 1987). Subject volunteers received cumulative intravenous diazepam at 8.8, 35.1 and 140.1 μg/kg. This would correspond to doses of 0.625, 2.5 and 10 mg in a 70 kg subject. Each subject was read a list of 18 words in the same semantic category at a rate of one word every 3 seconds. Six of the 18 were read twice, and six were presented only once. Subjects were asked to notify the examiner if a repeat was heard, as a test of attention. A distractor task followed in which subjects were given a semantic category and asked to generate a word list from that category. A recall and recognition task followed this distractor trial, and subjects were also asked whether the words they recognized had been presented once or twice, which the authors characterized as a measure of "automatic processing" (Wolkowitz *et al.*, 1987).

Main effects were found for diazepam on attention, recognition and automatic processing, with decreasing performance as a result of diazepam administration. Incorrect word intrusions into free recall were also significantly increased. While diazepam did not affect free recall *per se*, when the authors corrected for intrusions as guessing, they did find significantly decreased recall in the diazepam conditions. The authors noted anecdotally that the amnestic effects of diazepam were so marked that some subjects "did not even recall having heard a given memory list" (Wolkowitz *et al.*, 1987, p. 27).

In contrast to these impairments of episodic memory, subjects showed no deficits in their ability to generate semantic category words in the interference task. The authors interpreted their results as consistent with a model in which diazepam interferes with acquisition or consolidation of new memories, but does not affect memory or retrieval of previously acquired information. The authors further suggest that this pattern of memory dysfunction is similar to that found in Korsakoff's patients, and that diazepam may be a pharmacological model for certain organic amnesias. Unfortunately, since subjects' memory abilities were highly correlated with subjective ratings of sedation, the possibility cannot be ruled out that attention rather than memory function is impaired.

Chronic effects of benzodiazepine

There has been mixed support for chronic benzodiazepine-induced neuropsychological impairment. In what might be thought of as "experimental chronic" benzodiazepine administration, Bornstein, Watson and Pawluk (1985) gave normal college student volunteers without history of neurological or psychiatric illness nightly capsules of either triazolam, flurazepam or placebo for 7 days. Baseline, intermediate and final neuropsychological tests were administered, including Grooved Pegboard, Trails, Finger Tapping, Hand Dynamometer, Wechsler Memory Scale Logical and Figural Memory, the Knox Cube Test and a choice reaction time task. Subjects were also given a questionnaire to uncover possible side-effects. Although no significant differences on any neuropsychological measures were found when baseline differences were controlled, many more side-effects were reported by the experimental groups. While this study suggests that low-dose, intermediate-term use of certain benzodiazepines does not produce neuropsychological deficit, the study does not really address long-term sequelae of chronic use or abuse of minor tranquilizers.

A more recent and ecologically valid study that did investigate chronic neuropsychological effects of benzodiazepines, used a patient population which had been prescribed benzodiazepines for a mean of 60 months (Lucki, Rickels and Geller, 1986). Thirty-three of the experimental subjects were single-benzodiazepine users, four additional patients received two (flurazepam and triazolam) and one patient regularly received clorazepate dipotassium (Tranxene) and lorazepam (Ativan). Six of the total group received additional medications — four taking antidepressants and two receiving antihypertensives. Daily intake was in the therapeutic range "in nearly every case" (Lucki, Rickels and Geller, 1986, p. 427). Twenty-six drug-free controls were recruited from a patient group presenting with anxiety disorders at the same clinic. Control subjects were matched for sex, age and education with the norms of the experimental group. Tests administered included subjective mood scales, Digit Symbol Substitution Test, as well as tests involving symbol copying, letter cancellation, Critical Flicker Fusion and free recall of word lists. Only performance on Critical Flicker Fusion differentiated experimental subjects from controls, and since multiple comparisons were made without adjusting the alpha level, this single significant result may be artifactual. The same authors retested 17 of their subjects 4–8 days after termination of benzodiazepine. Again, only Flicker Fusion thresholds showed significant increases. Patients also reported significantly greater sedation and anxiety during withdrawal.

The results of the Lucki *et al.* (1986) study suggest that chronic use of benzodiazepines within therapeutic guidelines does not have neuropsychological effects on the functions tested by the authors. This lack of effect may be due to tolerance and drug adaptation in very long-term users, or else the possibility that more difficult neuropsychological tasks (e.g. those requiring divided attention or parallel processing) might be necessary to exhibit subclinical effects in this population. Given previously reported findings of benzodiazepine-induced memory dysfunction, it is regrettable that only a single test of memory was included in the battery.

Chronic use of benzodiazepines in combination with other medications may produce severe neuropsychological impairment. Brooker, Weins and Weins (1984) report the case study of a 53-year-old male attorney who showed severe (Average Impairment Rating of 1) neuropsychological impairment on the Halstead–Reitan battery after long-term use of diazepam (Valium) and meprobamate (Equanil/Miltown). The patient showed almost complete symptom reversal at $1\frac{1}{2}$ years post-initial assessment, when he had been abstinent for 6 months.

Tests used in benzodiazepine research

Wittenborn (1980) reviewed tests which discriminated benzodiazepine users from controls. He suggests that the following tests are most capable of discriminating the two groups: Critical Flicker Fusion, learning and memory tests, manipulation tests, time estimation, Digit Symbol Substitution Test and cancellation taks. In general, test batteries which load heavily on memory and attentional processes would appear to be the most sensitive to benzodiazepine-induced impairments.

Psychological and psychiatric effects

While the expected therapeutic effect of benzodiazepines is usually the reduction of anxiety, paradoxical changes in affect and behavior have also been reported. Hall and Zisook (1981) reviewed these paradoxical reactions which include depression, tremulousness, apprehension, insomnia, severe anxiety, suicidal ideation, hatefulness and rage. Gross cognitive disturbances linked to benzodiazepine use include psychosis, manic or hypomanic behavior, confusional states and visual hallucinations. Korsakoff-like syndromes have also been reported (Hall and Zisook, 1981).

DISULFIRAM (ANTABUSE)

Disulfiram is prescribed in the treatment of chronic alcoholism. Its daily use causes exaggerated and aversive sensitivity to ethanol. By blocking the enzyme aldehyde dehydrogenase, disulfiram causes an accumulation of acetaldehyde, with resulting autonomic reactions, including nausea, vomiting, headache and hypotension.

Sterman and Schaumberg (1980) find distal axonal breakdown resulting in peripheral neuropathy to be associated with standard therapeutic doses (250–500 mg daily). The course of impairment begins several months after initiating treatment and takes another several months to recover after the drug is stopped. Paresthesias, weakness and sensory impairment are characteristic, with rare episodes of optic neuritis. Disulfiram has also been linked to a reversible toxic encephalopathic syndrome with symptoms of delirium, psychosis and cerebellar signs. These central and peripheral symptoms may be related to accumulation of carbon disulfide, since disulfiram in the body is catabolized into this potent neurotoxin (Sterman and Schaumberg, 1980).

There is little neuropsychological research on the effects of Antabuse on neuropsychological functioning, but available data suggest that further studies are needed. Prigatano (1977) compared the neuropsychological functioning of 22 inpatient, recidivist alcoholics treated with disulfiram against an equal number of inpatient alcoholics involved in a 90-day inpatient milieu treatment program. Patients were matched "as closely as possible" on age, education, years of alcohol abuse and general intelligence. The subjects in the Antabuse group had been taking this medication somewhere between 14 and 21 days.

Disulfiram-treated alcoholics were significantly more impaired than the milieu treatment group in abstract reasoning (Category Test), speech perception (Speech Perception Test) and in their overall impairment indexes. Percentages of patients from each group who would be classified as impaired, using Reitan's norms, appear in Table VI.1. While it is tempting to ascribe such results to Antabuse administration, they are most likely a function of pre-existing differences in the two groups, particularly since the Antabuse group was composed of recidivists with a history of previous treatment failure. Support for this hypothesis was found in a preliminary follow-up study reported by Prigatano (1977) in the same paper. When six slightly younger and better-educated alcoholics were tested upon entry into treatment, and then again after 2 weeks of Antabuse treatment, they failed to show significantly increased impairment. The Category Test of these subjects was significantly impaired upon *entry* into the program, and thus not as a function of Antabuse. In fact, when tested after 2 weeks of Antabuse administration, these subjects improved significantly on the Category Test

TABLE VI.1. Neuropsychological impairment as a function of disulfiram treatment. (Reprinted, by permission of the publisher, from Prigatano, G. P. Neuropsychological functioning in recidivist alcoholics treated with disulfiram. *Alcoholism: Clinical and Experimental Research*, 1, 81–86. Copyright 1977 by The Am. Med. Sec. on Alcoholism, Res. Soc. on Alcoholism and Other Drug Dependencies, Inc.)

TEST	PERCENTAGE OF SUBJECTS RATED AS IMPAIRED	
	ANTABUSE ALCOHOLICS	MILIEU ALCOHOLICS
Category Test	91	59
TPT Total Time	82	68
TPT Memory	23	27
TPT Location	86	77
Seashore Rhythm Test	50	41
Speech Perception Test	91	36
Tapping Preferred Hand	91	55
Impairment Index	82	50

(75.2 versus 48.5 errors), TPT total time and the Impairment Index. There was a non-significant tendency for Speech Perception to be worse on the second testing, which the author speculates could achieve significance with a larger *N*. Thus, the issue of whether Antabuse causes neuropsychological impairment remains open at this time. Studies which test the effects of Antabuse on more completely matched groups controlling for recidivism would appear to be essential to answer the question.

NEUROLEPTICS

Neuroleptics or "major tranquilizers" are prescribed to manage and control symptoms of confusional states, schizophrenias, late Alzheimer's disease and other functional or structural disorders that cause a breakdown of cognitive and emotional functioning. Neuroleptic agents include the phenothiazines, thioxanthenes and butyrophenone.

Neurological effects

Neuroleptics can have various deleterious effects on the central nervous system. Acute intoxication from neuroleptic medications can produce nonspecific CNS changes, including cerebral edema, reversible neuronal swelling and vacuolation, secondary anoxic and vasocirculatory lesions (Jellinger, 1977). Acute behavioral changes from neuroleptic administration include *akasthesias* or states of intense restlessness coupled with anxiety, that are usually seen in the first days of neuroleptic therapy or when the dose of drug has been significantly increased. Symptoms can be reversed with anticholinergic treatment (Goetz, 1985) and can spontaneously resolve within several weeks. *Dystonias* are another potential side-effect seen early in the course of neuroleptic administration, and may occur with just one parenteral dose. The head and neck show abnormal positions, and eyes may maintain a fixed upward gaze. Piperazine derivatives are most likely to precipitate dystonias (Goetz, 1985).

Other neurological complications of neuroleptic therapy can include parkinsonian symptoms, and toxic confusional states that also may be related to the anticholinergic effects of these drugs.

Neuroleptic malignant syndrome (NMS)

The most serious acute reaction to neuroleptics is that of "neuroleptic malignant syndrome", a potentially fatal reaction to antipsychotic medication. The syndrome is characterized by extrapyramidal signs, including parkinsonian symptoms, muscle rigidity, dystonia, akinesia and tremor. Hypothermia and other signs of autonomic dysfunction are also present, including very high fever, dysarthria, seizures and deterioration of mental status.

NMS was thought to be rare; however, recent estimates suggest that more than 1.4% of patients exposed to neuroleptics will develop the syndrome each year (Sternberg, 1986). More than 150 cases have been reported thus far, with an approximately 22% mortality rate (Shalev and Munitz, 1986). NMS usually begins within a few days of drug administeration and develops quite rapidly. Termination of neuroleptic treatment usually reverses symptoms "within 4 to 40 days" (Shalev and Munitz, 1986, p. 339). While etiology is unknown, patients with existing neurological abnormalities including OBS, mental retardation and substance abuse (opiates and alcohol) are "over-represented among fatal cases, comprising 32% of fatalities (Shalev and Munitz, 1986, p. 340). The syndrome is apparently not dose-related.

Neuropsychological effects of NMS

There is little literature addressing the specific neuropsychological effects of NMS. In this regard, Rothke and Bush (1986) examined a 28-year-old female with post-partum psychotic depression. She developed NMS after receiving increasing doses of haloperidol over the course of 8 days at a final dosage of 70 mg/day(!). Neuropsychological examinations were performed approximately 4 months and 10 months after her initial hospitalization.

Initial evaluation suggested significant deficits in visuospatial functions and in memory. While immediate verbal memory was unimpaired, mild to moderate deficits in delayed recall were found. Severe impairments in immediate and delayed visual memory were also noted. The patient's overall memory quotient on the Wechsler Memory Scale was only 69. Her score on the Category Test was 103, suggesting significant impairment in abstract spatial reasoning. MMPI scores were not reported, but were described as unremarkable.

On the follow-up examination the patient showed some improvement in attentional and overall intellectual abilities. Her Memory Quotient increased to 101. In contrast, delayed verbal recall was severely impaired, more so than in the initial testing and delayed visual recall continued to be severely impaired. The patient's Category Test score continued to be in the range of clinical impairment. Since the patient's attentional abilities and non-pathological MMPI appear to rule out the influence of psychopathology on test scores, the authors suggest that NMS may have caused the patient lasting neuropsychological impairment. Neuropsychological investigation of other cases of NMS appear warranted to determine the typicality of Rothke and Bush's (1986) results.

Chronic effects of neuroleptics

Jellinger (1977) performed neuropathologic post-mortem examinations on patients with long-term use of neuroleptics. He found "neuronal swelling, glial satellitosis and neuronophagia" in patients' caudate nuclei with more frequently encountered changes in patients with symptoms of tardive dsykinesia. Christensen, Moeller and Faurbye (1970) performed post-mortem neuropathological examinations on schizophrenics with oral dyskinesia and found degeneration of the substantia nigra in 27 of the 28 patients, and gliosis of the midbrain in 25. Only seven of 28 unmedicated control subjects showed similar degeneration of the substantia nigra, and only four of 28 showed midbrain and brainstem abnormalities. Since neuroleptic drugs block both acetylcholine and dopamine in the central nervous system, it is possible that some of the neuropathological effects cited above are the result of prolonged alterations in levels of these neurotransmitters. It is unclear, however, whether premorbid neuropathology found in a subset of schizophrenics could also be responsible for autopsy findings like these.

Chronic behavioral effects of neuroleptic medication include extrapyramidal syndromes, behavioral and autonomic effects (Sterman and Schaumberg, 1980). The most well-known extrapyramidal effect of neuroleptic administration is tardive dyskinesia, a syndrome comprising involuntary choreiform movements of the face, lips and tongue. The syndrome is usually considered to be a potential side-effect of chronic neuroleptic administration, although short-term trials of medication have also been known to evoke symptoms. Tardive dyskinesia may be reversible on termination of the causative medication, although long-term sequelae have also been noted.

Neuropsychological effects — tardive dyskinesia
Response to neuroleptic drugs varies greatly among patients. Very little

research has been performed on neuropsychological differences as a function of neuroleptic response. An obvious research topic is the investigation of normal and abnormal (tardive dyskinesia) neuroleptic responders. Struve and Willner (1983) performed such a study and examined the scores on an analogical reasoning task of all patients who began neuroleptic treatment. Patients who would later develop TD were found to show significantly lower scores on this task than patients who would eventually become part of the "normal" non-TD controls (Struve and Willner, 1983). Additionally, TD patients' scores did not change as a function of medication over time, suggesting either abnormal but stable initial medication response, or else structural brain differences between the two groups. While this study's findings are obscured by failure to control for educational differences among patients, the goal of discovering a neuropsychological predictor of TD is worthy of further exploration.

Other neuropsychological effects

The same neuroleptic-induced alterations of dopamine and acetylcholine that may be related to long-term neuropathology may concomitantly produce neuropsychological side-effects. A review of relevant studies by Heaton and Crowley (1981) suggested that neuroleptics with little cholinergic activity, including the piperazine phenothiazines and haloperidol, "do not seem to impair cognitive function or motor speed . . . . However these agents are more likely to produce acute extrapyramidal and other side-effects and may thereby impair performance on some motor coordination tasks" (Heaton and Crowley, 1981, p. 501).

Those neuroleptics which do reduce central nervous system cholinergic activity have been associated with other types of neuropsychological deficits. Tune *et al.* (1982) tested the recent memory of 24 outpatient chronic schizophrenics, using a 10-item free recall word list. Subjects were taking the equivalent of 200 mg/day of chlorpromazine and also received anticholinergic medications (benztropine or trihexyphenidyl) for extrapyramidal symptoms. The authors report a "highly significant inverse correlation between increasing serum levels of anticholinergics and recall scores ($r = 0.51$, $p < 0.01$). Recall did not correlate with an estimate of IQ or the overall severity of schizophrenic symptoms (Tune *et al*, 1982, p. 1461).

The relationship between memory deficit and serum anticholinergic levels was further explored in a study which examined both free recall and recognition memory as a function of anticholinergic activity (Perlick *et al.*, 1986). The authors examined 17 chronic schizophrenics receiving either mesoridazine, haloperidol, chlorpromazine, thioridizine or fluphenazine. Subjects were administered a neuropsychological battery that included WAIS-R Vocabulary, Similarities, Block Design and Picture Completion Tests, the Associate Learning subtest of the Wechsler Memory Scale,

Benton's Revised Visual Retention Test (BVRT), and the Mattis–Kovner Memory Inventory — a test of verbal recall with periodic recognition memory "probes". Replicating the Tune *et al.* (1982) results, the authors found that, after controlling for IQ, subjects with anticholinergic serum levels (ASLs) above the group mean showed significantly impaired free recall compared to subjects below the mean ASL. Recognition memory for the "probes", however, was not affected by ASL. There was also no relationship between ASL and the other neuropsychological measures, nor between serum neuroleptic levels and memory.

While patients in the Tune *et al.* (1982) study had anticholinergic effects induced with antiparkinsonian drugs, the Perlick *et al.* (1986) subjects had the majority of their anticholinergic reductions produced by the neuroleptic medications themselves. The results of these studies taken together suggest that either anticholinergic neuroleptic medications or antiparkinsonian agents may produce memory impairment that is correlated with serum anticholinergic level.

Further investigation of anticholinergic memory deficits seems warranted since unimpaired recognition memory in the Perlick *et al.* subjects suggests that the anticholinergic "memory" deficits may not be in the encoding phase. Instead, retrieval may have been impaired in some way by faulty attentional, motivational or planning processes (Perlick *et al.*, 1986).

Not all neuropsychological functions of schizophrenics are impaired by neuroleptic medications. Strauss, Lew, Coyle and Tune (1985) showed beneficial effects of neuroleptic levels on distractibility. They examined 28 outpatients with a diagnosis of chronic undifferentiated schizophrenia on reaction time and an auditorally presented digit span test. This latter test was presented using a female voice alone, or with a male voice listing extraneous numbers between presentations by the female voice (distracting condition). In either case, subjects were asked to attend only to the numbers presented by the female voice. Neuroleptic levels showed significant negative correlation with auditory distractibility. Serum anticholinergic levels were not significantly correlated with test scores.

Similarly, Braff and Saccuzzo (1982) found improved speed of information processing in a tachistoscopic task for medicated schizophrenics compared with unmedicated schizophrenics. Since both groups performed significantly more poorly than depressed controls, the authors concluded that schizophrenic disorder, rather than medication, was responsible for slower information processing, and neuroleptic medication may even reverse certain information processing deficits.

Neuropsychological effects — children

Children are much less frequently prescribed neuroleptic medications, and there are correspondingly fewer studies of neuropsychological dysfunction in

210   *Neuropsychological Toxicology*

neuroleptic-medicated children. One example is Platt *et al.* (1984) who found mild effects on cognitive functions in 61 children with a diagnosis of undersocialized aggressive conduct disorder. A mean dose of 2.95 mg/day of haloperidol caused slowing in simple reaction time and worsened Porteus Maze scores. No effects were found in tests of memory, concept attainment, short-term recognition memory or the Stroop test.

LITHIUM

Lithium was discovered in 1817 and is classified as a group I alkali metal. Before its current use as a psychiatric medication it was first tried as a gout treatment, and then later as a salt substitute, the latter having toxic or fatal results. Lithium's utility in normalizing the psychiatric symptoms of mania and bipolar disorder were not known until 1949 when the first case reports were published (Sansone and Ziegler, 1983). Today, lithium is commonly accepted as the preferred treatment for bipolar disorder and unipolar manic disorder. It is also used to treat chronic cluster headaches (Sterman and Schaumberg, 1980). Individuals at risk for lithium neurotoxicity are those being treated for the aforementioned psychiatric disorders. Although lithium is used in several industrial capacities, including plastics and ceramic production, and in lubricants (Dempsey and Meltzer, 1977), lithium toxicity is not reported to be an industrial problem (Hamilton and Hardy, 1974).

Neurological effects

Lithium shows preferential toxicity for the central nervous system over the heart or kidney. Neurotoxic levels of lithium can induce abnormal EEG and dysarthria, as well as gait and limb ataxia; these appear to abate without permanent sequelae as lithium levels decline. Acute lithium overdose can precipitate coma, and long-term deficits from lithiuim-induced coma may be more a function of the coma itself than lithium (Sterman and Schaumberg, 1980). Overdose of lithium can be fatal and immediate hemodialysis is indicated to prevent death or permanent brain damage (Sansone and Zeigler, 1985).

Peripheral nervous system effects

Girkem, Krebs and Muller-Oerlinghausen (1975) found six of 17 bipolar patients on long-term lithium to show significant slowing of motor nerve conduction velocity; however, half of these patients were simultaneously taking other medications and one patient had cancer. In the same report the authors replicated their finding of lower nerve conduction velocity in a group of seven normal volunteers who received lithium for 1 week. NCVs remained significantly decreased 7 days after lithium withdrawal and may have been the cause of five volunteers' complaints of weakness or fatigue (Sansone and Zeigler, 1985; Girkem, Krebs and Muller-Oerlinghausen, 1975). Other peripheral nervous system effects of maintenance therapy with lithium include "fine rapid tremor of mild to moderate intensity (Sansone and Zeigler, 1985, p. 242). Parkinsonian symptoms and cogwheel rigidity have been infrequently observed.

Central nervous system effects

Lithium encephalopathy caused by overdose can be accompanied by "flaccid paralysis, proximal muscle weakness, fasciculations, and areflexia" (Sansone and Zeigler, 1985, p. 243). EEG patterns show dose-related slowing which may persist "for at least 11 days after the last dose of lithium" (Sansone and Zeigler, 1985, p. 245).

Severe and sometimes fatal reactions to lithium in the context of normal blood lithium have been linked to toxic brain accumulations of the metal. Animal studies suggest that brain lithium levels may be higher than serum concentration after steady-state blood levels are produced. Sansone and Zeigler (1985) report two studies in which autopsies showed elevated brain lithium compared to serum lithium. In one of these the pons showed $2\frac{1}{2}$ times the levels of serum lithium, while the second study found overall brain toxicity with highest accumulations in the white matter and brainstem (Sansone and Zeigler, 1985). A third study reports permanent damage to the basal ganglia and cerebellar connections as a consequence of lithium toxicity (von Hartitzsch *et al.*, 1972).

Neuroleptics in combination with lithium

Lithium, when used in combination with neuroleptics, may be more likely to produce neurological abnormalities than use of lithium alone. Fetzer, Kader and Danahy (1981) report three cases of organic brain syndrome produced when these two medications were combined. Withdrawing lithium ameliorated symptoms in two of these patients, although the authors cite a potential risk of irreversibility. Prakash, Kelwala and Ban (1982) reviewed 39 cases of lithium/neuroleptic neurotoxicity and observed that the syndrome was characterized by confusion, disorientation and unconsciousness. Extrapyramidal signs were often present and included tremor, akathisia, dyskinesia and dystonia. Also occasionally reported were cerebellar signs and slow wave EEG. The authors speculate that neuroleptics may somehow raise brain uptake of lithium to toxic levels.

Neuropsychological effects of lithium

Patients taking lithium typically do not "enjoy" the effects of the medication, and give subjective accounts of cognitive impairment. However, neuropsychological studies of lithium effects have produced contradictory findings, possibly because of the many potential confounds inherent to this type of research. First, neuropsychological impairment is exhibited by individuals with bipolar disorders (e.g., Savard, Rey and Post, 1980) and may be related to abnormal brain structure (Pearlson *et al.*, 1984). Other potential confounds that limit the interpretation of existing neuropsychological studies include failure to control for effects of age, inadequate assessment of pre- and postmorbid mood, not assessing serum lithium levels with consequent failure to rule out lithium toxicity, educational variation among subjects and inadequate statistical treatment (e.g. Lund, Nissen and Rafaelsen, 1982).

Lithium has been examined for its effects on memory in several studies. In general, the better-controlled studies have not found lithium to significantly affect memory. For example, Ghadirian, Engelsmann and Ananth (1983) attempted to determine whether duration of lithium treatment was related to memory function. When age, serum lithium, psychopathology and physical illness were controlled, there were no significant effects of lithium duration.

Another study eliminated affective or psychiatric disorder as a source of variance by examining the neuropsychological effects of lithium administration on normal college males (Weingartner, Rudorfer and Linnoila, 1985). Subjects were maintained on standard lithium doses of 1225 ± 300 mg/day until steady-state serum concentrations of 0.82 ± 0.17 mEq/l by the 8th day. Double-blind crossover experimental design was employed, with all subjects participating in both conditions and each subject matched as his or her own control. Subjects were asked to listen to sets of categorically related words, presented once or twice. They were required to identify word repetitions, attempt free recall, and then identify correct words among distractors in a recognition task. They were also asked to judge whether each identified word occurred once or twice.

No differences in free recall or recognition were found regardless of the number of word presentations. However, subjects produced more intrusion errors in the lithium condition than the control condition, both in recall and recognition. The authors suggest that while lithium does not affect number of items recalled or recognized, it may affect the "clarity" of what is remembered and therefore may be an analogue of the "cognitive blurring" that occurs in patients on lithium, and which may be responsible for their non-compliance (Weingartner, Rudorfer and Linnoila, 1985).

A third study which used psychiatric patients as their own controls, found no overall effects between patients before and after they began lithium treatment (Smigan and Perris, 1983). However, the authors also did not find effects of other drugs, age and serum lithium levels on performance; factors which have been implicated in neuropsychological impairment by many other studies. The overall sensitivity of their methodology is therefore somewhat suspect.

Examining the effect of age and lithium administration, Friedman, Culver and Ferrell (1977) found that patients below 55 years old did not exhibit neuropsychological impairment. Eight patients under age 55 who received prescription doses of lithium for bipolar affective disorder showed an average impairment index of 0.26 on the Halstead–Reitan Battery. Five older patients (mean age 62.4) receiving lithium for the same amount of time (mean 3.6 years) had an average impairment index of 0.72, suggesting that age alone — or a possible interactive effect of age, illness and lithium use — may have produced neuropsychological impairment.

Other neuropsychological functions may be more consistently affected by lithium than memory, particularly those involving motor and/or perceptual speed. For example, Squire *et al.* (1980) tested a mixed group of psychiatric patients in a double-blind, crossover design. Subjects who took an average dose of 0.94 mEq/l did not show learning or memory deficit, but were impaired in several speeded tasks, including Digit Symbol and a clerical copying task. Serum lithium levels correlated significantly with time to complete Trails B, suggesting a loss of cognitive efficiency or flexibility. This effect was also found by Small *et al.* (1972), who administered parts of the Halstead–Reitan Battery to a mixed group of affective and schizophrenic disorder patients. The authors reported high lithium levels to be correlated with poor performance on Finger Tapping, Block Design, Trails B, Digit Symbol, the Minnesota Paper Form Board Test and a verbal test. In addition, lithium also produced a significant decrement in scores on the Tactual Peformance Test. These effects may be related to peripheral nervous system abnormalities or yet-to-be-understood cortical mechanisms. Hopefully, further research will better clarify the nature and etiology of lithium's neuropsychological effects.

In conclusion, based on current data and on data reviewed earlier (e.g. Heaton and Crowley, 1981), neuropsychological evidence for lithium impairment is inconclusive. High serum lithium levels can be neurotoxic and can be correlated with acute effects on several neuropsychological tests, especially those which measure attention, cognitive efficiency and flexibility. It is not known whether these acute effects cause chronic, cumulative neuropsychological damage. The evidence for lithium-induced memory loss is contradictory at this time.

Continued neuropsychological studies using double-blind, crossover, counterbalanced designs would seem to be necessary to resolve the conflicting literature to date. Subject population variables must be addressed; individual differences in brain structure among bipolar patients must be controlled; subjects who receive lithium first must be allowed sufficient intervals for drug clearance, and practice effects must be addressed. Neuropsychological interactions, if any, of lithium and aging also require further exploration.

MUSCLE RELAXANTS

Baclofen has been linked to both toxic and withdrawal-related encephalopathy syndromes. Toxic encephalopathy is characterized by confusion, and somnolence and coma may ensue. Seizures, myoclonus and "combative hallucinatory agitation" during unconsciousness can occur (Goetz, 1985, p. 205). Abrupt withdrawal may also precipitate psychiatric and neurological symptoms, including hallucinations, seizures and mania. Dantrolene is another muscle relaxant cited by Goetz (1985) to have neurological effects. Muscle weakness, "euphoria, lightheadedness, dizziness and fatigue" have been reported (Goetz, 1985, p. 206).

STEROIDS

Corticosteroids (e.g. dexamethasone, prednisone) are employed on a spectrum of diseases in which their immunosuppressant or anti-inflammatory properties can be beneficial. Thus, dementias resulting from inflammatory processes with resulting increased intracranial pressure may show temporary or permanent remission with steroid administration. Paulson (1983) lists several dementing illnesses that respond positively to steroids, among them global encephalopathies, e.g. subacute sclerosing panencephalitis and Kreutzfeldt–Jacob disease. Lupus erythematosus, sarcoid meningitis and dementias with fluctuating mental states are also suggested to improve with steroids.

Steroids may also *worsen* central nervous system functioning and thus may *induce*, rather than ameliorate, dementing illness (Varney, Alexander and MacIndoe, 1984; Paulson, 1983). Varney *et al.* (1984) studied six patients who received 60–125 mg/day of prednisone for a variety of steroid-treatable diseases. Two of six patients had long-lasting cognitive sequelae subsequent to resolving steroid psychosis. The other four patients showed global but reversible deficits on follow-up (which varied from 80 days to 2 years). All patients were tested with a neuropsychological battery that included WAIS, parts of the Wechsler Memory Scale, several of Benton's tests (e.g. BVRT, Facial Recognition Test, 3D Constructional Praxis scale, and other tests). The authors characterized the deficits as disturbances in "memory retention, attention, concentration, mental speed and efficiency, and occupational performance" (Varney, Alexander and MacIndoe, 1984, p. 372). The authors note that the patients were not overtly toxic, intoxicated or demented, but rather that each was impaired relative to his own prior and subsequent functioning.

VINCRISTINE

Vincristine is an alkaloid that has been used in cancer chemotherapy since 1962. It is "predictably and uniformly neurotoxic" (Le Quesne, 1984).

Neurotoxic symptoms begin with paresthesias, with severe weakness ensuing. Extensor muscles of the fingers, wrists and legs become weak. There is partial recovery with elimination of paresthesias; however, ankle jerks usually failed to show recovery and superficial loss of sensation can persist (Le Quesne, 1983).

OTHER DRUGS

The medications listed in Table VI.2 have not been investigated with neuropsychological measures. However, their effects might be expected to produce abnormalities on such tests, especially in sensory and motor functions (from Schaumburg, Spencer and Thomas, 1983; Goetz, 1985).

TABLE VI.2. Selected drugs with neurotoxic effects

DRUG	USE	EFFECT
Aminoglycosides	Antibiotic	Eighth cranial nerve damage; ototoxic, vestibular toxicity, neuromuscular blockade
Chloramphenicol	Antibiotic	Distal symmetrical neuropathy, optic neuropathy
Clioquinol	Amebicide	CNS degeneration of optic tracts and long spinal cord tracts
Dapsone	Treatment of leprosy	Reversible motor neuropathy
Ethionamide	Treatment of tuberculosis	Symmetrical sensory polyneuropathy, paresthesias of the feet
Glutethimide	Sedative/hypnotic	Rarely — distal sensory axonopathy (reversible)
Isoniazid	Treatment of tuberculosis	Sensory paresthesias (numb fingers and toes); slow but complete recovery of peripheral neuropathy
Metronidazole (Flagyl)	Anti-bacterial/ protozoan	Peripheral distal neuropathy
Misonidazole	Radiosensitizing agent	Peripheral neuropathy, CNS pathology similar to thiamine deficiency syndrome (Wernicke's encephalopathy)
Nitrofurantoin	Antimicrobial	Peripheral neuropathy with paresthesias, rapid deterioration can occur with severe sensory loss
Nitrous oxide	Anesthetic	Mild, distal, symmetrical polyneuropathy, high levels of abuse may cause myelopathy
Perhexiline maleate	Angina pectoris	Peripheral neuropathy with 300–400 mg/day, 4 months to 1 year
Pyridoxine	Vitamin B_6	Distal sensory neuropathy
Sulfonamide	Treatment of urinary tract infections	Peripheral neuropathy, CVA, headache, fatigue, tinnitus, psychosis, focal CNS symptoms, e.g. aphasia (rare)

ABUSED DRUGS

Abused drugs are substances which have a high reinforcing potential in human beings. To some extent a category of abused drugs overlaps previously described neurotoxins (e.g. toluene, benzodiazepines); however, other abused drugs are prescription medicines with legitimate uses but which also induce physical and/or psychological addiction. Although not all highly reinforcing drugs are chronically neurotoxic, all produce acute neuropsychological impairment.

AMPHETAMINES

Amphetamines and related stimulants are prescribed appropriately for narcolepsy and for childhood hyperactivity. They are also highly reinforcing and thus have a high abuse potential. Neurological consequences of amphetamine abuse include arteritis, vasculitis and intracranial hemorrhage (Carlin, 1986). Psychiatric consequences of prolonged use of amphetamines include paranoid-schizophrenic-like psychosis. There is very little neuropsychological literature on the effects of amphetamine use or abuse. The few reports available have not found significant levels of impairment (e.g. Trites *et al.*, 1974). The long-term psychological effects of amphetamine use have yet to be addressed in a research study (Carlin, 1986).

COCAINE

History

Cocaine is derived from an alkaloid of the coca plant and has been used since at least 3000 B.C. for various sacramental, medical and recreational purposes. Cocaine was thought to be in common use before the Inca civilization, and the Incas themselves believed the plant to be divine, restricting its use to nobles and priests (Mulé, 1984). They may also have used cocainized saliva to prepare patients for trephining (Nicholi, 1984).

The psychological and pharmacological effects of cocaine were rediscovered by the medical community in the 1880s. Sigmund Freud enthusiastically recommended the drug for its anesthetic and mood-elevating properties. Freud prescribed cocaine for several of his patients and also self-medicated to relieve his own migraines and "neurasthenia".

Freud's experience with cocaine was probably similar to that of countless current users; initial moderate use and enthusiastic recommendations, followed by addiction, deterioration of affect, memory and attention. There is at least circumstantial evidence linking Freud's cryptic and opaque *Project for a Scientific Psychology* (1895) to a period of cocaine use, a year before he finally put "the cocaine brush aside" in 1896 (S. Freud, in Masson, 1985, p. 201).

The early twentieth century saw the production of many cocainized patent medicines, the most popular of which was Coca-Cola. The Pure Food and Drug Act of 1906 forced the removal of cocaine from "Coke" and the Harrison Narcotic Act made cocaine illegal in 1914 (Mulé, 1984).

There are still several legitimate medical uses of cocaine. Its primary medical application is as an anesthetic in nasal operations (Nicholi, 1984).

All available data indicate that cocaine use has reached epidemic proportions in the United States, with estimates of 33 million individuals who have used cocaine, up from about 9 million in 1972 (Nicholi, 1984). An increase of 10 million users in this decade alone suggests that it has become a major national health problem (Mulé, 1984). There has been more than a 200% increase in cocaine-related deaths and emergency room visits, and a 500% increase in admissions to federally funded cocaine treatment programs from 1976 through 1981 (Washton and Tatarsky, 1984). Cocaine use now spans all demographic groups with 9% of all professionals having tried cocaine (Siegel, 1982) and "considerable" spread into the middle and working classes as well (Washton and Tatarsky, 1984, p. 247). Even high school students have discovered cocaine; one recent study estimated that one in every six high school seniors had tried cocaine, and that almost 5% had used this drug in the month prior to the survey (O'Malley, Johnston and Bachman, 1985, cited in Melamed and Bleiberg, 1986).

Initially thought to be fairly benign and non-addictive, cocaine has become increasingly recognized for its addictive potential and its toxicity. Rats allowed to self-administer cocaine injections, and who in consequence developed severe tonic-clonic seizures, would reinitiate cocaine administration "as soon as the convulsions subsided" (Bozarth and Wise, 1985, p. 83). In the same study, rats were placed on a 30-day protocol of either cocaine or heroin self-administration. Group mortality of the cocaine-injecting rats was 90% compared with 36% for the heroin group (Bozarth and Wise, 1985).

Cocaine can be inhaled (snorted), smoked or injected. The drug is commonly available in a variety of forms: as a powder with various levels of purity, refined with ether to produce a more potent product (free-basing) or chemically refined in other ways ("crack"). For inhalation, low to average doses are about 25–150 mg. Toxicity depends upon route of administration. Reported toxic reactions to topical cocaine anesthesia in plastic surgery are uncommon, and a conservative estimate of maximum safe dose has been estimated from 100 to 300 mg (Jones 1984). Fatal dose is approximately 1g.

Neurophysiological effects

While topical anesthetic use of cocaine in modern plastic surgical procedures has been described as relatively safe, cocaine abuse has several frequently reported and potent neurotoxic effects. First, cocaine is a powerful central nervous system stimulant that mobilizes massive adrenergic discharge and simulates the neurophysiological response of a "fight or flight" reaction. EEG and ECG show general desynchronization after cocaine administration (Gold and Verebey, 1984).

Second, seizures, possibly tonic–clonic type (Cohen, 1984), have been reported by about one quarter of free-base and intravenous cocaine users interviewed on a cocaine hotline (Washton and Gold, 1984). Seizures caused by repeated cocaine administration may be related to the phenomenon of "kindling", an outward spread of electrical activity from the limbic system as a result of repeated stimulation (Melamed and Bleiberg, 1986). Experimental kindling paradigms in animals have resulted in reduced seizure threshold. A third neurotoxic effect of cocaine use has recently been demonstrated in animals. Altura, Altura and Gebrewold (1985) report the production of vascular spasms and subsequent cerebrovascular damage in animal experiments. It is probable that cocaine produces similar cerebrovascular damage in human abusers.

Cocaine's stimulatory effects also include the peripheral nervous system. Peripheral nervous system effects include vasoconstriction, pupil dilation, sinus tachycardia and ventricular arrhythmias (Goetz, 1985).

Cocaine seems to exert its potent reinforcing properties by blocking the re-uptake of dopamine, increasing the availability of dopamine at receptor sites and producing increased neurotransmission. Further, since re-uptake and re-use of dopamine cannot occur, dopamine production must be stepped up. This suggests that depression–depletion states following continued cocaine administration are the result of exhaustion of dopamine production sites (Dackis and Gold, 1985). Further support for cocaine's action upon the dopaminergic system is provided by animal and human studies which show reduction in reinforcement potential of cocaine and amphetamine when dopamine antagonists are administered (Wise, 1984).

Depletion states in thyroid axis hormones may also partially account for psychological symptoms of cocaine-induced depression, producing a state of drug-induced hypothyroidism (Dackis and Gold, 1985).

Psychological effects

The profile of psychological symptom onset varies with type of administration; inhalation or injection of cocaine produces almost instantaneous mood changes. Oral cocaine requires from 10 to 20 minutes to fully express its effects.

Clinical observations on the continued use of cocaine suggest systematic symptom progression. Initial acute reactions of low to average doses (25–150 mg) include euphoria, increased feelings of alertness, mental acuity and energy. Anorexia and decreased need for sleep are common. Elated mood slowly changes to irritation, restlessness, depression and psychomotor retardation. These are reversible with continued administration of cocaine, setting a cycle of positive and negative reinforcement that becomes a potent addiction (Gold and Verebey, 1984).

More serious psychological symptoms occur with increased use, including panic attacks in half the users reporting to a cocaine hotline (Washton and Gold, 1984). Paranoid ideation, depression, irritability, anxiety and loss of motivation are reported by more than half of other subjects, and memory difficulties are described by a third of all respondents (Washton and Tatarsky, 1984).

Cocaine psychosis occurs with toxic levels of cocaine use, and is characterized by delusions of persecution and auditory, visual or olfactory hallucinations. Parasitosis and formication, the sensation of snakes or insects crawling under the skin, are common, and addicts have been known to insert needles into their skin, looking for "cocaine bugs" (Nicholi, 1984). Similarities between the toxic psychosis produced by cocaine and that resulting from amphetamine use are said to be "far more striking than their differences" (Fischman, 1984, p. 86).

Withdrawal

Depressive disorders of various types are common and prolonged in cocaine withdrawal. An "abstinence" syndrome has been postulated by Gawin and Kleber (1986), who noted an initial depressive "crash" with lethargy, extreme dysphoria, suicidal ideation, intense cocaine craving, paranoia and hypersomnia, lasting from 1 to 40 hours after termination of cocaine administration. These symptoms were followed by a subphase of hypersomnolence, intermittent awakenings and hyperphagia, lasting 8–50 hours.

Phase two, withdrawal, consisted of 1–5 days of normalized affective response, which progressed to anxiety, increased cravings and anhedonia. These symptoms lasted an additional 1–10 weeks until cravings ceased. If subjects remained abstinent, baseline emotional functioning returned in this third phase, characterized by more limited cyclic cravings, possibly triggered by environmental cues. These cravings may be indefinite (Gawin and Kleber, 1986). Lithium and antidepressants may increase ability to abstain.

Neuropsychological effects

Very little information is available on specific neuropsychological concomitants of cocaine use. Most of the literature extant has relied on questionnaires of subjectively experienced symptoms without accompanying neuropsychological validation. For example, a recently survey of cocaine users suggested that 57% experience memory problems (Washton and Gold, 1984).

Press (1983) studied the neuropsychological effects of either cocaine or opiate use on the Luria–Nebraska Battery. Sixteen subjects had either a 2-year history of regular heavy cocaine use, or else a 3-year history of semiannual bingeing. All cocaine users had been abstinent for at least 2 months prior to testing. This group was compared to 16 opiate abusers with a 5-year history–5-month abstinence user profile. An equal number of matched non-drug-using subjects formed the control group. Polydrug abusers and heavy alcohol users were excluded from the study.

Results on the Luria–Nebraska approached but did not achieve significance ($p = 0.068$), with the opiate users performing more poorly than the cocaine users. In post hoc comparisons the controls appeared to perform better than either drug group on the Rhythm and Expressive Speech Scales. Drug users also showed a trend toward having more scales on the LNNB in the impaired range. Factor-analytic studies further suggested that verbal memory was significantly more impaired in both heroin and cocaine abusers. In reviewing the records of several subjects the author suggests that high-dose chronic users of free-base cocaine may be more likely than snorters to show "severe generalized deficits in memory" (Press, 1983, p. 119).

Melamed and Bleiberg (1986) studied free-basing cocaine users after psychiatric nursing staff in a drug treatment hospital noted an anecdotal impression that free-base cocaine users seemed far more likely than other patients to injure themselves while participating in patient baseball games (Melamed, 1986, personal communication). The authors subsequently examined a group of these young adult subjects who reported an average of 32.5 months use of free-base cocaine. For their initial assessment, subjects were tested 48–72 hours after their last reported use of free-base cocaine. Design of the experiment involved the use of multiple *t* tests; however, Bonferoni's test corrected for multiple comparisons.

Results of the study, although somewhat inconsistent, suggested impaired neuropsychological functioning. Both Trails A and B were within the range of impairment, with Trails B showing "serious" impairment on Reitan and Wolfson's (1985) norms. On the Paced Auditory Serial Addition Test (PASAT), free-base users showed impairment only on the *easier* 2.4- and 2-second, but not on the shorter, more difficult 1.6- and 1.2-second trails. This latter result is difficult to understand as a function of neuropsychological impairment, although Melamed (personal communication) hypothesizes that the easier subtest PASAT may be a more sensitive measure than the more difficult version. Otherwise motivational or functional factors, rather than the authors' hypothesis of neuropsychological factors, may provide a better explanation for the authors' data.

A second assessment conducted after 10 days of abstinence showed significant improvement in both Trails tests and in the PASAT 2.4 and 2.0 conditions. However, Trails B and PASAT 2.4-second trial continued to be performed at a significant level of impairment relative to normative data.

The Melamed and Bleiberg (1986) study is not without methodological problems, including the use of published norms in lieu of a matched control group. It is unclear whether Reitan and Wolfson's (1985) neuropsychological norms are an appropriate control for the performance of Melamed and Bleiberg's mostly middle- and upper-middle-class subjects.

If these findings are replicated they may prove to be related to neurotransmitter depletion. Additional abnormalities on neuro-psychological tests may become apparent when larger cohorts of patients are studied using neuropsychological methods. Melamed and Bleiberg's (1986) findings could also be explained as a function of the long-standing changes in psychological status noted by Gawin and Kleber (1986) following withdrawal from cocaine. Results are consistent with neuropsychological dysfunctions elicited from individuals with endogenous forms of depression (Newman and Sweet, 1986).

The results of these two studies, while very preliminary, do suggest that neuropsychological deficits of unknown etiology may be present in both the acute and abstinent phases of withdrawal from cocaine. However, further neuropsychological studies using matched controls and larger subject samples would be necessary to validate these early findings.

"DESIGNER DRUGS"

The proposed Analogue Enforcement Act defines "designer drugs" as substances that have a substantial similarity in either structure or effect to substances already regulated by the Controlled Substances Act (Ziporyn, 1986). In practice, designer drugs are usually narcotics that have been synthesized in clandestine laboratories to imitate or "improve upon" existing drugs of abuse. Toxicity and potency are often vastly increased. For example, 3-methyl fentanyl, a synthetic heroin analogue, requires only 2 micrograms per dose, and an amount placed on the head of a pin is sufficient to kill 50 people (Ziporyn, 1986).

Synthesis of these compounds has been lucrative and also initially legal, since the Food and Drug Administration cannot currently ban synthetic drugs in advance of their creation. The consciousness-enhancing drug MDMA (N,alpha-dimethyl-1,3-benzodioxole-5-ethanamine), also known as "Ecstasy", is of this class, as are the fentanyls, a group of drugs widely used in anesthesiology. Both are now controlled substances; the former was recently banned because of its similarity to another compound shown to cause brain damage in animals.

Perhaps the most striking observation of neurotoxicity resulting from designer drug use was the recent appearance of a severe Parkinson's disease syndrome in users of the synthetic heroin substitute MPPP (methyl-4-phenyl-4-propionoxy-piperidine). When distilled at the wrong temperature or pH, another compound, "MPTP" (1-methyl-4-phenyl-1,2,4,5-tetrahydro-pyridine) is also created (Campagna, 1985). MPTP selectively destroys dopamine-producing neurons in the substantia nigra. The unfortunate victims of this drug, most of whom were under 35, developed symptoms characteristic of advanced Parkinson's disease, including rigidity, stooped posture and speaking difficulty. Paradoxically, the irreversible consequences visited on these drug abusers may prove valuable to researchers looking for causes of Parkinson's. Since this is the first time that Parkinson's has been traced to an exogenous poison, researchers are now investigating incidences of Parkinson's disease which have occurred where certain herbicides similar in composition to MPTP (e.g. Paraquat) have entered the water supply (A bad drug's benefit, 1985).

The future of designer drug use is "bleak", according to one source, with predictions of increasing occurrences of neurodegenerative disease resulting from use of these synthetic neurotoxins (Roberton, cited in Ziporyn, 1986). While no neuropsychological studies of designer drug effects have entered the literature thus far, such investigations would seem strongly indicated, from both a theoretical standpoint, and for the possibility of further delineating the dangerous and toxic effects of these substances.

GLUE SNIFFING

See Chapter 4 – Neuropsychological Toxicology of Solvents.

LSD AND PSYCHEDELIC DRUGS

Substances which induce "altered states" of consciousness, which distort cognitive, sensory and perceptual awareness, are ancient intoxicants. Naturally occurring hallucinogenic substances have been used for thousands of years, and are mentioned in ancient Vedic scriptures. Despite an ancient lineage, abuse of these compounds is reported to have been relatively rare, perhaps because they served religious or cultural functions that strictly delimited proper use. (Strassman, 1984).

LSD (lysergic acid diethylamide) was discovered to be an hallucinogen in 1943 by researcher Albert Hoffman, who accidentally ingested it. The fact that it was an inexpensively synthesized and powerful psychedelic stimulated widespread use, both among scientists and abusers. Research applications of

LSD included experimental trials with advanced cancer patients to expand their awareness and increase acceptance of their condition. Such research was terminated in the late 1960s as the drug's abuse potential came to national attention.

While other psychedelics have been widely available and abused (e.g. psilocybin, mescaline, STP), only LSD has been neuropsychologically investigated. Evidence for neuropsychological impairment is mixed in the available literature, and is hampered by lack of premorbid test data, poor methodology of existing studies and the fact that LSD use rarely occurs in isolation from abuse of other drugs.

One of the more unusual reports is Abraham's (1982) finding of chronic color vision deficit in a group of 46 individuals who averaged 88 LSD experiences. The authors suggest their result is consistent with abnormal color persistence along the neuro-ophthalmic pathway caused by LSD's competitive inhibition of serotonin. The duration of color vision deficit is apparently prolonged, although it is not known whether it is permanent. Replication and validation of the Abraham study seems indicated.

McGlothlin, Arnold and Freedman (1969) studied LSD users with a median of 75 LSD experiences. The authors employed an elaborate battery of neuropsychological tests including the Halstead–Reitan Neuropsychological Battery. The sole significant finding was that, compared to controls, LSD users were more impaired on the Category Test. However, absolute level of impairment was not, in itself, in the impaired range and did not correlate with number of exposures.

Cohen and Edwards (1969) compared LSD users who took LSD at least 50 times to controls matched on age, education IQ and SES. They excluded glue sniffers, but not other types of drug taking from the experimental group. Drug subjects performed significantly more poorly on Trails A and a test of spatial abilities. Impairment on Trails A and The Raven Progressive Matrices Test correlated with number of LSD "trips". Unfortunately, lack of information on other drug use, and the exclusion of an unknown number of obviously impaired patients, mitigates the conclusions of this study.

Wright and Hogan (1972) studied a small group of LSD users with less LSD experience (average number of experiences 30). No differences between experimental and control groups were found on the Halstead–Reitan battery and the Aphasia Screening Test. It is unclear whether negative results simply reflect inadequate exposure history. Culver and King (1974) found that users of LSD performed somewhat less well on Trails Tests, though their scores were not in the impaired range.

In a review of studies prior to 1975, Grant and Mohns (1975) concluded that there was mixed evidence for neuropsychological impairment in LSD users but that there was no consistent evidence to suggest that LSD caused permanent neuropsychological disturbance. Strassman (1984) concurred in a more recent review, stating "the most carefully performed studies to date do not . . . support the contention that frequent LSD use is associated with permanent brain damage" (p. 588). Carlin (1986) has criticized all prior LSD researchers for their reliance on univariate statistical procedures, and for failing to correct for multiple t or F tests. He also speculates that central tendency research designs may wash out individual-specific patterns of impairment (Carlin, 1986).

MARIJUANA

Marijuana is an intoxicant consisting of the leaves and flowers of the female *Cannibis sativa* plant. Citations of marijuana use date back to 2737 B.C. in China, where it was termed "the liberator of sin" (Abel, 1976a). Marijuana was one of the most popular intoxicants for the counterculture of the 1960s but recent estimates suggest that its use may have declined somewhat. A 1984 *New York Times* poll suggested that the proportion of teenagers who had tried marijuana declined from 51% in 1979 to 42% by 1982. Daily use dropped from 10.7% in 1978 to 5.5% in 1983 (Murray, 1986).

The active ingredient in marijuana is delta-9-tetrahydrocannabinol, or THC. In addition to its psychoactive effects, experimental use of THC has suggested several beneficial medical applications, including treatment of open angle glaucoma and asthma. In addition, its antiemetic and antianorexic effects make it potentially useful in cancer radiation therapy and chemotherapy (Cohen, 1980).

Neurological effects

In addition to well-known euphoriant effects, marijuana intoxication may produce tremor, brief periods of muscle rigidity, or myoclonic muscle activity. High doses cause "hyperexcitability of knee jerks with clonus" (Jones, 1980, p. 67). Surface EEG recordings typically do not reveal significant alterations, in sharp contrast with results from primate studies using deep electrode implant recordings. These latter studies showed "marked alterations" in the septal and amygdala regions; alterations which persisted for up to 8 months after inhaling smoke equivalent to three marijuana cigarettes per day for a period of 3–6 months (Jones, 1980, p. 68).

Only a single study using neurologically compromised individuals found cerebral atrophy in marijuana users (Campbell *et al.*, 1971). This finding has not been replicated in studies of healthy long-term marijuana users.

Neuropsychological effects

Acute

Used recreationally, marijuana smoke has a rapid 1–10-minute onset and duration of about 3–4 hours (Abel, 1976a). Feelings of intoxication are affected by context of administration and are prone to placebo effects. Acute intoxication appears to induce global changes in neuropsychological functioning. Memory, speech, cognitive efficiency and flexibility, attention and spatial abilities are all disrupted, and the degree of this disruption is dose-dependent (Ferraro, 1980). For example, Dornbush, Fink and Freedman, (1976) found measures of short-term memory and reaction time to be affected at an unspecified "high dose" but not at a similarly unspecified "low dose". Similarly, several studies by Abel and his co-authors (1976b,c) suggest acute memory changes immediately after smoking marijuana. In one study, Abel (1976b) had eight subjects serve as their own counterbalanced controls. Each was asked to read Bartlett's "War of the Ghosts" and recall it 15 minutes later in writing. While under the influence of marijuana, seven of eight subjects recalled significantly fewer words overall, and fewer content words compared to their test results while sober. Similar results were reported by Miller, Drew and Kiplinger (1976) in the same volume. However, since neither study had a recognition condition, the results could be explained either as a function of memory or motivational impairment.

Impairments in recognition memory appear to be primarily related to the tendency of marijuana-intoxicated subjects to make false positive identifications of material not previously learned. Abel (1976c), for example, found that marijuana-intoxicated subjects make more intrusion errors in a recognition task. Dornbush (1974) found a small decrease in memory and an increase in false alarms for subjects tested for recognition memory while using marijuana. The effect was found whether subjects learned material while intoxicated or "sober". Other studies have not found marijuana-induced recognition deficits (e.g. Darley *et al.*, 1974; Miller *et al.*, 1977).

New learning, as well as memory, is impaired with marijuana use. Rickles *et al.* (1973) found results suggesting that moderate doses of marijuana interfered with and increased the difficulty of learning new material.

Such acute impairments appear limited to material learned under the influence of the drug. Recall or recognition of material learned while 'sober' is not affected when recalled or recognized later in an intoxicated state (Ferraro, 1980; Darley *et al.*, 1973, 1977; Stillman *et al.*, 1974).

Other effects

Marijuana has also been shown to affect reaction time, motor coordination in machinery operation, accuracy, and hand steadiness. In one German study, driving impairment was stated to be found for as long as 6 hours post-THC intake (Kielholz *et al.*, 1972, cited in Yesavage *et al.*, 1985). Several ecologically relevant and disturbing studies have examined the effects of marijuana on the complex perceptual-motor and decision-making abilities of airline pilots. The first asked certified pilots to maintain holding patterns on a flight simulator after smoking marijuana. Significant effects on performance were found up to 4 hours after smoking compared to placebo (Janowsky *et al.*, 1976).

A second study examined ten experienced licensed private pilots who were trained for 8 hours on a flight simulator, allowed to smoke one marijuana cigarette, and then retested at 1, 4 and 24 hours later on the simulator (Yesavage *et al.*, 1985). Subjects were significantly less able to align and land at the center of the runway after ingesting marijuana; impairments which persisted over the 24-hour testing period. Unfortunately the authors did not include a control condition that would allow potential confounds (e.g. fatigue, regression toward the mean, etc.) to be addressed.

If valid, these simulator studies suggest that subtle effects of marijuana may seriously impair complex psychomotor and decision-making behavior long after subjective intoxication ends. Even highly trained subjects are apparently unable to compensate for marijuana-induced perceptual-motor dysfunction. The results are particularly unsettling in light of several highly publicized train and plane accidents during this decade where operators have subsequently tested positive for marijuana.

Chronic effects

Several studies suggest that long-term use of marijuana may affect processing of complex cognitive operations, including both short-term memory and mental operations (Melges *et al.* 1970a, b; Casswell and Marks, 1973). Carlin and Trupin (1977) compared a sex-, age- and education-matched group of individuals who had smoked marijuana for an average of five years with controls, and found that smokers performed significantly more poorly on Trails B.

Alternatively, a number of other studies have failed to find consistent deficits as a function of chronic marijuana intoxication. For example, Schaeffer, Andrysiak and Ungerleider (1981) examined a group of 10 subjects who reported using between 2 and 4 ounces of marijuana mixed with tobacco for an average of 7.4 years. When tested with a comprehensive neuropsychological battery, including the WAIS, the Benton VRT, the Rey Auditory Verbal Learning Test, Trails, and other tests, subjects showed no impairment in cognitive functioning. In fact, IQ scores were all in the Superior to Very Superior range. All this despite the fact that most of the experimental volunteers continued to use marijuana during the period of neuropsychological testing. Similar negative results have also been obtained by earlier researchers (e.g. Grant *et al.*, 1973; Rochford, Grant and LaVigne, 1977).

To summarize, while acute effects of marijuana have been demonstrated by a number of studies, chronic neuropsychological effects of long-term marijuana use have yet to be consistently demonstrated. Major research questions remain unanswered, including questions of individual differences in chronic use, the long-term effect of marijuana on personality functioning (e.g. an "amotivational syndrome"), and whether structural brain changes are produced in long-term marijuana users.

OPIATES

Opiates, particularly heroin, do not appear to have chronic neurotoxic effects. Rounsaville *et al.* (1982) found few significant differences when using a brief battery to test 72 opiate addicts compared with epileptics and CETA workers. Addicts actually outperformed CETA controls on finger tapping. The authors' choice of control groups must be questioned, since all groups performed in the mildly impaired range for Trails A and B, Digit Symbol and a pegboard task. There was also no relationship between recent drug use and neuropsychological status, suggesting that the tests employed may not have been sensitive to drug-related impairments. However, Fields and Fullerton (1975), using the complete Halstead–Reitan battery, also failed to find significant differences between addicts and controls.

While the current literature does not suggest chronic neuropsychological impairment from direct effects of opiates, injection of opiates is not without neuropsychological risk. Secondary infections which penetrate the blood–brain barrier are easily introduced via contaminated needles or conditions of injection. Acquired Immune Deficiency Syndrome (AIDS) has been shown to be transmitted in this way to produce neurotoxic bacterial, fungal and viral infection.

PHENCYCLIDINE (PCP)

Phencyclidine was created in 1956 with the intention of creating a new analgesic (Maddox, 1981). Human clinical trials were conducted after animal studies suggested that the material had potent analgesic properties. Over 3000 research patients received PCP for local surgical procedures or preparatory to general surgery. The first side-effect noted was that all patients experienced complete amnesia for the operation and postoperative phase of recovery, a consequence considered beneficial by some. The second, termed "emergence phenomena", were "excitation reactions most frequently encountered in young or middle-aged males", reactions that eventually caused the termination of human clinical studies (Maddox, 1981, p.5). PCP became a "street drug" in 1967 and was immediately put into wide usage by a polydrug abusing population which either injects, "snorts", eats, or smokes it on marijuana (Fauman and Fauman, 1981).

Neuropsychological effects

Unfortunately, there is very little information on the long-term neuropsychological effects of PCP use. PCP abusing populations are likely to be polydrug abusers, which makes the unique contribution of PCP to neuropsychological impairment difficult to determine. Further, one-third to one-half of sampled "street" PCP has been found to contain other chemical agents with dissimilar pharmacological structure but similar behavioral effects (Lewis and Hordan, 1986).

Acute effects of PCP, however, are clear. Impairments in judgment, logical reasoning, abstraction and attention have been noted, as has "extreme" loss of ability to sustain organized thought (Domino and Luby, 1981, p. 405).

Chronic effects of phencyclidine have been addressed by Carlin *et al.* (1979), who compared 12 chronic PCP users with normal controls and 12 polydrug abusers who did not use PCP. Both PCP users and polydrug abusers were significantly impaired, suggesting that chronic neuropsychological effects of PCP may be similar to that of polydrug abuse.

Another recent study used a screening battery approach to study 30 adolescents and young adults who were referred to drug abuse counseling (presumably PCP from the context of the article) (Lewis and Hordan, 1986). Mean Full Scale IQ of this sample was 92.5, with Performance IQ being several points higher (96.2) than Verbal IQ (91.7). The tests most sensitive to impairment in this population included Trails B, where 30% showed scores above the brain-damage cutoff, and the Category Test, where "more than 70 percent of the sample were in the mild, moderate or severe impaired range" (Lewis and Hordan, 1986, p. 198). Almost 60% of the sample also performed "below normal" on the finger tapping test, a finding suggestive of impaired fine motor performance or motivational deficit.

As in any non-controlled study, conclusions cannot be drawn as to whether population effects or drug effects produce these neuropsychological impairments. Replication in a controlled design is indicated.

Emotional effects

In one study, 19 of 24 PCP users reported having bad reactions to PCP, including loss of sensation or motor control, paralysis, confusion, sensory distortion or unconsciousness. Twenty-three of 24 subjects admitted to losses of judgment and memory during PCP intoxication, sometimes disposing them to accidents. Unfortunately, these reactions were not discouraging to this group, almost all of whom continued to abuse PCP (Fauman and Fauman, 1981).

Violent behavior has been associated with PCP abuse, but it is unclear whether PCP has unique violence-inducing properties or whether individuals who abuse PCP are more likely to have histories of violent acting out. Psychosis is a common concomitant of PCP abuse and is of a toxic confusional type that does not resemble schizophrenia.

POLYDRUG ABUSE

Polydrug abuse is characteristic of many heavy drug users. Users will often simultaneously or sequentially use alcohol, cocaine, opiates, barbiturates and other drugs in various combinations.

Of all abused drug effects, polydrug abuse seems to show the most research support for neurotoxicity. Two out of three studies for which an Impairment Index could be compiled were in the impaired range (Parson and Farr, 1981). For example, Grant *et al.* (1978), reporting the results of a 3-month multi-site study, found 37% of polydrug abusers to show neuropsychological impairment on the Halstead–Reitan Battery. Three-month follow-up testing saw impairment in 34% of the 91 subjects who completed the second battery (Grant *et al.*, 1978).

A later study compared the likelihood of neuropsychological impairment in young (mean age 30) alcohol versus polydrug abusers (Grant *et al.*, 1979). Half of the polydrug abusers were impaired on a clinician's rating of Halstead–Reitan Battery scores, compared to only 20% of the alcohol abusers. Equivalent verbal IQ scores between the two groups argues against educational differences accounting for these results, but the relatively small sample size in each group ($n = 20$) limits the generalizability of these conclusions.

CONCLUSIONS — NEUROPSYCHOLOGICAL TOXICOLOGY OF DRUGS

Neuropsychologists who work with medical patients, or who are asked to evaluate impairment in drug-abusing individuals, must be aware that acute neuropsychological effects are possible under almost all medications, and that chronic effects have been seen for many others. Some drugs apparently produce quite specific neuropsychological impairments (e.g. verbal memory deficit in patients receiving antihypertensives). Others may produce non-specific encephalopathies (e.g. steroids). A careful medical, educational and demographic history is a necessary addition to the neuropsychological test results in such cases. Sometimes it is only with such information that the clinical neuropsychologist can evaluate test results in the context of potentially confounding influences.

It is unfortunate that drug abuse studies typically fail to include such information in their experimental designs, thereby lessening their utility for clinicians and researchers. The majority of neuropsychological studies on drug effects have methodological or statistical design flaws which make their conclusions difficult to interpret. Some of these flaws are within the control of the experimenter, including use of small numbers of subjects, inadequate or missing control groups, and failure to control for premorbid abilities.

230 Neuropsychological Toxicology

Other less than optimal conditions are beyond the control of the researcher. For example, some types of drug abuse do not exist in isolation from other factors, e.g. underclass membership, alcohol abuse, head injury or poor nutrition.

For health researchers, both abused and prescription drug effects are increasingly understood to be multifactorial in nature. Alcohol researchers have come to a similar conclusion. As the clinical complexity of drug effects becomes apparent, experimental design considerations become salient, and neuropsychological researchers have been increasingly called upon to design drug experiments, develop and administer tests and implement interventions based upon test results. This should have the effect of increasing the quantity and quality of drug research in the next decades.

VII
Neuropsychological Toxicology of Pesticides

INTRODUCTION

Most commonly used pesticides, including the chlorinated hydrocarbons (e.g. DDT), the organophosphates (e.g. Malathion, Diazinon, Ronnel) and the carbamates (e.g. Baygon, Maneb, Sevin, Zineb) are lethal to insects via neurotoxic action (Morgan, 1982). Studies using higher mammals have also demonstrated pesticide neurotoxicity (e.g. Vandekar, Plestina and Wilhelm, 1971; Aldridge and Johnson, 1971; DuBois, 1971). It is not surprising, therefore, that neurotoxic effects of pesticides are also found in human exposure victims, and that both cognitive and emotional functions are affected. What may be surprising is the extent of the potential problem, since of all neurotoxic substances produced by civilization, pesticides probably vie with lead for the widest distribution in the environment. In the United States, where there has been a government-mandated ban of leaded fuels, pesticides may well have taken the place of lead as the most ubiquitous neurotoxic material released into the ecosystem.

The actual amount of pesticide put into the environment is staggering. In 1975, for example, approximately 1.3 *billion* pounds of pesticides were utilized by the United States alone (Ecobichon and Joy, 1982). An estimated 340,000 workers are involved in some aspect of pesticide production in the United States (Moses, 1983). An additional estimated 2.5 million migrant or seasonal workers come into contact each year with pesticides (Moses, 1983). Combining these figures would still underestimate total number of exposed subjects, since they do not include those involved in the commerce, transportation and distribution of pesticide.

Considering the magnitude of potential exposure, it is all the more startling to find less neuropsychological research on pesticide effects than for almost any other neurotoxic substance in common use. There are probably several reasons why pesticide-exposed individuals and neuropsychologists do not encounter each other more often, reasons that depend upon both individual

231

and sociocultural factors. For example, many exposed workers in the United States are migratory, or seasonal transient, workers. Medical facilities are not always provided; California is the only state where medical surveillance of organophosphate workers is mandated by law (Coye *et al.*, 1986). Even if access to treatment were available, seasonal workers without union representation might justifiably fear job loss if physical illness is reported. In addition, poisoning episodes may not be recognized as such by itinerant agricultural employees not apprised of local pesticide spraying schedules or expectable toxic exposure symptoms. Fourth, few industrial employees of pesticide manufacturers have access to, or awareness concerning the value of, neuropsychological examination as part of a health screening. Finally, neuropsychologists, as a group, are not yet an active presence in industrial settings or occupational medicine clinics.

For whatever reason, the limited numbers of clinical and research personnel engaged in neuropsychologically related pesticide investigations cannot even begin to address the complexity and magnitude of the problem, the potential dangerousness of these materials, or the frequency of human toxic reactions. With worldwide accidental poisonings from pesticides numbering 500,000 per year and mortality in excess of 1% (Ecobichon and Joy, 1982), it is clear that adverse consequences of pesticide use are a common and serious danger. It can be hoped that growing interest in toxicology by neuropsychologists will also be reflected in increased attention to the cognitive and affective consequences of pesticide exposure.

ROUTES OF EXPOSURE AND INDIVIDUALS AT RISK

Most patients who present with pesticide poisoning are involved in the formulation of the compounds, or in their agricultural application. However, individuals not connected with agricultural industries can also be at risk. Exposure has been reported accidentally, as a result of eating pesticide-contaminated, unwashed fruit (Ratner, Oren and Vigder, 1983), drinking contaminated residential water (Dean *et al.*, 1984) or through the misuse of home insecticide products (Reichert *et al.*, 1977). Deliberate pesticide ingestion as a suicide attempt has also been reported (Lerman, Hirshberg and Shteger, 1984). Hospital personnel may be a high-risk group for pesticide exposure because of frequent and routine applications of insecticide in the hospital's physical plant. Hospital staff exposed to professional applications of insecticide have developed mental confusion, nausea and other symptoms in consequence (Biskind and Mobbs, 1972).

Even office workers are not protected against accidental exposure. One study describes subjective symptoms and neurochemical alterations experienced by a group of five office workers who were exposed to chlorpyrifos (Dursban) and methylcarbamic acid (Bendiocarb 1%) dusted on the outside of the building to kill termites, but presumably carried into the office by an air-intake vent (Hodgson, Block and Parkinson, 1986). It is not known how many of such outbreaks go unreported, since office and professional staff may be unaware of routine insecticide applications and hence may attribute pesticide-induced symptoms to other factors (Biskind and Mobbs, 1972).

ORGANOPHOSPHATE COMPOUNDS

Pesticide	Exposure limits
Malathion	15 mg/m^3
	15 mg/m^3 (NIOSH)
	10 h TWA (ACGIH)
	10 mg/m^3
IDLH level	5000 mg/m^3
Parathion	0.1 mg/m^3
	0.05 mg/m^3
	10 h TWA
IDLH level	20 mg/m^3

There has been more research on *organophosphate* (OP) compounds than other pesticides, perhaps because they were originally developed for their neurotoxic properties as "nerve gases" during World War II. *Soman, Sarin* and *Tabun* are all organophosphate products, differing from their insecticidal counterparts mainly in potency and function (Duffy and Burchfiel, 1980). An organophosphate compound, tri-*o*-cresyl phosphate (TOCP), was responsible for the highly publicized late 1920s and early 1930s epidemic of severe peripheral neuropathy called "Ginger Jake" paralysis, a syndrome that was eventually linked with TOCP-adulteration of the "Jamaica Ginger" beverage.

Organophosphate compounds are more acutely toxic than other types of pesticides (Stopford, 1985). Parathion is the most toxic with a lethal dose as low as 100 mg/kg, while malathion (LD of 858 mg/kg) is one of the least toxic organophosphate products (Namba, 1971). Most incidences of significant organophosphate poisoning have involved exposure to parathion or methylparathion. Organophosphate poisoning has been less frequent in the United States compared to India, Egypt and Mexico, where mass epidemics have been reported (Goetz, 1985).

OP insecticides may be absorbed from "all possible routes" including skin, lungs, gastrointestinal tract and conjunctiva (Namba, 1971, p. 290). Once absorbed, their principal action is to inhibit acetylcholinesterase, possibly irreversibly (Arian, cited in Gershon and Shaw, 1961). Lesion or change in CNS acetylcholine receptors may occur (Duffy *et al.*, 1979), through "accumulation of acetylcholine at neuroeffector junctions and autonomic ganglia" (Morgan, 1982, p. 12). This has been hypothesized to be the major cause of OP's toxicological effect (Rodnitzky and Levin, 1976).

Presumptive diagnosis of organophosphate poisoning can be made when serum cholinesterase activity is reduced by 10–50% in the context of OP exposure (Goetz, 1985). Mild behavioral symptoms can include fatigue, headache, dizziness and abdominal complaints. More severe symptoms include miosis and muscle fasciculations, although these signs may not be present "even in severe poisoning" (Namba, 1971, p. 295). Extreme weakness or paralysis may result from acute exposure (Stopford, 1985). Bulbar signs may be seen, including difficulty speaking and swallowing, and shortness of breath (Goetz, 1985). Other characteristic physical symptoms include sweating, emesis and excessive tearing (Namba, 1971). Finally, a "garlic" odor on the patient's breath may be indicative of organophosphate poisoning.

Neurological effects

Neurological effects of organophosphate poisoning can be divided into *clinical* effects, visible upon casual physical examination, and *subclinical* symptoms which are available only upon laboratory or neuropsychological evaluation. Clinically observable symptom patterns were reported by Whorton and Obrinsky (1983), who examined or reviewed the records of 19 farm workers who entered a field too soon after application of phosphamidon (Dimecron) and mevinphos (Phosdrin), two highly toxic organophosphates.

Initial complaints included weakness, blurring of vision and nausea. Visual complaints of eye discomfort in reading or watching television were the longest-lasting symptoms, persisting at least 5 months post-exposure. One month post-exposure, 11 of the subjects continued to report headaches and weakness. Anxiety was reported by approximately one-third of the subjects, but these symptoms might have been reactive to fear of income loss or future medical disturbance rather than a function of neurotransmitter abnormalities. Three children who were part of this group exhibited the same pattern of symptoms as exposed adults, including weakness, fatigue and inability to keep up with peers in play activity or sports. Symptom constellation in children was said to resolve within 2–3 months (Whorton and Obrinsky, 1983).

Subclinical effects "can be found with great regularity in exposed subjects, notwithstanding the absence of any clinically apparent signs and in the face of normal cholinesterase levels in these same individuals" (Rodnitzky, 1973). Subclinical neurological symptoms of OP exposure include decreased sensory nerve conduction velocities, and increased fiber density (Stalberg *et al.*, 1978). Lasting neurological effects may be produced. One study followed 77 industrial workers exposed to the organophosphate *Sarin*. Although the workers were clinically asymptomatic, and did not have reductions in cholinesterase activity during the year prior to the investigation, their EEGs were significantly different from controls from the same plant. Exposed subjects displayed increased high-frequency beta activity (12–30 Hz) on spectral analysis and visual inspection of the EEG record suggested increased amounts of slow activity, non-specific abnormalities and increased amounts of REM in the sleep EEG (Duffy *et al.*, 1979; Duffy and Burchfiel, 1980).

Recent investigations have also located small, but statistically significant, signs of subclinical neuropathy in otherwise asymptomatic individuals exposed to organophosphate compounds, although peripheral and polyneuropathies reported from OP have also been suggested to be unrelated to cholinesterase inhibition (Namba, 1971).

Neuropsychological effects of organophosphates

Neuropsychological symptoms of OP poisoning include a variety of cognitive and affective symptoms including "impaired vigilance and reduced concentration, slowing of information processing and psychomotor speed, memory deficit, linguistic disturbance, depression, anxiety, and irritability" (Ecobichon and Joy, 1982, p. 171). One study which injected volunteers with an organophosphate found slowed responses to motor and intellectual tasks, inability to sustain attention and concentration, as well as poorer learning and memory. One subject described his experiences:

> Several things are strange. Anything I think goes from big to small . . . . My arms feel strange to touch . . . . I can't seem to keep my mind on what I'm trying to think about . . . . I just go blank . . . . what were we talking about? . . . . I just kind of forget everything (Bowers, Goodman and Sim, 1964, p. 385).

While subjects' descriptions are consistent with other clinical reports of pesticide intoxication, the authors regrettably did not include a placebo condition, or specify the OP dosage level.

In an unpublished study, neuropsychological testing with the Halstead–Reitan battery has been reported by Savage *et al.* (1980), which corroborated neurological findings. The authors found 24% of the exposed individuals to perform in the impaired range, twice the number of impaired controls. The authors reported a main effect of pesticide exposure on 34 neuropsychological subtest scores. Finally, subjects showed deficits in coordination and fine motor speed after acute organophosphate pesticide poisoning. Visual retention and constructional deficits have also been reported (Jusic, 1974) and memory dysfunctions are frequently cited.

Metcalf and Holmes (1969) found impaired performance on the WAIS, the Benton Visual Retention Test and a story recall task in a group of agricultural and industrial workers chronically exposed to pesticides. "Mental confusion" is also a frequently reported finding as a consequence of intoxication, and has apparently resulted in aerial accidents by crop sprayers who became unable to fly. The latter, however, has not been validated with appropriate neuropsychological tests (Levin and Rodnitzky, 1976).

Korsak and Sato (1977) administered part of the Halstead–Reitan battery to 59 male volunteers who had varying (unspecified) degrees of exposure to OP and other pesticides. High-OP exposure subjects performed significantly more poorly on Bender–Gestalt and Trails B compared to low-OP subjects. Unfortunately the authors did not include information about subject matching procedures, if any — leaving the results potentially subject to educational or other confound.

Effects on personality and emotional functioning

Many changes in personality variables have also been reported as a function of exposure to OP and other pesticides. Although early case studies describing "schizophrenic" and depressive reactions to organophosphate poisoning (e.g. Gershon and Shaw, 1961) have been disputed for being impressionistic and non-quantifiable (e.g. Barnes, 1961; Bidstrup, 1961), recent reports continue to note increased tension, restlessness, anxiety and apprehension as a function of exposure to OP and other pesticides (Russell, 1983; Ecobichon and Joy, 1982; Levin, Rodnitzky and Mick, 1976; Levin, 1974; Namba, 1971).

Emotional effects of OP exposure are consistent with what is known about the cholinesterase-inhibiting properties of pesticides, since percutaneous injections of anticholinesterase in human volunteers produced initial feelings of fatigue, followed by subjective feelings of "jitteriness or tenseness inside". Subjects became depressed, irritable and "listless" (Bowers, Goodman and Sim, 1964, p. 384).

Levin, Rodnitzky and Mick (1976) investigated the possibility of subclinical personality disturbance in 24 individuals exposed to organophosphates in agricultural or commercial settings. Controls included a mixed group of farmers tested out of spraying season, or those who did not participate in insecticide application. Controls were matched with experimental subjects for age and education. Compared to controls, pesticide-exposed subjects exhibited significantly higher anxiety on the Taylor Manifest Anxiety Scale, an effect determined by the scores of the 13 commercial pesticide applicators, rather than the farmers. Commercial pesticide workers also had lower plasma cholinesterase than controls. Other measures, e.g. the Beck Depression Inventory, did not show differential effects of pesticide exposure or type of employment.

It is possible, of course, that depressed plasma cholinesterase is simply coincidental with higher stress levels inherent to the job of commercial pesticide applicator rather than a direct result of pesticide exposure. The authors rightly suggest replication of their study using larger and more diverse subject populations.

Emotional symptoms may be better correlated with plasma cholinesterase levels than blood ChE, though symptoms may persist beyond recovery of blood and plasma ChE levels, possibly for 6 months or more following exposure (Levin, Rodnitzky and Mick, 1976).

CHLORINATED HYDROCARBONS

DDT

DDT ($C_{14}H_9Cl_5$)   1 mg/m^3
lowest detectable limit (NIOSH)
0.5 mg/m^3 TWA by NIOSH- validated method

DDT (dichlorodiphenyltrichloroethane) is a chlorinated hydrocarbon that, until recently, was one of the most widely used pesticides. It was the first synthetic insecticide to achieve widespread use, and was extensively employed during the 1940s and 1950s (Stopford, 1985). In recent years, however, the use of DDT has tapered off in developing countries because it is very stable in the environment and increases in concentration along the food chain. Like all organochlorine pesticides, DDT is highly lipid-soluble and accumulates in fatty tissues. It is also a potential carcinogen. DDT is still sold in developing countries where insect predation and disease risks outweigh environmental concern.

DDT's neurotoxic action is to interfere with transmission of nerve impulses by blocking normal repolarization of the axon after transmission of an impulse. The result is "a more or less continuous train of impulses along the fiber following a single impulse" leading to "severe disruption of nervous system function" (Morgan, 1982, p. 7).

DDT changes electrical activity in the brain, including "the cerebellum, cortex, limbic system and various subcortical structures" (Ecobichon and Joy, 1982, p. 107). Acute ingestion of DDT causes nystagmus, hyperesthesias and motor impairment, in dose-dependent severity. In mild cases most symptoms disappear within several days, although severe, possibly allergic reactions have also been reported. Doses as low as 6 mg/kg per day are associated with moderate poisoning. Two common symptoms of such poisoning are apprehensive excitement and persisting weakness in hands and feet. Chronic DDT exposure cases are rare and neuropsychological examinations of exposure cases have not entered the literature. Polyneuropathies have been reported in individual cases, though DDT's role has been disputed.

"AGENT ORANGE" (DIOXIN)

Over 100 million pounds of this potent herbicide were applied by the United States Air Force as a defoliant in Vietnam. Agent Orange has been linked to a variety of toxic effects, including chloracne, porphyrea cutanea tarda, liver disorders and immune system abnormalities. However, psychological and neuropsychological measures have thus far failed to validate neurotoxic effects on exposed Vietnam veterans. For example, Korgeski and Leon (1983) evaluated 100 veterans who participated in the Vietnam war. The authors used both neuropsychological and personality tests, including the Wechsler Logical Memory Subtest of the Wechsler Memory Scale with delayed recall, the Porteus Maze Test, the MMPI, a psychological problem self-report and other (unspecified) tests of spatial memory, problem solving and learning.

Korgeski and Leon (1983) analyzed their subjects' data twice; once to determine the relationship between subjects' *belief* of their exposure and test performance, and a second time to see whether Defense Department computer records of herbicide spraying correlated with subjects' performance. Veterans who believed they had been exposed reported significantly more subjective psychological difficulties, both on the MMPI and self-report inventory. Problems reported included depression, anxiety, rage attacks, and irritability. However, when subjects' proximity to actual sprayings were extrapolated from Defense Department records, all differences between exposed and unexposed individuals disappeared. No differences whatsoever were found in the veterans' neuropsychological performance, whether they were classified by objective or subjective criteria. Finally, while general medical problems were diagnosed equally in each group, skin problems were significantly associated only in the group which *believed* it was exposed. The authors suggested that the belief of exposure to Agent Orange may be more associated with psychological difficulties than actual exposure, although there is always the possibility that subject report is a more accurate index of exposure than Defense Department records.

Another study investigated Dioxin exposure in a non-military population and reported similar findings (Hoffman *et al.*, 1986). The authors examined a set of households exposed to 2,3,7,8- tetrachlorodibenzo-*p*-dioxin (the active ingredient in Agent Orange) when it was combined with waste oil and sprayed on residential, commercial and recreational lands to control dust. Households in a mobile home park were the focus of study.

While depressed immune system reaction to Dioxin was detected in the exposed group, no neuropsychological abnormalities were shown on Trails, Grip Strength and reaction time. The exposed group did show significantly elevated tension/anxiety and anger/hostility scores on the Profile of Mood States (POMS), but the etiology of these symptoms is unclear.

To summarize, there does not appear to be any current support for neuropsychological impairment as a result of exposure to dioxin, a pesticide with other undisputed toxic effects. However, since legal and medical controversies continue unresolved, the final verdict on this substance has probably not been delivered. From current evidence it may prove more useful to employ conventional psychological evaluations on individuals exposed to dioxin, since what little evidence that exists for psychological effects has been measured with tests of personality and emotional function.

KEPONE

Chlordecone, trade-marked as Kepone, has produced one of the most recent and severe outbreaks of pesticide poisoning. In 1975, workers at the Life Sciences Products Company in Hopewell, Virginia, showed an attack rate of up to 70%, since "workers walked regularly through a slurry of the pesticide without boots or protective clothing, . . . a powdery residue . . . soiled workers' clothing [and] caked their skin . . . [and] the few protective masks provided were rarely used" (Taylor, Selhorst and Calabrese, 1980, p. 411). Exposed workers developed the "Kepone shakes" with tremor and ocular trembling. Irritability and memory loss were reported in 13 of 23 patients, although no tests or statistics are cited (Taylor, Selhorst and Calabrese, 1980).

TELONE (1,3-DICHLOROPROPENE)

Telone is used as a pesticide and a nematocide, and is manufactured by Dow Chemical Company. Several neuropsychological and neuropsychiatric effects of Telone exposure have been described. One exposed individual developed personality changes in the course of several weeks, becoming anxious and fearful, and 4 years later developed weakness, inability to concentrate, and anhedonia (Peoples, Maddy and Thomas, 1976). The same authors also recounted the history of 36 fireman who developed headaches, anxiety, and memory and concentration problems, as a probable result of exposure to a 1200-gallon spill of Telone on the roadway. Russell (1983) tested 11 California highway workers exposed to Telone and compared them with seven non-exposed workers on a screening battery consisting of the Wechsler Memory Scale, Trail-Making Tests and the Minnesota Multiphasic Personality Inventory. Significant differences were found only for MMPI personality variables, with Depression, Maladjustment and Manifest Anxiety scales elevated compared to controls.

OTHER PESTICIDES

Carbamates, like organophosphate pesticides, also inactivate acetylcholinesterase. Acute symptoms include lightheadedness, blurred vision, salivation, weakness and muscle fasciculations (Stopford, 1985). There have been no reports of formal neuropsychological examination performed on carbamate-poisoned individuals. However, Ecobichon and Joy (1982) described a case of carbamate exposure in a 55-year-old farmer who hand-sprayed a vegetable garden with carbaryl. Acute symptoms included severe vertigo, visual impairments, paresthesias, fatigue and memory loss. Photophobia, mild paresthesia and memory loss continued to be experienced 1 year after the exposure, with the patient reportedly needing to continually compensate for memory impairment with written reminders. Personality changes may also occur, with one case report noting uncontrolled aggressive behavior in both a man and his pet cat, to which the subject applied a commercial tick powder composed of 5% carbaryl (Bear, Rosenbaum and Norman, 1986).

Chlorinated cyclodienes, including chlordane, heptachlor, aldrin, dieldrin, endrin and endosulfan, cause convulsions as a primary manifestation of exposure (Stopford, 1985). Other neurological effects are similar to those found for pesticides as a group, including headache, dizziness and fasciculation.

Paraquat is an herbicide that gained recent public attention when it was chosen by the U.S. government to destroy clandestine marijuana crops. While there are no neuropsychological studies available, autopsy brain studies of two fatal paraquat poisonings suggest alterations in cell contents which are consistent with effects of aging, vitamin E deficiency, hypoxia and other causes. Cerebrovascular changes and marked alteration of myelin were also found (Grcevic, Jadro-Santel and Jukic, 1977). Investigations of paraquat continue since it was found to be chemically similar to an incorrectly manufactured 'designer drug' linked to Parkinsonian abnormalities (A bad drug's benefit, 1985).

VIII
Other Neurotoxins

ANESTHETIC GASES

Introduction

The first anesthetic inhalant was diethyl ether, used by an American physician in 1842 (Edling, 1980). Many compounds have been used since then for their anesthetic properties, including halothane (2-bromo-2-chloro-1,1,1-trifluorethane), nitrous oxide, chloroform, trichloroethylene and methyoxyflurane (Edling, 1980; Bach, Arbit and Bruce, 1974; Patterson *et al.*, 1985). Today as many as 200,000 persons are routinely exposed to waste anesthetic gases. Seventy-five thousand of these individuals work in hospitals (Patterson *et al.*, 1985). Operating room staff, in particular, may be chronically subjected to low-level ambient exposure of anesthesia; up to 500 ppm of halothane in the working field of the anesthetist, and from 1 to 85 ppm throughout the larger area of the operating room (Dudley *et al.*, 1977).

Since anesthetic gases, by definition, have been developed for their consciousness-altering properties, it is not surprising that acute exposure to anesthetics can alter neuropsychological test behavior. However, despite the *a priori* neurotoxicity of solvent/anesthetics, most available surveys of anesthetic-exposed personnel have been epidemiologic in nature and have relied on questionnaire data rather than neuropsychological test results (Patterson *et al.*, 1985). There are few studies of exposed groups using neuropsychological measures, and no longitudinal investigations of groups at risk. No studies of chronically exposed OR personnel are available; however, animal experiments have documented CNS damage after continuous exposure to halothane.

Neuropsychological effects — acute

There is obviously no disputing the consciousness-altering effects in clinical applications of anesthesia. The effects of smaller, subclinical exposures typically found in operating theaters are more controversial. Several studies by Bruce and his colleagues support the notion that very low doses of anesthesia can produce certain neuropsychological impairments. For example, Bach, Arbit and Bruce (1974) subjected volunteers to 500 ppm nitrous oxide mixed with 15 ppm halothane in air. Subjects showed significant decrements in choice reaction time, several subtests of the Wechsler Memory Scale and memory for tachistoscopically presented patterns. Bruce and Bach (1975) exposed subjects to 500 ppm nitrous oxide and 15 ppm enflurane for 4 hours and then administered a 35-minute neuropsychological battery. Two tests showed impairment: Digit Span and a divided attention decision-making task. Other tests were unaffected, including memory subtests from the Wechsler Memory Scale, a tachistoscopic task and five subtests from the WAIS. In subjects receiving only 500 ppm N_2O, only Digit Span was significantly decremented.

Bruce and Bach (1976) tested 100 male subjects who were exposed to either nitrous oxide alone, or in combination with halothane. There were five independent groups:

1. 500 ppm nitrous oxide + 10.0 ppm halothane
2. 50 ppm nitrous oxide + 1.0 ppm halothane
3. 25 ppm nitrous oxide + 0.5 ppm halothane
4. 500 ppm nitrous oxide alone
5. 50 ppm nitrous oxide alone

Each subject was tested once with air exposure alone and once after 2 hours exposure to anesthetic. All subjects received a tachistoscopic test of visual short-term memory, the Raven's Progressive Matrices Test, the O'Connor Dexterity Test, an audiovisual choice reaction time task, a test of vigilance and the Digit Span test. While logical reasoning tasks like the Raven's and manual dexterity were resistant to anesthetic effects, significant decrements in performance were found in all conditions. Subjects in the lowest-dose condition (50 ppm nitrous oxide alone) showed significant decrements only in the most complex task, the audiovisual divided attention test. Volunteers exposed to the highest amount of anesthetic also performed significantly more poorly on the tachistoscope and Digit Span tests. Digit Span proved sensitive to all but the lowest (50 ppm N_2O–no halothane) group. The authors use their results to speculate that even very low levels of waste gas available in operating rooms may be capable of impairing the neuropsychological functioning of operating room staff.

There are, however, some inconsistencies in the Bruce and Bach (1976) study. Results include an unexplained (probably chance) improvement in vigilance in the 50 ppm N_2O–1 ppm halothane group. Also, subjects who received high-dose nitrous oxide alone were impaired on more tasks than those receiving high-dose nitrous oxide plus halothane, a result that seems explainable only in terms of preexisting differences among subject groups.

The findings of Bruce and his colleagues have also been called into question by several studies which failed to replicate their results. Cook *et al.* (1978) exposed subjects to twenty times the amount of halothane of the former's study — 200 ppm halothane and from 1000 to 4000 ppm of nitrous oxide. Though the dose of anesthetics was many times larger than in the Bruce and Bach (1976) study, no evidence of neuropsychological impairment was found.

In the study which most resembled Bruce's paradigm (naive subjects and similar tests), Cook *et al.* (1978) compared subjects' performance on air-to-anesthetic on the same day, while Bruce and Bach waited a week between air and anesthetic trials. Thus, subjects in the Cook *et al.* study may have remembered their performance on the first trial more clearly than subjects in the Bruce and Bach study, and may have attempted to equalize performance between trials. Also, Bach and Bruce (1976) tallied 100 responses to complex reaction time stimuli per trial, while Cook *et al.* used 50 responses per trial, suggesting that fatigue or vigilance failures over trials could have made Bruce and Bach's subjects perform more poorly in the latter 50 trials, thereby degrading overall performance.

Smith and Shirley (1977) also failed to find neuropsychological effects of anesthesia exposure in subjects who were exposed either to halothane 100–150 ppm, or to a mixture of halothane 15 ppm and nitrous oxide 500 ppm. However, the latter study employed anesthetists or anesthetic technicians who spent "a major part of the working day in an operating theater" (Smith and Shirley, 1977, p. 65), suggesting the possibility that adaptation or selection for high tolerance for anesthetics may have occurred in this group.

Thus, neuropsychological effects of low-level anesthesia inhalation are equivocal. Hopefully, future studies will resolve the discrepant results reported in these studies. An observation by Cook *et al.* (1978) suggests that variations between subjects may be an important factor in researching the neuropsychological effects of anesthetic exposure. They noted wide variation in subject responses to *clinical* amounts of anesthesia, which suggests that perhaps the stronger responders to clinical doses may be the only subjects who show impairments with subclinical exposures.

Developmental neurotoxic effects of anesthetics

Dudley *et al.* (1977) documented unexpected and prolonged learning disability in rat pups exposed to trace levels of halothane *in utero*. Based upon their findings, the authors warn female operating room personnel to transfer to other medical services at least 1 month before conception. There is no evidence at this time to link post-natal exposure to operating room anesthetic gases to permanent neuropsychological disability (Edling, 1980). Neither, however, is there a study which addresses the question. Longitudinal neuropsychological studies of operating room personnel and their children would seem to be strongly indicated.

Nitrous oxide

Nitrous oxide was discovered by Priestly in 1779 and was first used as an anesthetic in 1844. No time was lost among the recreational drug users of that era, who immediately experimented with nitrous oxide and made it a popular abused drug during the 1840s. Since nitrous oxide is approved by the Food and Drug Administration as a food additive, and is on the GRAS (Generally Recognized As Safe) list, it has been legally used as a propellant aerosol in whipped-cream cans. These cans contain approximately 3 liters of 87–90% N_2O. Nitrous oxide gas chargers for commercial whipped-cream contain 4.3-5 liters of 93-98% N_2O (O'Donoghue, 1985).

O'Donoghue (1985) reported there have been at least 22 cases of myeloneuropathy and/or polyneuropathy from chronic use of nitrous oxide. All but two of these cases involved voluntary, recreational abuse. The remaining patients were exposed to N_2O in badly ventilated areas. Early symptoms included sensory paresthesias, loss of balance, gait ataxia and impotence. Personality alterations have also been reported. Neurological examination results were consistent with sensorimotor neuropathy, involving the spinal cord and possibly the cerebellum (O'Donoghue, 1985).

Neuropsychological effects

Greenberg *et al.* (1985) tested the acute neuropsychological effects of 20% nitrous oxide on 12 male subjects who served as their own controls. Subjects received nine tests from an automated neuropsychological battery presented on a COMPAQ microcomputer (Baker, Letz and Fidler, 1985). Three tests were significantly affected by nitrous oxide, including: Finger Tapping; a Continuous Performance Test which required subjects to press a button whenever they saw a large "S" that randomly appeared in a string of other letters; and a Symbol Digit test where numbers were matched to abstract symbols presented on the screen. Nitrous oxide slowed subject performance in each case.

CARBON MONOXIDE

CO:

OSHA	50 ppm (55 mg/m^3)
NIOSH	35 ppm, 8 h TWA
	200 ppm ceiling (no minimum time)
IDLH level	1500 ppm

The poisonous properties of carbon monoxide (CO) have been utilized as far back as the time of Cicero (106–43 B.C.) where charcoal fumes were used by suicide attempters and in the execution of criminals (Shepherd, 1983). Ramazini, a seventeenth-century physician, wrote of the miners who inhaled carbon monoxide vapors which "pervert and pollute the natural composition of the nervous fluid, and the result is palsy, torpor, and the maladies above mentioned" (cited in Shephard, 1983, pp. 3-4).

Carbon monoxide is produced both as a natural oxidation product of methane, and from man-made sources such as auto exhaust emissions and the burning of waste material (World Health Organization, 1979). Carbon monoxide occurs anywhere that incomplete combustion occurs, including gasworks, garages and service stations. Tobacco smoke is also a significant source of carbon monoxide in a closed environment (World Health Organization, 1979b).

Because the hemoglobin molecule binds preferentially with CO over oxygen, it has special toxic affinity for both the brain and the heart, "the most susceptible organs in the body to an oxygen deficit" (Grandstaff, 1973, p. 292). Severity of organ damage is largely dependent upon blood concentration of carboxyhemoglobin.

Neurological effects

Carbon monoxide is capable of causing such a variety of neurological sequelae as to provoke Garland and Pearce's (1967) observation that CO poisoning is associated with almost every known neurological syndrome. One such frequently reported result of acute CO intoxication is the phenomenon of delayed neuropsychological and psychiatric sequelae. Typically, the pattern consists of several days to weeks of apparent recovery, followed by acute-onset dementia, deterioration of neurological status and sometimes permanent disability or death. From 2.7% to 30% of patients exposed to toxic amounts of CO have been reported to exhibit this pattern of "pseudorecovery" followed by rapid deterioration. There do not appear to be any predictors useful in determining who will develop this syndrome of delayed neurotoxicity, although the syndrome seems to occur more frequently in patients with histories of neurologically related illness (e.g. diabetes mellitus, hypertension) (Min, 1986).

The most complete record of CO-induced delayed neurotoxicity was compiled by Min (1986), who examined the records of 738 patients admitted to hospital with accidental CO poisoning. Of these, 86 (12%) were diagnosed as having delayed-onset CO neurotoxicity. The majority of these patients appeared to recover for 2 weeks to 1 month and then rapidly deteriorated. All patients were said to show a mixture of psychiatric and neurological symptoms, including "apathetic mask-like facial expression, symptoms of dementia, such as amnesia and disorientation, urinary incontinence and hypokinesia" (Min, 1986, p. 82). Other frequent symptoms included irritability, distractibility, various types of apraxia and behavioral abnormalities, including silly smiles, frowns or repetitive behaviors. On follow-up of 56 patients, 34 were said to recover to "almost premorbid levels", 11 showed slight weakness and memory impairment, eight had moderate memory impairment, five patients did not show cognitive recovery from initial demented state and six died of infections. Regrettably, neuropsychological testing, if performed, was not reported.

Acute effects

O'Donoghue has summarized the effects on behavior at various levels of CO exposure (see Table VIII.1).

Acute neuropsychological effects

While it has been suggested that levels of 3–4% of carboxyhemoglobin produce detectable loss of psychomotor function, support for this hypothesis has been inconsistent and contradictory. For example, Ramsey (1972) found an increase in simple reaction time after 45 minutes exposure to CO (carboxyhemoglobin 4.5%) while Fodor and Winneke (1972) were unable to show slowing of either arm, wrist or finger movements with carboxyhemoglobin levels as high as 20%. The subject of Bender *et al.* (cited in Shephard, 1983) were said to show deterioration of performance on the Purdue Pegboard Test after $3\frac{1}{2}$ hours exposure to 10 Pa CO (CHb = 7.2%) while Stewart *et al.* (1970) report no decrements. Shephard (1983) has suggested that the sensitivity of various tasks to CO exposure is related to task difficulty, as research subjects appear to be able to draw on "spare mental capacity" and maintain performance by increasing concentration (Shephard, 1983).

Minimal acute experimental effects were found in healthy subjects exposed to 100 ppm of CO for $2\frac{1}{2}$ hours and required to perform single or dual information-processing tasks (Mihevic, Gliner and Horvath, 1983). Subjects showed mild impairment in performing simultaneous tasks only when CO exposure was combined with secondary tasks of moderate difficulty. No decrements in motor performance were found.

In severe acute CO poisoning (about half of which in a recent survey were attempted suicides), half of the total group displayed abnormal mental status. Depression was common, although this symptom probably existed premorbidly. Other alterations in emotional function, including delirium, persisted up to 4 weeks. Permanent dementing process occurred in 4% of these patients (Ginsberg, 1980).

Chronic neuropsychological effects

Chronic CO poisoning at lower exposure levels produces several CNS effects, initially on auditory and visual vigilance, and also in peripheral vision. Johnson *et al.* (1974) found highway toll collectors (who may also

TABLE VIII.1. Human toxic effects of carbon monoxide. (Reprinted with permission from O'Donoghue, J. L. (1985). Carbon monoxide, inorganic nitrogenous compounds and phosphorous. In J. L. O'Donoghue (Ed.), *Neurotoxicity of Industrial and Commercial Chemicals*, Volume 1, 193–203. Copyright CRC Press, Inc., Boca Raton, FL.)

CARBOXYHEMOGLOBIN BLOOD SATURATION (% COHb)	APPROXIMATE CO CONCENTRATIONS PRODUCING STATED COHb SATURATION (PPM)	HUMAN TOXIC RESPONSE
0.3–0.7	1–3	Normal range due to endogenous CO production
1–5	5–30	Selective increase in blood flow to compensate for reduced blood oxygen carrying capacity; with advanced cardiovascular disease, cardiac reserve may be insufficient to compensate; major urban expressway CO levels may reach 25 ppm during peak traffic levels
5–9	30–60	Visual light threshold increased; chest pain occurs with less exertion in patients with angina pectoris; one- to three-pack-a-day smokers have similar COHb levels
10–20	65–150	Slight headache; visual evoked response abnormal; may be lethal for those with severely compromised cardiac function; CO levels may exceed 100 ppm during weather inversions
20–30	150–300	Throbbing headache; fine manual dexterity abnormal; dizziness, hyperpnea, and palpitations with exertion
30–40	300–700	Severe headache; nausea; vomiting, confusion, increased heart and respiratory rates especially with exertion; syncope
40–50	500–700	Progressive worsening of all symptoms: vision, hearing, and intellect impaired; incoordination
50–60	700–1000	Coma and convulsions
60–70	1000–2000	Coma, cardiorespiratory depression, lethal if untreated
94	10,000	Coma without headache, nausea and vomiting
99	50,000	May induce fatal cardiac arrhythmias and death without significantly elevating carboxyhemoglobin

have been exposed to lead) to perform more poorly on parallel processing tasks as a function of carbon monoxide levels.

NT—I

A case study of acute and chronic effects of carbon monoxide has been reported by Vincente (1980), who administered serial neuropsychological evaluations to a patient 4 and 13 months post-CO intoxication. Deficits were noted in cognitive efficiency and flexibility, rhythm, short-term verbal and visual memory, orientation and complex learning. At 13 months post-trauma the patient displayed patchy areas of recovery, e.g. normal performance on Trails A and B, but continued having memory and spatial deficits.

The following case is unfortunately rather typical of many neurotoxicity referrals in its complex and possibly confounding medical history. Ms. Y, reported here, had documented carbon monoxide intoxication but also a history of several closed-head injuries. The patient's low level of education further contributes to the difficulty of accurate assessment. However, despite such a checkered neurological history, she maintained an unbroken work history until her carbon monoxide exposure.

Case example: Carbon monoxide intoxication
Tests administered:
    Shipley Institute of Living Scale
    Finger Tapping Test
    Wechsler Memory Scale:
        Logical and Figural Memory, Immediate and Delayed Recall
    Trail-Making Test A and B
    Stroop Color–Word Test
    Digit Symbol Test
    Luria–Nebraska Pathognomonic Scale
    Spatial Relations Test
    Grooved Pegboard Test
    Minnesota Multiphasic Personality Inventory (MMPI)
    Personal Problems Checklist for Adults
    Clinical Interview

Background information:
The patient was a black female in her 40's with an 8th grade education. Her most recent job was that of a stockroom clerk/manager which she performed responsibly with good supervisory evaluations. She was referred for neuropsychological evaluation from the Occupational Medicine Clinic at Cook County Hospital to determine the cognitive and emotional sequelae of carbon monoxide intoxication induced by a defective space heater in her apartment.

Two days prior to her hospitalization, Ms. Y. stated that she awakened in the morning with stomach pains, but when she visited a physician that day, she was apparently sent home. The following day, the patient awakened in the morning reportedly unable to control the movement of her arms and legs. Ms. Y. then attempted to dress herself, enlisting the aid of her twelve year old son, but their combined efforts were not successful and the patient gave up and went back to sleep. Ms. Y. remembered awakening at noon and returning to sleep. She was discovered unconscious by her adult daughter at 5:30 p.m. that same day. Ms. Y. remained in coma for approximately one week, but has no personal recollection of how long she was unconscious.

The patient believed that her memory had deteriorated since the accident, and indeed, she had forgotten her initial testing appointment the week before. She also admitted to forgetting that she is cooking on the stove and frequently burns her food. Prior to CO exposure, accidental burning of food would occur at most 2–3 times per year. In contrast, the patient reportedly has burned her cooking "almost every day" since she was discharged from the hospital. Ms. Y. also stated that she forgets where she hides her money, with resulting permanent loss of 60 dollars several months ago. In addition, the patient stated that she has been unable to adequately continue in her employment as a supply clerk, having returned to work for three days and finding she could no longer perform the functions of her job. She denied any periods of disorientation.

The patient's medical history included two closed-head injuries, the first when she was struck in the occipital region with a stick brandished by her fiancé. The second, more recent head injury occurred in the 1970s where the patient struck her head in an auto accident, cracking the windshield. Ms. Y. remained conscious in both cases, did not seek medical attention and was able to return to work without incident. There was no reported history of seizures, high fevers or other periods of unconsciousness. Ms. Y. denied alcohol or drug abuse.

Discussion:

The patient's current test results (Table VIII.2) suggested mild to moderate neuropsychological dysfunction consistent with carbon monoxide intoxication. Ms. Y.'s most significant deficits involved both visual memory (Fig. VIII. 1–2) and her ability to organize, plan, self-monitor and maintain attention. For example, Ms. Y. showed poor memory for abstract designs, and when required to match simple patterns to numbers, performed slowly and reversed many patterns. She also performed poorly and made several errors when attempting to draw lines between alternating letters and numbers (Trails B).

Some areas of poor performance may be more easily tied to the patient's relatively low education (8th grade). For example, Ms. Y. did poorly on an IQ screening measure which suggested that her vocabulary and abstract abilities were well below average. However, the patient's reportedly good record of employment prior to her accident suggests that non-verbal memory and organizing abilities necessary for effective performance as a stockroom distributor are significantly decremented as a result of her recent exposure to carbon monoxide.

Personality evaluation suggested that Ms. Y. is coping poorly with the stress of her injury and subsequent unemployment. She reported feelings of depression, poor sleep, tension, social isolation and low self-esteem. Ms. Y. attempted to handle current life stressors with inflexible and probably ineffective coping strategies. She may have had periods where her defenses deteriorated and she appeared disorganized and unable to cope. The patient's current personality functioning may be due to structural sequelae of carbon monoxide intoxication and coma, as depression and poor coping are commonly reported neuropsychological consequences of these types of cases.

Summary and recommendations:

This is a black female in her early 40s rendered unconscious for approximately

TABLE VIII.2. Neuropsychological effects of carbon monoxide intoxication

Test scores

1. *Finger Tapping:* RH mean: 42.4 Russell 2
   (Dom. hand: R) LH mean: 32.4 Russell 3
2. *Wechsler Memory Scale:*
   (a) *Logical*
   Immediate recall: A: 12 B: 8.5 Total: 20.5 Russell 2
   Delayed recall: A: 11 B: 4.0 Total: 15.0 Russell 2
   (b) *Figural*
   Immediate recall: A: 2 B: 1 C: 0 Total: 3 Russell 4
   Delayed recall: A: 3 B: 1 C: 1 Total: 5 Russell 3
3. *Trail Making Test:* A: 34 (seconds) Russell 2
   B: 149 (seconds) Russell 3
4. *WAIS-R Digit Symbol Test:* Raw score: 21 Scaled score 3
5. *Stroop Test:*
   No. of Words: 81 + age corr.: 0 Total: 81 T score 36
   No. of colors: 68 + age corr.: 0 Total: 68 T score 42
   No. of colored words: 20 + age corr.: 0 Total: 20 T score 25
6. *Luria-Nebraska Pathognomonic Scale:* Critical level 65.80
   No. of errors: 21 T score 58.0
7. *Spatial Relations:* (Greek Cross) Best: 2 + Worst: 3 = 4 Russell 2
8. *Pegboard:* (Grooved) RH: 84" T 35 LH: 84" T 43
9. *IQ Estimate:* Shipley Institute of Living ("doubtful validity")
   Raw score: (V:16 A:8) CQ: 86
10. *Personality Tests:*
    MMPI:

L: 3 T: 43	PD: 26 T: 67	MA: 16 T: 48
F: 8 T: 62	MF: 34 T: 72	SI: 46 T: 73
K: 12 T: 49	PA: 11 T: 59	A: 20 T: 56
HS: 21 T: 66	PT: 43 T: 79	R: 20 T: 55
D: 32 T: 74	SC: 43 T: 81	ES: 27 T: 29
HY: 27 T: 64		MAC: 16 T: 16

Note: 0–5 Russell ratings are from Russell (1975) and Russell, Neuringer and Goldstein (1970) where higher scores indicate greater impairment.

one week due to carbon monoxide intoxication from a faulty space heater. The patient exhibited deficits in visual memory, non-verbal abstraction, planning, attention and concentration, all of which are consistent with known effects of CO intoxication and coma. Lower than average intellectual screening results are probably more attributable to education than with CO exposure. The patient is coping poorly with social and psychological consequences of her disability; she is depressed, isolated, tense and does not cope well emotionally.

Ms. Y. will most likely not be able to resume her employment in the near future. Cognitive rehabilitation of what appear to be right hemisphere deficits in non-verbal memory and abstraction may allow the patient to return to work in the future. Supportive psychotherapy to increase self-image and coping skills is also indicated; a referral to the patient's local mental health center would be desirable.

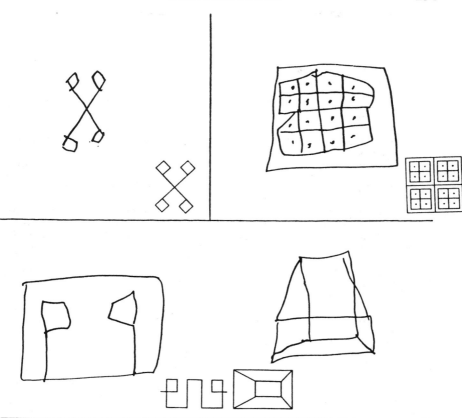

FIGURE VIII.1. Carbon monoxide poisoning. WMS: Figural memory — immediate recall. For reader comparison, card images were inset subsequent to the evaluation.

ETHYLENE OXIDE

C_2H_4O:

OSHA	1 ppm (1.8 mg/m^3)
NIOSH	0.1 ppm, 8 h TWA
	5 ppm, 10 minute ceiling
ACGIH	1 ppm
IDLH	800 ppm

Ethylene oxide is a gas primarily used to disinfect materials that would be damaged by heat sterilization. Because the gas readily penetrates cellophane and other wrappings, it is used by manufacturers of medical supplies to disinfect pre-packaged materials. Because ethylene oxide is the preferred (and sometimes the only) way to sterilize these materials, exposure is

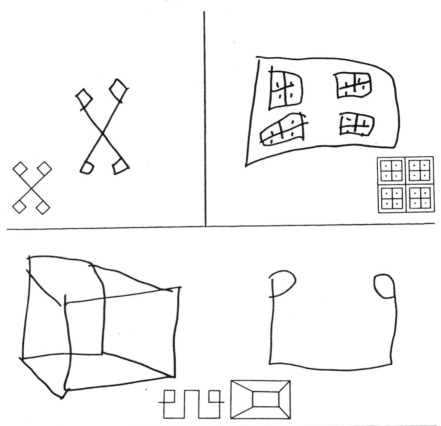

FIGURE VIII.2. Carbon monoxide poisoning. WMS: Figural memory — 30-minute delayed recall. For reader comparison, card images were inset subsequent to the evaluation.

widespread. It has been estimated that over 100,000 workers are exposed to ethylene oxide in the health care industries alone (Gross, Haas and Swift, 1979). Many more individuals may come into contact with the gas during other industrial processes involving ethylene glycol, including fumigation, as well as production of pigments, rocket propellants and ethylene glycol (Gross, Haas and Swift, 1979).

Dermatological, conjunctival and mucosal irritation are consequences of exposure to ethylene oxide. Pulmonary edema, nausea and vomiting have also been noted (Finelli *et al.*, 1983). Central and peripheral nervous system sequelae have been reported, including headache, abnormal EEG, seizures and generalized sensorimotor polyneuropathy. Neurological examinations have showed substantial recovery at a 2-week interval post-exposure (Gross, Haas and Swift, 1979). Clinical examination and electrophysiological

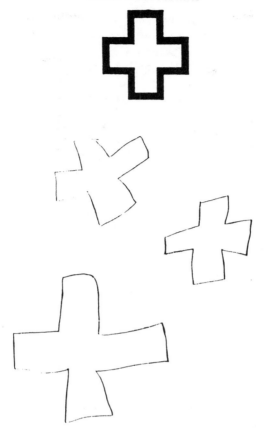

FIGURE VIII.3. Carbon monoxide poisoning. Spatial Relations Test (direct copy).

measures are usually, but not always, normal after 6 months (Finelli *et al.*, 1983).

Neuropsychological effects

Estrin *et al.* (1986) used a computerized neuropsychological battery to compare the performance of eight female hospital workers with chronic ethylene oxide exposure to controls matched for age, sex and education. Ethylene oxide subjects were exposed for a mean of 11.6 years. Subjects were administered several neurological tests and a computerized neuropsychological battery that included the Continuous Performance Test, Simple Reaction Time, Digit Span forward, Symbol Digit, Pattern Memory and Horizontal Addition and Hand-Eye Coordination.

Exposed subjects performed significantly more poorly on the Hand–Eye

Coordination Test, and the Symbol Digit Test also approached significance ($p = 0.06$). While no other test result achieved significance, the exposed group showed poorer performance on all tests. Unfortunately the authors analyzed their data with multiple t tests and significance levels were not corrected for multiple comparisons.

There was also a significant dose–response relationship between scores on the Continuous Performance Test and years of exposure to ethylene oxide that persisted after controlling for age. The only neurological test correlated with ethylene oxide exposure was a significant (age corrected) dose–response relationship between years of exposure and diminished sural nerve conduction velocity (Estrin *et al.*, 1986).

Case report: Ethylene oxide
Tests administered:
    Finger Tapping Test
    Wechsler Memory Scale Subtests:
        Logical and Figural Memory: Immediate and Delayed Recall
        Digits Forward and Backward
        Associate Learning Test
    Trail-Making Test A and B
    WAIS-R Digit Symbol Subtest
    Stroop Color-Word Test
    Luria–Nebraska Pathognomonic Scale
    Spatial Relations Test
    Grooved Pegboard Test
    Grip Strength Test
    Shipley Institute of Living Scale
    Profile of Mood States
Background information:
The patient was a black male in his late 30s referred for neuropsychological testing to evaluate cognitive and emotional sequelae of chronic ethylene oxide exposure. Mr. N. reported that he operated a sterilizer of plastic hospital materials for five years, ending in 1985 when he was switched to the operation of a UPS machine. The sterilizer used ethylene oxide gas as part of the sterilization process. Mr. N. stated that for the first four years of his exposure, the sterilizing machines had no exhaust systems, thereby allowing the gas to escape in his direction whenever he opened the door to remove the equipment.

Mr. N. first noted physical symptoms during his third year of employment; these included dry, damaged hair and greyish skin discoloration. He remembered wondering about the effects of sterilizer chemicals, especially as they appeared corrosive to his clothing and shoes. Subsequently, the patient developed "rough headaches". In addition, Mr. N. claimed to have "passed out" about 10–12 times during his period of exposure for periods of up to a minute.

Mr. N. denied any history of head injury, high fevers or seizure disorder. There was no current or past history of alcohol or drug abuse. The patient reported an episode of hypertension occurring in February 1985, but stated that it had

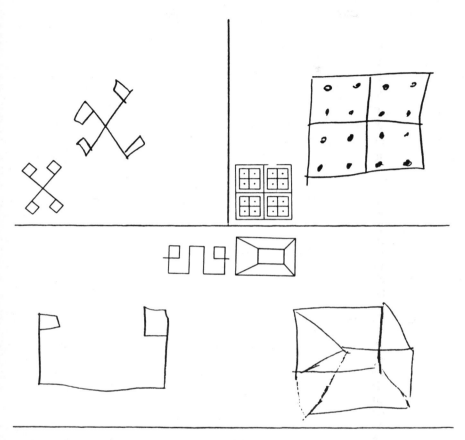

FIGURE VIII.4. Chronic ethylene oxide exposure. WMS: Figural memory — immediate recall. For reader comparison, card images were inset subsequent to the evaluation.

resolved in a subsequent evaluation. He is currently prescribed ergotamine for headache.

Discussion:

Current neuropsychological test results (Table VIII.3) suggest a pattern of deficits attributable to both ethylene oxide exposure and pre-existing learning disability. The patient shows severe deficits in visual memory, learning new verbal material, and significant difficulties in sustaining attention and concentration; deficits probably not attributable to low education alone.

Other areas of poor performance are more likely attributable to pre-existing learning disability, including very poor reading and spelling skills, and the manipulation of abstract verbal concepts. Mr. N. admitted to school difficulties that limited his achievement in school and which may have caused him to leave high school before graduation.

Personality evaluation in clinical interview did not suggest any remarkable difficulties. Mr. N. denied symptoms of depression and had no history of psychiatric hospitalization or use of mental health services. The patient

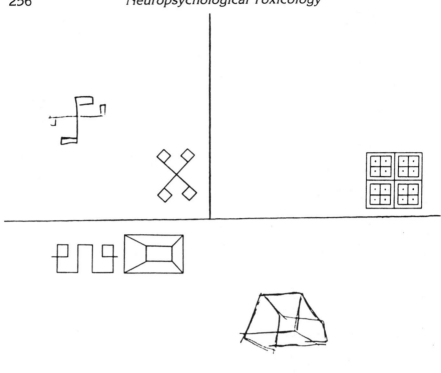

FIGURE VIII.5. Chronic ethylene oxide exposure. WMS: Figural memory — 30 minute delayed recall. For reader comparison, card images were inset subsequent to the evaluation.

admitted to feeling angry and abused by his employers who, he believes, withheld information that would have allowed him to make a knowledgeable decision about continuing to work with ethylene oxide. However, he showed no evidence of unusual suspicion or delusion concerning his exposure.

Summary and recommendations:
This is a male in his 30s referred for neuropsychological evaluation after a 5-year history of work-related ethylene oxide exposure. The patient showed educational deficits which by pattern and history appear to pre-date exposure. Other dysfunctions seem consistent with published literature on ethylene oxide neurotoxicity. Central nervous system effects of ethylene oxide have also been reported and the patient's poor visual memory and inability to sustain attention and concentration may be CNS sequelae of exposure.

TABLE VIII.3. Neuropsychological effects of ethylene oxide exposure

Test scores

1. *Finger Tapping:*   RH mean: 45   Russell 2
   (Dom. hand: R)   LH mean: 47.8   Russell 1
2. *Wechsler Memory Scale:*
   (a) *Logical*

Immediate recall:	A: 12	B: 1.5	Total: 13.5	Russell 3
Delayed recall:	A: 6.5	B:0.0	Total: 6.5	Russell 4

   (b) *Figural*

Immediate recall:	A: 1	B: 1 C: 1	Total: 3	Russell 4
Delayed recall:	A: 2	B: 0 C: 0	Total: 2	Russell 5

3. *Trail Making Test:*   A: 30 (seconds)   Russell 1
                                B: 145 (seconds)   Russell 3
4. *WAIS-R Digit Symbol Test:*   Raw score: 44   Scaled score 7
5. *Stroop Test:*

No. of Words: 100 + age corr.: 0	Total: 100	T score 46
No. of colors: 58 + age corr.: 0	Total: 58	T score 35
No. of colored words: 25 + age corr.: 0	Total: 25	T score 30

6. *Luria-Nebraska Pathognomonic Scale:*

                                                      Critical level 60.55
                                 No. of errors: 17   T score 51

7. *Spatial Relations:* (Greek Cross) Best: 1 + Worst: 1 = 2   Russell 1
8. *Pegboard:* (Grooved) RH: 85 T 35   LH: 96 T 32
9. *Grip Strength:* RH: (1) 85   (2) 59   LH: (1) 61   (2) 56
   (kg)   Mean RH: 72   Mean LH: 58.5
10. *IQ Estimate:* Shipley Institute of Living Scale
                        Raw score: (V: 6 A: 6)
11. *Digits Forward:* 7   *Digits Backward:* 4
12. *Associate Learning Test:* 1;0   6;0   6;0
13. *Personality Tests:* POMS
14. *Personal Problems Checklist for Adults*

Note: 0–5 Russell ratings are from Russell (1975) and Russell, Neuringer and Goldstein (1970) where higher scores indicate greater impairment.

FORMALDEHYDE

(HCHO):
Exposure limits:

OSHA	3 ppm
	5 ppm (ceiling)
	10 ppm, 30 min ceiling
NIOSH	lowest feasible limit
ACGIH	1 ppm
IDLH level	100 ppm

Formaldehyde is a highly irritating and potentially carcinogenic liquid or gas used in germicides, fungicides, embalming fluids, artificial fibers and dyes (Anger and Johnson, 1985). It is a byproduct of cigarette smoke, auto and

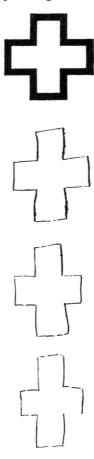

FIGURE VIII.6. Chronic ethylene oxide exposure. Spatial Relations Test (direct copy).

diesel exhaust and is gradually emitted from urea foam insulation, particle board and other construction materials (Kilburn *et al.*, 1985). Formaldehyde is also employed in histology laboratories to fix animal and human tissue for pathological diagnosis (Kilburn, Seidman and Warshaw, 1985). Occupational exposure to formaldehyde occurs in histology technicians, fiberglass batt makers and other occupations where formaldehyde is produced. NIOSH estimates that 1.7 million workers are exposed to formaldehyde in their jobs (Anger and Johnson, 1985).

Non-occupational exposure to formaldehyde occurs primarily in homes insulated with urea-formaldehyde insulation. Workers and tenants in these residences have reported symptoms of eye irritation, chest tightness and neuropsychological symptoms, including memory loss, irritability and headache (Kilburn *et al.*, 1985).

Neuropsychological effects

What little information is available on the neuropsychological effects of formaldehyde exposure is descriptive rather than quantitative. For example, Kilburn *et al.* (1985b) surveyed neurobehavioral symptoms among histology technicians and formaldehyde batt makers. Reported symptoms included sleep disorder, altered sense of balance, loss of concentration and memory deficit. Mood alterations were also present. Greater numbers of symptoms were reported by workers employed in higher exposure occupations.

Kilburn, Seidman & Warshaw (1985a) examined female histology technicians who had daily exposure to formaldehyde but who were also exposed to xylene and toluene. Neuropsychological symptoms claimed by the technicians included recent memory loss, loss of concentration, dizziness and lightheadedness. Reported symptoms of decreased concentration and recent memory were "three times as frequent" in a group exposed to formaldehyde for 4 hours per day compared to controls. The authors' analysis suggested that neuropsychological symptoms increased with duration of exposure to formaldehyde rather than to toluene or xylene.

JET FUELS

These lead-free fuels consist of aromatic, olephin and saturated hydrocarbons, including small amounts of benzene and toluene (Knave *et al.*, 1978). Acute neuropsychological effects on fuel workers include dizziness, headache and fatigue. Chronic exposure appears to produce symptoms of "neuraesthenia, anxiety and/or mental depression". Simple reaction time showed an increasing linear trend over time that was significantly greater for exposed individuals than for controls (Knave *et al.*, 1978, p.29). Performance decrements relative to matched controls were also found in a modified version of the Bourdon–Wiersma Vigilance Test where subjects were required to draw lines over groups of four dots. The authors characterized these results as effects on attention and sensorimotor speed. No differences in memory function or dexterity were found (Knave *et al.*, 1978).

In a more recent study, Struwe, Knave and Mindus (1983) found significantly increased use of medical service for emotional problems among jet fuel-exposed workers compared to matched controls. Of the most severely symptomatic subjects, seven of 14 were judged to have mild organic brain syndrome. Unfortunately, while the authors listed the neuropsychological tests employed (i.e. "SRB, Benton, dots, digit symbol, blot and pins") (Struwe, Knave and Mindus 1983, p. 58), they did not provide data, criteria or statistics related to the diagnosis.

POLYCHLORINATED BIPHENYLS (PCBs)

OSHA   42% chlorine: 1 mg/m^3, 8 h TWA
                54% chlorine: 0.5 mg/m^3, 8 h TWA

NIOSH   occupational carcinogen, reduce exposure to lowest feasible
             limit

Polychlorinated biphenyls are used in high-voltage electrical and electronic applications, and in the production of paint, plastics and carbonless copying paper. They are "counted among the most toxic chemicals", do not degrade in the environment, and exhibit increasing concentration in body tissues along the food chain (Regiani and Bruppacher, 1985, p. 225).

There have been two major episodes of mass poisoning with PCB, the first during 1968 in western Japan. About 1600 people were exposed to a mixture of PCBs and other polychlorinated compounds after they ingested rice oil contaminated with these substances (Regiani and Bruppacher, 1985).

The second incident was similar to the first. It occurred during 1978 in Taiwan where approximately 2000 people were poisoned by using PCB-contaminated cooking oil. PCB had been used as a heat conductor in the cooking oil processing plant, and a pipe containing PCBs had leaked into the cooking oil (Cia and Chu, 1984). This unfortunate epidemic has given researchers most of the currently available information about the neurotoxic properties of PCB.

PCB exposure has been found to cause a variety of symptoms, the most obvious being severe acne-like eruptions. Early-stage exposure symptoms include eye discharge, disturbance of vision and fatigability, malaise and non-specific symtoms such as cough, poor appetite, sore limbs, pruritus and abnormal menstruation (Lu and Wong, 1984).

Neurological manifestations of PCB poisoning

Cia and Chu (1984) examined 35 consecutive dermatological admissions to their hospital and report that 31 (88.6%) had had one or more neurological complaints. Headaches and dizziness were found in about one-third of the patients. Paresthesias in fingers and toes were reported in 65.7% of patients. Hypoesthesia or hyperesthesia were found in 37% of the cases. Deep tendon reflexes were characterized as absent or sluggish in 17% of patients, and another one-third reported back and limb pain.

EEG examinations of six cases (22%) were abnormal in individuals with no prior seizure history. Mean nerve conduction velocity was significantly slower in the exposed group compared to a control group. The authors found evidence of peripheral neuropathy in 28.6% of their patients. Despite the finding of abnormal EEG in one-fifth of the sample, and headache or dizziness in two-fifths, the authors suggested their evidence did not support evidence for CNS dysfunction. Unfortunately, neuropsychological measures were not applied to test that hypothesis. Further, there do not appear to be any neuropsychological studies of PCB poisoning in the literature at this time. Available evidence strongly suggests the need for such a project, and it can be hoped that neuropsychologists who see PCB-exposed patients will attempt relevant research.

IX
Research and Diagnostic Issues

The development of research protocols in neuropsychological toxicology is not simply a matter of choosing the subject population and administering appropriate tests. There are unique problems that complicate the study of toxic effects on psyche and behavior, problems which require organizational skill as well as good experimental design.

INDUSTRIAL STUDIES

These are difficult studies to perform from an organizational standpoint. Most companies are simply not willing, on the basis of a phone call, to open their doors for experimentation. Adversarial relationships between labor and management, legal liability for any neurotoxic effects that are found, and the loss of employee productivity while tests are being conducted all mitigate against easy research access to these sites. For neuropsychologists, working through existing governmental and medical agencies probably provides the best avenue of access to industrial plants.

NIOSH

One of the most important of these agencies is NIOSH, the National Institute for Occupational Safety and Health. NIOSH is the research counterpart of the Occupational Safety and Health Administration (OSHA) and was created by the same regulatory act which created OSHA. Local NIOSH offices may be of help to neuropsychologists in several ways. First, the agency has already published a number of studies addressing the neuropsychological effects of individual toxic substances. These studies may be obtainable from a regional NIOSH office, or from the publication clearinghouse in Washington, DC.

Second, since NIOSH is empowered by law to conduct health hazard evaluations, neuropsychologists with an interest in adding neurobehavioral methods to those evaluations might make that interest known to their local or regional NIOSH office. If neuropsychological services are needed, that office may put them in touch with the outside contractors used by NIOSH to perform evaluation services. These are usually university hospitals or what are called educational resource centers (ERCs), which train occupational health physicians (Bingham, 1983). These agencies may already have established liaisons with neuropsychologists, in which case it may be possible to collaborate or participate in a local interest group.

DRUG STUDIES

Compared to industrial plants, neuropsychological researchers may find hospital sites to be a much more familiar research environment. Neuropsychologists affiliated with university hospitals may find them especially receptive to ongoing research projects. Most university hospitals will have research committees already in place to approve and oversee new projects. Project approval becomes easier if patient populations already require medications of interest. Approval is also made easier by the non-invasive, low-risk nature of neuropsychological testing, there being essentially no risk over and above that of the medication to be studied. Drug studies can also be performed through the office of a private practitioner. Although much easier from an organizational point of view, finding receptive private clinicians and relevant patient populations may require perseverance and investigative skills.

Common design considerations apply, whether neurotoxicology research is conducted in the hospital, the private practitioner's office, or the industrial plant. Several of these important considerations warrant discussion in this chapter.

RESEARCH DESIGN

Neuropsychological testing results from toxicity research are not diagnostic in the same way as medical laboratory tests. With few exceptions, toxic exposures do not tend to produce consistent and focal patterns of neuropsychological impairment. Since impairments tend to be non-specific, the study must be constructed as carefully as possible to rule out potential confounding influences.

Subject selection and potential confounds

To enable the selection of a homogeneous experimental group, a careful and detailed history of each patient is a necessity. For example, current and prior employment of subjects must be described in detail. Job title alone is not an adequate indicator of specific duties. A company's title of "engineer" could mean "nuclear physics Ph.D." at one worksite and "janitor" in another. In addition, every effort should be made to find objective evidence of premorbid functioning (e.g. previous psychological tests, school grades, or selective service examinations).

A detailed history is also necessary to rule out confounding influences on neuropsychological performance. These potential confounds can be *internal* and unique to the individual (e.g. simultaneous neurological illness coincident with neurotoxin exposure). They can also be *external* and shared by the population. For example, suppose a significant discrepancy in grip strength is noted in a population of factory employees under study for neurotoxic exposure. Before neurotoxicity is blamed for unequal grip, the possibility should be entertained that other factors caused the discrepancy (e.g. machinery used by the subjects which exercises their arms unequally, thereby producing unusually strong grip in the exercised hand).

Some confounding influences are *acute*; for example, subject fatigue at the time of test administration. Others are *chronic*, including illnesses with nervous system or orthopedic sequelae, e.g. diabetes, hypertension, arthritis, alcoholism or Alzheimer's disease.

Age, if uncontrolled, can be a major confound. Many of the neuropsychological tests commonly employed in toxicology research are the same tests which are most sensitive to age-related losses of efficiency or performance. In addition, older subjects have usually received greater life-time exposure to neurotoxic materials.

In general, acute confounds can be reduced by controlling details related to test administration and by including questions related to potential confounds (e.g. fatigue, affect, etc.) in the study design. Data from subjects with chronic or severe confounding influences on their neuropsychological performance should probably be excluded from the study.

Control groups

When a neuropsychological toxicology research design includes a control group, it is important that this control group is selected with the same care as the subject population. Failure to do so essentially invalidates any conclusions based on comparison to the control group. Ideally, control subjects should have identical histories in every area except that of toxic exposure. While such an ideal is not realizable in practice, basic variables of age, education, race, gender, medical history and job classification should be equated.

Selection biases

Careful attention must also be paid to the inevitable biases that result from the selection of a research population. For example, tests on a population of active, working individuals could underestimate potential neurotoxic effects of a particular toxin on that group because of what has been termed the "healthy worker" phenomenon. It is assumed that workers, by virtue of their active and current employment, are healthier than the general population; a population which differs in age, illness and other parameters from the healthy worker. In addition, workers who are most adversely affected by neurotoxic exposure may quit (e.g. Seppäläinen *et al.*, 1983) or be fired from the job because of toxin-induced impairment. Workers retained may be self-selected for minimal sensitivity to a particular neurotoxin, predisposing the researcher to make a Type II error (false acceptance of the null hypothesis) in the event of negative findings.

The opposite error (Type I) can occur in the study of workers already identified as having a neurotoxin-induced syndrome, or in patients who must receive a certain drug due to illness. In the workplace the possibility of bias in the direction of overestimating industrial toxicity might be termed a "sick worker" effect. For example, workers who are referred to an occupational medicine clinic with symptoms of "solvent poisoning" may be unusually sensitive to a particular toxin and not typical of the population response to that toxin.

In drug studies, patients receiving medication are, by virtue of the illness for which they receive drugs, also not representative of the general, unmedicated population. For example, patients receiving anticonvulsants are also usually diagnosed with brain injury or seizure disorder. Their pattern of neuropsychological response to anti-seizure medication may be affected by health variables that led to their treatment with anticonvulsants rather than by the drug.

Potential biases inherent in research population selection suggest that special care must be taken to correctly sample the population under study. If circumstances or design limit the types of subjects selected to a particular subset of a population, cognizance should be taken of that fact when the results are finally interpreted.

EXPERIMENTAL DESIGN STRATEGIES

Sound statistical practice and procedures inhere as much in neuropsychological toxicology as in conventional psychological research. Among the methodological problems capable of distorting results are data snooping, conducting many tests without correcting for Type I error rate, having too many dependent variables, using tests with low power and violating a test's statistical assumptions (Muller and Benignus, 1984).

Causality must always be cautiously inferred in neuropsychological toxicology studies. Interpretation of the data must be made in the context of known exposure preceding neurotoxic illness, and results should be credible in relation to known biological factors and previous research. The most definitive evidence would be a change in toxic exposure that also alters morbidity (Hernberg, 1980, p. 169).

Schoenberg (1982) lists the following experimental designs which may have application to behavioral neurotoxicology.

In *case-control* studies, individuals who have been identified as neurotoxin-exposed are compared against matched controls. The design may allow comparison of present characteristics with a cross sectional design or past exposure history (if data are available) using retrospective data. Advantages of case–control designs include low cost, relatively fast data collection and no need for follow-up testing. Difficulties include finding appropriately matched controls, and problems verifying past exposure history.

Prospective or *cohort* studies follow groups of exposed and control individuals to measure changes over time. In prospective studies, unlike case–control studies, absolute risk can be measured. Another important consideration is that individuals can be assessed *before* they begin exposure to neurotoxic substances, and can be followed after exposure ceases. Cohort designs cannot, however, add new testing procedures or diagnostic techniques retrospectively. Additionally, volunteers for cohort studies may not be representative of non-volunteering workers (Schoenberg, 1982).

Quasi-experimental designs

An important innovation in single case research has been the use of quasi-experimental designs. Single case experimental designs may be a practical (and in some instances the only possible) alternative to group research when investigating neuropsychological effects of neurotoxic exposure. Individuals exposed to neurotoxic medicines or industrial substances can be followed before, during and after neurotoxic exposure with these designs (Barlow and Hersen, 1984). The quasi-experimental individual case study design includes use of repeated measures, baseline behavior assessment and manipulation of only one variable at a time (e.g. changing a subject's time in contact with a particular industrial agent, but not the total number of hours worked). For example, the one variable rule in a neuropsychological study of drug effects might produce the following sequence "(1) no drug, (2) placebo, (3) active drug, (4) placebo and (5) active drug" (Barlow and Hersen, 1984, p. 87).

Individual case study designs have advantages and limitations. Individual subjects exposed to rare neurotoxicants may be easier to locate than large cohorts subject to conventional experimental procedures. On the other hand, generality of toxic effects will always be an unresolved issue in individual case designs. Individual differences in neurotoxic susceptibility and neuropsychological responses clearly exist. Further, since there is usually a publication bias against negative case results, publication of positive case studies may collectively encourage acceptance of a "Type I" error (inappropriate rejection of the null hypothesis). The tendency of journals to publish only positive cases is unfortunate. Hernberg (1980) observes that evaluation and publication of negative results is as crucial for the understanding of neurotoxic effects as positive results.

Statistical procedures

Because toxic exposure may be the product of individual effects, multivariate analyses may be preferred over univariate statistics. Scaling procedures may also help determine whether neurotoxic sequelae form an ordered sequence based on exposure, or whether individual patterns of susceptibility are more common (Fein *et al.*, 1983).

PRACTICAL CONSIDERATIONS

Practical considerations apply in the design of neurotoxicity research. For example, since many neurotoxicology evaluations are conducted on site, rather than at the psychologist's office, care must be taken to select a quiet, comfortable testing room, away from high traffic areas, workplace noise and distracting activity. Requiring some level of confidentiality among members of the research population is necessary in order to prevent subjects tested early from giving information to later subjects. Where possible, researchers (but not clinicians) should attempt to test "blindly"—that is, to evaluate subjects without knowing their experimental or control group membership. Blind testing reduces the possibility of conscious or unconscious researcher influence on test results. Biases can be further reduced by having all test instructions and materials presented in as standardized a manner as possible. Materials should be administered in a specific order, and instructions should be read, rather than ad libbed.

Test selection

Assessment devices must be sensitive to the detection of subclinical neurotoxicity. Many neuropsychological tests commonly used for general psychological evaluations would not be chosen for neurotoxicology studies. For example, the Wechsler Intelligence Tests (e.g. WAIS-R), the Luria–Nebraska Neuropsychological Battery and tests of linguistic dysfunction are all comparatively insensitive to subclinical toxicity.

Selected neuropsychological tests should also be capable of detecting effects specific to the neurotoxic agent under study. *n*-Hexane, a peripheral nervous system neurotoxin, might require a different battery than lead, a metal which affects both central and peripheral nervous system functions.

Personality, affect, and "personal problem" inventories are essential additions to neurotoxicology studies. Many toxins cause emotional abnormalities as part of their neurotoxic profile (e.g. pesticide-induced irritability or depression etiologically related to lead poisoning).

Use of affect and problem inventories can also aid in ruling out unrelated or pre-existing psychopathology and psychosocial stressors (e.g. schizophrenic disorder; death in the family), that may influence neuropsychological performance. Many patients will present with approximately normal test performance but nevertheless complain about perceived inadequacies. Since initial phases of neurotoxic symptomatology may only be diagnosable by questionnaire and history rather than abnormal neuropsychological examination, it is especially important to undertake extensive interviews and historical information collection. This might include speaking to collaterals and co-workers where permitted, obtaining employment records and medical history, and observing the patient's coping skills and personality dynamics.

The following case is presented as an example of one in which stress and psychological dynamics, rather than neurotoxic exposure, appear to be the predominant influences on neuropsychological presentation.

Case study: Neuropsychological evaluation of a patient referred for possible cyanide exposure

The patient is a college-educated, white male in his mid-50s whose work history was a textbook example of entrepreneurial achievement leading to executive management. The patient had led a "fast track" lifestyle with workaholic hours. He "relaxed" by speed-boat racing. In his latest job, Mr. C. had been hired to help manage a small corporation that produced cyanide as part of a manufacturing process. Because of a change in priorities by plant owners, Mr. C.'s job was eliminated and he was given a lower status position at the company. The company eventually folded because of bad management.

Mr. C. was referred for neuropsychological evaluation because of his worry that he had been exposed to harmful doses of cyanide in his capacity as plant manager. Complaints included tingling in his fingers and feeling "not 100%".

The patient's test results (Table IX.1) were interpreted as suggesting essentially unimpaired cortical functioning. Clinical interview and personality evaluation suggested that the patient had been coping very poorly with serious personal, legal and professional stressors. He was acutely depressed and had focused on his medical difficulties as an obsessive defense against more threatening personal problems. In the clinical interview, Mr. C. expressed fears of growing older, and viewed normal age-related decreases in speed and agility as incompatible with his past performance and lifestyle. He was reassured that any perceived neuropsychological impairments could be better explained by factors other than cyanide exposure. Outpatient psychotherapy was recommended to enable Mr. C. to improve his coping strategies and aid him in accepting minor changes related to aging.

TABLE IX.1. "Organic versus functional?" Possible cyanide exposure.

1. *Finger Tapping:* (Dom. hand: R)	RH mean: 47.5 LH mean: 49.5		Russell 2 Russell 0
2. *Wechsler Memory Scale:* (a) *Logical*			
Immediate recall:	A: 10.5 B: 10.5	Total: 21	Russell 2
Delayed recall:	A: 7 B:10	Total: 17	Russell 2
(b) *Figural*			
Immediate recall:	A: 2 B: 4 C: 5	Total: 11	Russell 1
Delayed recall:	A: 1 B: 4 C: 2	Total: 7	Russell 2
3. *Trail Making Test:*	A: 22 (seconds)		Russell 1
	B: 55 (seconds)		Russell 0
4. *WAIS-R Digit Symbol Test:*		Raw score: 52 Scaled score 8	
		(age corrected): 11	
5. *Stroop Test:*			
No. of Words: 87 + age corr.: 8		Total: 95	T score 43
No. of colors: 66 + age corr.: 4		Total: 69	T score 43
No. of colored words: 33 + age corr.: 5		Total: 38	T score 43
6. *Luria-Nebraska Pathognomonic Scale:*			
			Critical level 56.6
	No. of errors: 7		T score 35
7. *Spatial Relations:* (Greek Cross) Best: 1 + Worst: 1 = 2			Russell 1

8. *Pegboard:* (Purdue) RH: 15 (T 59)   LH: 14 (T 56)   BH: 13 (T 64)
   (other pegboard scores): Purdue pegboard assemblies: 9 completed
   Grip Strength: RH: (1) 48 (T 55)   (2) 52 (T 57)   Mean: 50
   (kg)   LH (1) 48 (T 58)   (2) 51 (T 59)   Mean: 49.5
10. *IQ Estimate:* Kent EGY Scale   Raw score: 27   1Q est.: 104
11. *Personality Test:* MMPI:

L T43	PD + 0.4k T57	SI T58
F T70	MF T64	A T68
K T51	PA T56	R T56
HS + 0.5k T93	PT + 1k T84	ES T37
D T92	SC + 1k T83	MAC T43
HY T89	MA + .2k T67	

Note: 0–5 Russell Ratings are from Russell (1975) and Russell, Neuringer and Goldstein (1970) with higher scores indicating greater impairment.

OTHER INFLUENCES UPON NEUROPSYCHOLOGICAL PERFORMANCE

Regardless of sensitivity, completeness and accuracy of the tests used, *a priori* neurotoxicity of the substances under investigation, and adequacy of experimental method, researchers and clinicians should not assume that impairment of neuropsychological performance is isomorphic with neurotoxic damage. There are many reasons for impaired test behavior, including those which have nothing to do with actual impairments. Some of these "impairments" may be severe and thus may mislead the examiner. A few examples are described below.

Behavior which imitates structural or metabolic brain dysfunction is called *pseudodementia*. Pseudodemented patients may or may not produce such impairments under voluntary control. If the impairment is under voluntary control the disorder is called *malingering*. Subjects may malinger for various reasons, often for secondary gain. *Litigation* can be a predisposing factor, and the test results of a litigating patient should always be interpreted very cautiously and carefully.

The number of patients who use neuropsychological examination in the search for secondary gain is probably underestimated. Gade, Mortensen and Udesen (1984) note an "almost exponential rise" in Danish cases of solvent-induced toxic encephalopathy in the past 4 years. Gade (personal communication) hypothesizes that this increase may be the result of legal and regulatory factors. He notes that the solvent-syndrome is a legitimate diagnostic entity in Denmark, and that when it is claimed as a disability by a worker the burden is on the State to prove otherwise. While the amount of pension from solvent disorders is not great, neither is it insignificant, and it is an obvious source of secondary gain for predisposed subjects. Similarly, while the United States has no official diagnostic category of "neurotoxic syndrome", government disability funds and legal damage suits provide reinforcement to those in search of secondary gains.

Other patients may perform in a pseudodemented fashion for reasons more connected with psychopathology than secondary gain. One such patient in our experience was exposed to pesticides when her father sprinkled the basement with a carbamate insecticide. She presented for testing with a formidable knowledge (and memory) of anticholinesterase effects of pesticides, gleaned from extensive readings. Despite her demonstrated retention of this complex knowledge, her test profile showed exaggerated memory deficits as well as an interesting pattern on Finger Tapping.

In averaged 10-second trials this patient was only able to produce a mean number of taps in the teens with her dominant hand. After several normal trials with her non-dominant hand the patient announced that her non-dominant hand was now impaired, and that the previously tested hand was normal. Subsequent testing confirmed a "shift" of impairment; her non-dominant hand was newly "impaired" and retesting of the dominant hand now showed normal fine motor speed. The patient was diagnosed as pseudodemented with probable parental conflicts contributing to her behavior. However, when psychotherapy was suggested the patient firmly insisted upon the "organicity" of her behavior.

Recognizing the patterns of pseudodemented performance is worth a monograph in itself; however, a pattern useful to neuropsychologists has been identified by Oberg *et al.* (1985). These authors examined a group of 14 patients who had been diagnosed as "pseudodemented" based on the following criteria:

1. Subjective complaints of severe cognitive difficulties.
2. Poor neuropsychological test performance.
3. Areas of clearly proficient functioning by history or conduct.
4. Normal neurological examination.
5. Normal CT scan.
6. No history of subnormal intelligence, alcohol abuse, neurological or major psychiatric illness.
7. No family history of presenile dementia.

These patients were compared with groups of psychiatric (psychotic/ borderline) patients, normal pressure hydrocephalus patients, and equal numbers of education-matched patients with documented mild or severe cortical atrophy.

Pseudodemented patients performed significantly better than the severely atrophic group in block designs and visuospatial learning but worse in WAIS Verbal IQ items (Information, Similarities and Vocabulary). Pseudodemented patients were also more impaired than the *severely* atrophic group in various memory tests. This pattern was substantially similar for the pseudodemented group in comparison with the other groups. Pseudodemented patients showed much more impairment on recognition memory, memory span and verbal IQ tests than other subjects. They tended to perform normally on block design and a task of visuospatial learning. This pattern is rarely, if ever, seen in actual organic brain disease (Oberg *et al.*, 1985).

Psychological impairments of function may occur in groups as well as individuals. One report described a shoe factory where 50–75 workers complained of headache, lightheadedness and dizziness "in response to a strange odor in the workplace" (Murphy and Colligan, 1979, p. 133). No known toxins were found by representatives of OSHA and state health officials. Instead, symptoms were found to be highly correlated with use of stimulant medication, perception of the workplace as too crowded, witnessing other workers become ill, and other symptoms indicating emotional arousal, psychosocial stressors or dissatisfaction with the workplace. Other, similar reports of mass psychogenic illness in an industrial setting have also been reported (Smith, Colligan and Hurrell, 1978; Stahl and Lebedun, 1974; Kerchkoff and Back, 1968).

Attention to these individual and group patterns, and, in the case example provided earlier, to the patient's testing behavior and the context of presenting complaints, will maximize the potential for researchers and clinicians to detect functional impairments of neuropsychological performance.

FUTURE RESEARCH ISSUES

The future of neurotoxicity research in part depends upon multidisciplinary cooperation and sharing of research successes and difficulties. A recent conference on the neurobehavioral effects of solvents, held in North Carolina, U.S.A., was a good example of such international, multidisciplinary cooperation. At the conference, entitled "The Neurobehavioral Effects of Solvents", physicians, neuropsychologists, animal researchers, industry representatives, biostatisticians and others came together to publish a consensus that would direct further scientific and industrial inquiry in the area of solvent neurotoxicity. While the conference and the consensus summary was specific to solvent-related issues, the issues raised by the group are applicable to neurotoxicology research generally.

First, limitations in the current state of knowledge about toxic effects formed a pervasive backdrop to the consensus summaries generated at the conference. Very basic questions remained about the nature, frequency and symptoms of neurotoxic disorders. Neither the overall patterns of intoxication syndromes nor the exceptions to those patterns were known. Very little, for example, was known about the overall progression of neuropsychological or neurological impairments as a result of solvent exposure. Even less was known about individual variations in that progression; who is most susceptible and why, what are the synergistic effects of exposure to multiple solvents, and what is the relationship between involuntary (workplace) and voluntary (alcohol, drug abuse) neurotoxic exposure.

Answering such questions will require both epidemiologic investigations as well as ipsative studies of individuals. Epidemiological data are needed to discover overall patterns of incidence, prevalence and dose–exposure relationships of solvent disorders, both for individual solvents and mixtures. Large-scale group investigations of solvent-using industries are needed, including painting and solvent manufacture, printing, electronics, degreasing, dry-cleaning and some military industries.

Multiple potential confounds complicate the determination of these patterns and therefore must be addressed by neurotoxicity researchers. The confounding influences noted by the "Neurobehavioral Effects" participants were similar to those which complicate neuropsychological research generally, including age, sex, ethnicity, brain injury, hobby exposure, alcohol, drugs and other hereditary and environmental factors.

Several issues unique to the multidisciplinary nature of neurobehavioral toxicology were also addressed. For example, the workshop participants noted a lack of common theoretical focus between animal and human researchers. Urging information-sharing and cooperation between disciplines, the participants recommended that animal model developers familiarize themselves with human neurotoxic symptoms and design experiments that have more direct relevance to human exposure effects. Because of the difficulty of intraspecies comparison, primate studies were also recommended.

In turn, human exposure researchers were likewise encouraged to design experiments for which animal analogues could be developed, e.g. psychomotor, visual memory and neurological function. The advantages of utilizing animal research include precise dose/exposure control, study of irreversibly toxic materials in an experimental context, and parallel investigation of neuropathology, biochemistry and metabolism.

Both experimental and quasi-experimental studies were deemed necessary to select and validate sensitive neurological and neuropsychological test procedures on relevant populations. Increased attention to experimental design variables was deemed to be a crucial aspect of these future studies.

Standardization of experimental technique, neuropsychological measures, questionnaires and methods of monitoring neurotoxic effects were called for to facilitate international comparisons and cooperative efforts. This latter recommendation was not universally accepted, since any prescribed battery trades off originality and potential improvement in the interests of comparability. Undoubtedly, as research becomes more widespread, sensitive tests will become more widely available and comparisons will be more easily performed without the use of a "mandatory" set of instruments. New tests will be subject to validation much as is already done in the field of psychology.

CONCLUSION

If there is a conclusion possible from the diverse information presented in this volume, it must be that it has taken several hundred pages to barely "introduce" a field ripe for study, that of neuropsychological toxicology. The task of training knowledgeable experts in the clinical and research facets of this field must be the next step in its development. At present such training is often gotten on an ad-hoc basis, through readings, practicums and clinical practice. Training opportunities may broaden, however, as neuropsychologists and other health care professionals begin to recognize the pervasive influence of neurotoxic substances on human health, health care and the quality of life. When this occurs, neuropsychological toxicology will have reached a third, extended stage of development. We will finally be able to answer the questions that, until recently, no one knew enough to ask.

References

A bad drug's benefit (9 December 1985), *Newsweek*, 84.

Abel, E. L. (1976a). *The Scientific Study of Marihuana*. Chicago: Nelson-Hall.

Abel, E. L. (1976b). Marijuana and memory. In E. L. Abel (Ed.), *The Scientific Study of Marihuana*. Chicago: Nelson-Hall, 113-116.

Abel, E. L. (1976c). Retrieval of information after use of marihuana. In E. L. Abel (Ed.), *The Scientific Study of Marihuana*. Chicago: Nelson-Hall, 121-124.

Abraham, H. A chronic impairment of color vision in users of LSD. *British Journal of Psychiatry*, **140**, 518-520.

Acker, C. (1986). Neuropsychological deficits in alcoholics: the relative contributions of gender and drinking history. *British Journal of Addiction*, **81**, 395-403.

Acker, W., Aps, E. J., Majumdar, S. R. Shaw, G. K., and Thomson, A. D. (1982). The relationship between brain and liver damage in chronic alcoholic patients. *Journal of Neurology, Neurosurgery and Psychiatry*, **45**, 984-987.

Adams, K. M., Grant, I., and Reed, R. (1980). Neuropsychology in alcoholic men in their late thirties: One year follow-up. *American Journal of Psychiatry*, **137**, 928-931.

Aldridge, W. N., and Johnson, M. K. (1971). Side effects of organophosphorus compounds: Delayed neurotoxicity. *Bulletin of the World Health Organization*, **44**, 259-263.

Allison, W. M., and Jerrom, D. W. A. (1984). Glue sniffing: A pilot study of the cognitive effects of long-term use. *International Journal of the Addictions*, **19**, 453-458.

Alterman, A. I., and Tarter, R. E. (1985). Assessing the influence of confounding subject variables in neuropsychological research in alcoholism and related disorders. *International Journal of Neuroscience*, **26**, 75-84.

Alterman, A. I., Tarter, R. E., Petrarulo, E. W., and Baughman, T. G. (1984). Evidence for impersistence in young male alcoholics. *Alcoholism: Clinical and Experimental Research*, **8**, 448-450.

Altura, B. M. (1984a). Introduction and overview. *Alcohol*, **1**, 321-323.

Altura, B. M., and Altura, B. T. (1984b). Alcohol, the cerebal circulation and strokes. *Alcohol*, **1**, 325-331.

Altura, B. M., Altura, B. T., and Gebrewold, A. (1983). Alcohol-induced spasms of cerebral blood vessels: Relation to cerebrovascular accidents and sudden death, *Science*, **220**, 331-333.

American Psychiatric Association (1980). *Diagnostic and Statistical Manual of Mental Disorders—DSM-III*. Washington, DC: American Psychiatric Association.

Andersen, I., Lundquist, G. R., Molhave, L., Find Petersen, O., Proctor, D. F.,

Vaeth, M., and Wyon, D. P. (1983). Human response to controlled levels of toluene in six-hour exposures. *Scandinavian Journal of Work Environment and Health,* **9,** 405–416.

Anderson, A. (1982). Neurotoxic follies. *Psychology Today,* July, 30–42.

Anger, W. K. (1984). Neurobehavioral testing of chemicals: Impact on recommended standards. *Neurobehavioral Toxicology and Teratology,* **6,** 147–153.

Anger, W. K. (1985). Neurobehavioral tests used in NIOSH-supported worksite studies, 1973–1983. *Neurobehavioral Toxicology and Teratology,* **7,** 359–368.

Anger, W. K., and Johnson, B. L. (1985). Chemicals affecting behavior. In J. L. O'Donoghue (Ed.), *Neurotoxicity of Industrial and Commercial Chemicals,* Volume I. Boca Raton: CRC Press, 52–148.

Angotzi, G., Camerino, D., Carboncini, F., Cassitto, M. G., Ceccarelli, F., Cioni, R., Paradiso, C., and Sartorelli, E. (1982). Neurobehavioral follow-up study of mercury exposure. In R. Gilioli, M. G. Cassitto, and V. Foa (Eds), *Neurobehavioral Methods in Occupational Health.* New York: Pergamon Press, 247–253.

Annau, Z. (1981). The neurobehavioral toxicity of trichlorethylene. *Neurobehavioral Toxicology and Teratology,* **3,** 417–424.

Annest, J. L., Pirkle, J. L., Makuc, D., Neese, J. W., Bayse, D. D., and Kovar, M. G. (9 June 1983). Chronological trend in blood lead levels between 1976 and 1980. *New England Journal of Medicine,* **308,** 1373–1377.

Antti-Poika, M. (1982a). Prognosis of symptoms in patients with diagnosed chronic organic intoxication. *International Archives of Occupational and Environmental Health,* **51,** 81–89.

Antti-Poika, M. (1982b). Overall prognosis of patients with diagnosed chronic organic solvent intoxication. *International Archives of Occupational and Environmental Health,* **51,** 127–138.

Araki, S., and Honma, T. (1976). Relationships between lead absorption and peripheral nerve conduction velocities in lead workers. *Scandinavian Journal of Work Environment and Health,* **4,** 225.

Arlien-Søberg, P. (1985). Chronic effects of organic solvents on the central nervous system and diagnostic criteria. In *Chronic Effects of Organic Solvents on the Central Nervous System and Diagnostic Criteria.* Copenhagen: World Health Organization, 197–218.

Arlien-Søberg, P., Bruhn, P., Gyldensted, C., and Melgaard, B. (1979). Chronic painters' syndrome: Toxic encephalopathy in house painters. *Acta Neurologica Scandinavica,* **60,** 149–156.

Arlien-Søberg, P., Henriksen, L., Gade, A., Gyldensted, C., and Paulson, O.B. (1982). Cerebral blood flow in chronic toxic encephalopathy in house painters exposed to organic solvents. *Acta Neurologica Scandinavica,* **66,** 34–41.

Arlien-Søberg, P., Zilstorff, K., Grandjean, B., and Pedersen, L. (1981). Vestibular dysfunction in occupational chronic solvent intoxication. *Clinical Otolaryngology,* **6,** 285–290.

Astrand, I. (1975). Uptake of solvents in the blood and tissues of man. A review. *Scandinavian Journal of Work Environment and Health,* **1,** 199–218.

Aub., J.C., Fairhall, L.T., Minot, A.S., and Reznikoff, P. (1926). *Lead Poisoning* (Medicine monographs 7). Baltimore: Williams & Wilkins.

Axelson, O., Hane, M., and Hogstedt, C. (1976). A case-referent study on neuropsychiatric disorders among workers exposed to solvents. *Scandinavian Journal of Work Environment and Health,* **2,** 14–20.

Bach, M.J., Arbit, J., and Bruce, D.L. (1974). Trace anesthetic effect on vigilance. In

C. Xinitaras, B.L. Johnson, and I. deGroot (Eds), *Behavioral Toxicology: Early Detection of Occupational Hazards*, HEW Publication No. (NIOSH) 74-126, Washington, DC, US. Government Printing Office, 41-50.

Baker, E.L. (1983a). Neurologic and behavioral disorders. In B. S. Levy and D. H. Wegman (Eds), *Occupational Health: Recognizing and Preventing Work-Related Disease*. Boston: Little, Brown and Company, 317-330.

Baker, E. L. (1983b). Neurological disorders. In W. N. Rom (Ed.), *Environmental and Occupational Medicine*. Boston: Little, Brown and Company, 313-327.

Baker, E.L., and Fine, L.J. (1986). Solvent neurotoxicity: The current evidence. *Journal of Occupational Medicine*, **28**, 126-129.

Baker, E.L., and Letz, R. (1986). Neurobehavioral testing in monitoring hazardous workplace exposures. *Journal of Occupational Medicine*, **28**, 987-990.

Baker, E.L., and Seppäläinen, A.M. (1986). Human aspects of solvent neurobehavioral effects. In J. Cranmer and L. Golberg (Eds), Proceedings of the workshop on neurobehavioral effects of solvents. *NeuroToxicology*, **7**, 43-56.

Baker, E. L., Feldman, R. G., White, R. F., and Harley, J. P. (1983a). The role of occupational lead exposure in the genesis of psychiatric and behavioral disturbances. *Acta Psychiatrica Scandinavica*, **67**, Suppl. 303, 38-48.

Baker, E. L., Feldman, R. G., White, R. F., Harley, J. P., Dinse, G. E., and Berkey, C. S. (1983b). Monitoring neurotoxins in industry: Development of a neurobehavioral test battery. *Journal of Occupational Medicine*, **25**, 125-130.

Baker, E. L., Folland, D. S., Taylor, T. A. *et al.* (1977). Lead poisoning in children of lead workers: Home contamination with industrial dust. *New England Journal of Medicine*, **296**, 260-261.

Baker, E. L., Letz, R. E., and Fidler, A. T. (1985b). A computer-administered neurobehavioral evaluation system for occupational and environmental epidemiology. *Journal of Occupational Medicine*, **27**, 206-212.

Baker, E. L., Letz, R. E., Fidler, A. T., Shalat, S., Plantamura, D., and Lyndon, M. (1985a). A computer-based neurobehavioral evaluation system for occupational and environmental epidemiology: Methodology and validation studies. *Neurobehavioral Toxicology and Teratology*, **7**, 369-378.

Baker, E. L., Smith, T. J., and Landrigan, P. J. (1985c). The neurotoxicity of industrial solvents: A review of the literature. *American Journal of Industrial Medicine*, **8**, 207-217.

Baker, E. L., White, R. F., Pothier, L. J., Berekey, C. S., Dinse, G. E., Travers, P. H., Harley, J. P., and Feldman, R. G. (1985d). Occupational lead neurotoxicity: Improvement in behavioral effects after reduction of exposure. *British Journal of Industrial Medicine*, **42**, 507-516.

Baker, R., and Woodrow, S. (1984). The clean light image of the electronics industry: Miracle or mirage? In W. Chavkin (Ed.), *Double Exposure: Women's health hazards on the job and at home*. New York: Monthly Review Press, 21-36.

Baker, S. J., Chrzan, G. J., Park, C. N., and Saunders, J. H. (1986). Behavioral effects of 0% and 0.05% blood alcohol in male volunteers. *Neurobehavioral Toxicology and Teratology*, **8**, 77-81.

Baloh, R., Sturm, R., Green, R., and Gleser, G. (1975). Neuropsychological effects of chronic asymptomatic increased lead absorption. *Archives of Neurology*, **32**, 326-330.

Bank, W. J., (1980). Thallium. In P. S. Spencer and H. H. Schaumberg (Eds), *Experimental and Clinical Neurotoxicology*, Baltimore: Williams and Wilkins, 570-577.

Barlow, D. H., and Hersen, M. (1984). *Single Case Experimental Designs*. New York:

Pergamon Press.

Barnes, G. E. (1979). Solvent abuse: A review. *International Journal of the Addictions.* **14**, 1-26.

Barnes, J. M., (1961). Psychiatric sequelae of chronic exposure to organophosphorus insecticides. *Lancet*, **2**, 102-103.

Bass, M. (1970). Sudden sniffing death. *Journal of the American Medical Association*, **212**, 2075-2079.

Bear, D., Rosenbaum, J., and Norman, R. (1986). Aggression in cat and human precipitated by a cholinesterase inhibitor. *Psychosomatics*, **27**, 535-6.

Beck, A. T., Ward, L. H., Mendelson, M., Mock, J., and Erbaugh, J. (1961). An inventory for measuring depression. *Archives of General Psychiatry*, **4**, 561-571.

Beckett, W. S., Moore, J. L., Keogh, J. P., and Bleecker, M. L. (1986). Acute encephalopathy due to occupational exposure to arsenic. *British Journal of Industrial Medicine*, **43**, 66-67.

Beckmann, J., and Mergler, D. (1985). Symptomatology questionnaires. In P. Grandjean (Ed.), *Neurobehavioral Methods in Occupational and Environmental Health: Symposium Report*, Coperhagen: World Health Organization, 26-28.

Begleiter, H., Porjesz, B., and Tenner, M. (1980). Neuroradiological and neuropsychological evidence of brain deficits in chronic alcoholics. *Acta Psychiatrica Scandinavica*, **62**, Suppl. 286, 3-13.

Behse, F., and Carlson, F. (1978). Histology and ultrastructure of alterations in neuropathy. *Muscle and Nerve*, **1**, 368.

Bellinger, D. C., Needleman, H. L., Leviton, A., Waternaux, C., Rabinowitz, M. B., and Nichols, M. L. (1984). Early sensory motor development and pre-natal exposure to lead. *Neurobehavioral Toxicology and Teratology*, **6**, 387-402.

Bellinger, D., Leviton, A., Needleman, H. L., Waternaux, C., and Rabinowitz, M. (1986). Low level lead exposure and infant development in the first year. *Neurobehavioral Toxicology and Teratology*, **8**, 151-161.

Benignus, V. A. (1981). Neurobehavioral effects of toluene: A review. *Neurobehavioral Toxicology and Teratology*, **3**, 407-415.

Benson, M. D., and Price, J. (1985). Cerebellar calcification and lead. *Journal of Neurology, Neurosurgery, and Psychiatry*, **48**, 814-818.

Berglund, M. (1981). Cerebral blood flow in chronic alcoholics. *Alcoholism: Clinical and Experimental Research* **5**, 295-303.

Berglund, M., Bliding, G., Bliding, A., and Risberg, J. (1980). Reversibility of cerebral dysfunction in alcoholism during the first seven weeks of abstinence — a regional cerebral blood flow study. *Acta Psychiatrica Scandinavica*, Suppl. 286, **62**, 119-127.

Bergman, H. (1984). The Halstead-Reitan neuropsychological test battery. *Scandinavian Journal of Work Environment and Health*, **10**, Supp. 1, 30-32.

Bergman, H., Borg, S., Hindmarch, T., Ideström, C.-M., and Mützell, S. (1980a). Computed tomography of the brain and neuropsychological assessment of male alcoholic patients and a random sample from the general male population. *Acta Psychiatrica Scandinavica*, Suppl. 286, **62**, 47-56.

Bergman, H., Borg, S., Hindmarsh, T., Ideström, C.-M., and Mützell, S. (1980b). Computed tomography of the brain, clinical examination and neuropsychological assessment of a random sample of men from the general population. *Acta Psychiatrica Scandinavica*, Suppl. 286, **62**, 77-88.

Bergman, H., Borg, S., and Holm, L. (1980c). Neuropsychological impairment and exclusive abuse of sedatives or hypnotics. *American Journal of Psychiatry*, **137**, 215-217.

Berndt, D. J., Berndt., S. M., and Kaiser, C. F. (1984). Multidimensional assessment of depression. *Journal of Personality Assessment*, **48**, 489–494.

Berry, G. J. (1976). Neuropsychological assessment of solvent inhalers. Final report to the National Institute on Drug Abuse. Washington, DC: U.S. Government Printing Office.

Berry, G. J., Heaton, R. K., and Kirby, M. W. (1977). Neuropsychological deficits of chronic inhalant abusers. In B. H. Rumack and A. R. Temple (Eds), *Management of the Poisoned Patient*, Princeton: Science Press, 9–31.

Bidstrup, P. L. (1961). (Letter to the Editor). *Lancet*, **2**, 103.

Bigler, E. D. (1984). *Diagnostic Clinical Neuropsychology*. Austin: University of Texas Press.

Bingham, E. (1974). Worker exposure to metals: metals seminar keynote address. In C. Xintaras, B. L. Johnson, and I. deGroot (Eds), *Behavioral Toxicology: Early detection of occupational hazards*. Washington, DC: Department of Health, Education and Welfare. Publication No. (NIOSH) 74–126, 199–206.

Biskind, M. S., and Mobbs, R. F. (29 May 1972). Psychiatric manifestations from insecticide exposure. *Journal of the American Medical Association*, **220**, 1248.

Blake, D. R., Winyard, P., Lunec, J., Williams, A., Good, P. A., Crewes, S. J., Gutteridge, J. M. C., Rowley, D., Halliwell, B., Cornish, A., and Hider, R. C. (1985). Cerebral and ocular toxicity induced by desferrioxamine. *Quarterly Journal of Medicine,* new series, **56**, 345–355.

Bleecker, M. L. (1984). Clinical neurotoxicology: detection of neurobehavioral and neurological impairments occurring in the workplace and the environment. *Archives of Environmental Health*, **39**, 213–218.

Bleecker, M. L., and Bolla-Wilson, K. (1985). Neuropsychological impairment following inorganic arsenic exposure. Unmasking a memory disorder. *Neurobehavioral Methods in Occupational Health*, Document 3, Copenhagen: World Health Organization. 172–176.

Bleecker, M. L., Agnew, J., Keogh, J. P., and Stetson, D. S. (1982). Neurobehavioral evaluation in workers following a brief exposure to lead. In R. Gilioli *et al.* (Eds), *Neurobehavioral Methods in Occupational Health*. New York: Pergamon Press, 255–262.

Block, R. I., and Berchou, R. (1984). Alprazolam and lorazepam effects on memory acquisition and retrieval processes. *Pharmacology, Biochemistry and Behavior*, **20**, 233–241.

Boeckx, R. L. (1979). The clinical chemistry of lead poisoning: new approaches to an old problem. Special review article. *Clinical Proceedings, CHNMC*, **35**, 216–231.

Bolla-Wilson, K. (1986). Neuresthenia vs. depression. Common presentation of CNS toxicity in the workplace. Paper presented at the *American Academy of Neurology*, New Orleans, April 1986, Annual Course 108, Occupational and Environmental Neurology.

Bolter, J. F., and Hannon, R. (1986). Lateralized cerebral dysfunction in early and late stage alcoholics. *Journal of Studies on Alcohol*, **47**, 213–218.

Bolter, J. F., Stanczik, D. F., and Long, C. J. (1983). Neuropsychological consequences of acute, high level, gasoline inhalation. *Clinical Neuropsychology*, **5**, 4–7.

Bornstein, R. A., McLean, D. R., and Ho, K. (1985). Neuropsychological and electrophysiological examination of a patient with Wilson's disease. *International Journal of Neuroscience*, **26**, 239–247.

Bornstein, R. A., Watson, G. D., and Kaplan, M. J. (1985). Effects of flurazepam and triazolam on neuropsychological performance. *Perceptual and Motor Skills*,

60, 47–52.

Bornstein, R. A., Watson, G. D., and Pawluk, L. K. (1985). Effects of chronic benzodiazepine administration on neuropsychological performance. *Clinical Neuropharmacology*, **8**, 357–361.

Bowers, M. B., Goodman, E., and Sim, V. M. (1964). Some behavioral changes in man following anticholinesterase administration. *Journal of Nervous and Mental Disease*, **138**, 383.

Boxer, P. A. (1985). Occupational mass psychogenic illness. *Journal of Occupational Medicine*, **27**, 867–872.

Bozarth, M. A., and Wise, R. A. (5 July 1985). Toxicity associated with long-term intravenous heroin and cocaine self-administration in the rat. *Journal of the American Medical Association*, **254**, 81–83.

Bracy, O. L. (1984). Using computers in neuropsychology. In Schwartz, M. D. (Ed.), *Using Computers in Clinical Practice*. New York: Haworth Press, 257–268.

Braff, D. L., and Sacuzzo, D. P. (1982). Effect of antipsychotic medication on speed of information processing in schizophrenic patients. *American Journal of Psychiatry*, **139**, 1127–1130.

Branconnier, R. J. (1985). Dementia in human populations exposed to neurotoxic agents: a portable microcomputerized dementia screening battery. *Neurobehavioral Toxicology and Teratology*, **7**, 379–386.

Brandt, J., and Butters, N. (1986). The alcoholic Wernicke–Korsakoff syndrome and its relationship to neuropsychological functioning. In I. Grant and K. M. Adams (Eds), *Neuropsychological Assessment of Neuropsychiatric Disorders*. New York: Oxford University Press, 441–477.

Brandt, J., and Provost, D. G. (1985). On the dissimilar effects of alcohol and aging on the perception of cognitive failings. *Alcohol*, **2**, 633–635.

Brandt, J., Butters, N., Ryan, C., and Bayog, R. (1983). Cognitive loss and recovery in long-term alcohol abusers. *Archives of General Psychiatry*, **40**, 435–442.

Bravaccio, F., Ammendola, A., Barruffo, L., and Carlomagno, S. (1981). H-Reflex behavior in glue (*n*-hexane) neuropathy. *Clinical Toxicology*, **18**, 1369–1375.

Breggin, P. R. (1983). *Psychiatric Drugs: Hazards to the Brain*. New York: Springer.

Brizer, D. A., and Manning, D. W. (1982). Delirium induced by poisoning with anticholinergic agents. *American Journal of Psychiatry*, **139**, 1343–1344.

Brooker, A. E., Wiens, A. N., and Wiens, D. A. (1984). Impaired brain functions due to diazepam and meprobamate abuse in a 53 year old male. *Journal of Nervous and Mental Disease*, **172**, 498–501.

Bruce, D., (1985). On the origin of the term "neuropsychology". *Neuropsychologia*, **23**, 813–814.

Bruce, D. L., and Bach, M. J. (1975). Psychologic studies of human performance as affected by traces of enflurane and nitrous oxide. *Anesthesiology*, **42**, 194.

Bruce, D. L., and Bach, M. J. (1976). Effects of trace anesthetic gases on behavioral performance of volunteers. *British Journal of Anaesthesiology*, **48**, 871–876.

Bruhn, P., Arlien-Søberg, P., Gyldensted, C., and Christensen, E. L. (1981). Prognosis in chronic toxic encephalopathy. *Acta Neurologica Scandinavica*, **64**, 259–272.

Buckholtz, N. S., and Panem, S. (1986). Regulation and evolving science: Neurobehavioral toxicology. *Neurobehavioral Toxicology and Teratology*, **8**, 89–96.

Buge, A., Supino-Viterbo, V., Rancurel, G., and Pontes, C. (1981). Epileptic phenomena in bismuth toxic encephalopathy. *Journal of Neurology, Neurosurgery, and Psychiatry*, **44**, 621–627.

Butters, N. (1985). Alcoholic Korsakoff's syndrome: Some unresolved issues concerning etiology, neuropathology and cognitive deficits. *Journal of Clinical and Experimental Neuropsychology*, 7, 181-210.

Butters, N., and Cermak, L. S. (1976). Neuropsychological studies of alcoholic Korsakoff patients. In G. Goldstein and C. Neuringer (Eds), *Empirical Studies of Alcoholism*. Cambridge, Mass.: Ballinger, 153-195.

Byrne, J. M., Camfield, P. R., Clark-Tovesnard, M., and Hondas, B. J. (1987). Effects of phenobarbital on early intellectual and behavioral development: A concordant twin case study. *Journal of Clinical and Experimental Neuropsychology*, 9, 393-398.

Byrne, R. (1982). *The 637 Best Things Anybody Ever Said*. New York: Fawcett Crest.

Cala, L. A., and Mastaglia, F. L. (1981). Computerized tomography in chronic alcoholics. *Alcoholism: Clinical and Experimental Research*, 81, 283-294.

Cala, L. A., Jones, B., Wiley, B., and Mastaglia, F. L. (1980). A computerized axial tomography (CAT) study of alcohol induced cerebral atrophy: In conjunction with other correlates. *Acta Psychiatrica Scandinavica*, 62, Suppl. 286, 31-40.

Calabrese, E. J. (1985). *Toxic Susceptibility: Male/female differences*. New York: John Wiley & Sons.

Calabrese, E. J. (1986). Sex differences in susceptibility to toxic industrial chemicals. *British Journal of Industrial Medicine*, 43, 577-579.

Campagna, K. D. (1986). Drug information forum: what are designer drugs? *U.S. Pharmacist*, 16-17.

Campbell, D. D., Evans, M., Thomson, J. L., and Williams, M. J. (1971). Cerebral atrophy in young cannabis smokers. *Lancet*, 2, 1219-1224.

Campbell, D. D., Lockey, J. E., Petajan, J., Gunter, B. J., and Rom, W. N. (1986). Health effects among refrigeration repair workers exposed to fluorocarbons. *British Journal of Industrial Medicine*, 43, 107-111.

Caprio, R. J., Margulis, H. L., and Joselow, M. M. (1974). Lead absorption in children and its relation to urban traffic densities. *Archives of Environmental Health*, 28, 195-197.

Carlen, P. L., Penn, R. D., Fornazzari, L., Bennett, J., Wilkinson, D. A., and Wortzman, G. (1986). Computerized tomographic scan assessment of alcoholic brain damage and its potential reversibility. *Alcoholism: Clinical and Experimental Research*, 10, 226-232.

Carlen, P. L., Wortzman G., Holgate, R. C., Wilkinson, D. A. and Rankin, J. G. Reversible cerebral atrophy in recently abstinent chronic alcoholics measured by computed tomography scans. *Science* 1978 200, 1076-1078.

Carlen, P. L., and Wilkinson, D. A. (1980). Alcoholic brain damage and reversible deficits. *Acta Psychiatrica Scandinavica*, Suppl. 286, 62, 103-118.

Carlen, P. L., Wilkinson, D. A., Wortzman, G., Holgate, R., Cordingley, J., Lee, M. A., Huszar, L., Moddel, G., Singh, R., Kiraly, L., and Rankin, J. G. (1981). Cerebral atrophy and functional deficits in alcoholics without clinically apparent liver disease. *Neurology*, 31, 377-385.

Carlin, A. S. (1986). Neuropsychological consequences of drug abuse. In I. Grant and K. M. Adams (Eds), *Neuropsychological Assessment of Neuropsychiatric Disorders*. New York: Oxford University Press, 478-497.

Carlin, A. S., and Trupin, E. (1977). The effects of long-term chronic cannabis use on neuropsychological functioning. *International Journal of the Addictions*, 12, 617-624.

Carlin, A. S., Grant, K., Adams, K. M., and Reed, R. (1979). Is phencyclidine (PCP) abuse associated with organic brain impairment? *American Journal of Drug and*

Alcohol Abuse, **6**, 273-281.

Carroll, J. B. (1980). Individual difference relations in psychometric and experimental cognitive tasks. In L. L. Thurstone Psychometric Laboratory Report No. 163. Chapel Hill N.C.: The University of North Carolina (NTIS Document AD-A086 057).

Cassitto, M. G. (1983). Current behavioral techniques. In R. Gilioli, M. G., Cassitto, and V. Foa (Eds), *Neurobehavioral Methods in Occupational Health*. New York: Pergamon Press, 27-38.

Casswell, S., and Marks, D. F. (1973a). Cannabis and temporal disintegration in experienced and naive subjects. *Science*, **179**, 803-805.

Casswell, S., and Marks, D. F. (1973b). Cannabis-induced impairment of performance on a divided attention task. *Nature*, **241**, 60-61.

Cavalleri, A., Trimarchi, F., Minoia, C., and Gallo, G. (1982). Quantitative measurement of visual field in lead exposed workers. In R. Gilioli, M. G. Cassitto, and V. Foa (Eds), *Neurobehavioral Methods in Occupational Health*. New York: Pergamon Press, 263-269.

Cavanaugh, J. B. (1983). Some clinical and neuropathological correlations in four solvent intoxications. In N. Cherry and H. A. Waldron (Eds), *The Neuropsychological Effects of Solvent Exposure*. Havant, Hampshire: Colt Foundation, 7-22.

Cavanaugh, J. B. (1985). Mechanisms of organic solvent toxicity: Morphological changes. In *Chronic Effects of Organic Solvents on the Central Nervous System and Diagnostic Criteria*. Copenhagen: World Health Organization, 110-135.

Cawte, J. (1985). Psychiatric sequelae of manganese exposure in the adult, foetal and neonatal nervous systems. *Australian and New Zealand Journal of Psychiatry*, **19**, 211-217.

Center for Disease Control (1983). NIOSH recommendations for occupational health standards. *Morbidity and Mortality Weekly Report*, **32**, Supplement. Atlanta: U.S. Department of Health and Human Services. 1S-24S.

Center for Disease Control (January 1985). *Preventing Lead Poisoning in Young Children*. United States Department of Health and Human Services. Document No. 99-2230.

Chaffin, D. B., and Miller, J. M. (1974). Behavioral and neurological evaluation of workers exposed to inorganic mercury. In C. Xintaras, B. L. Johnson, and I. deGroot (Eds), *Behavioral Toxicology: Early detection of occupational hazards*. Washington DC: Department of Health, Education and Welfare, Publication No. (NIOSH) 74-126. 213-239.

Chandra, S. V. (1983). Psychiatric illness due to manganese poisoning. *Acta Psychiatrica Scandinavica*, Suppl. 303, **67**, 49-54.

Chang, L. W. (1980). Mercury. In P. S. Spencer and H. H. Schaumburg (Eds), *Experimental and Clinical Neurotoxicology*. Baltimore: Williams and Wilkins, 508-526.

Chang, L. W. (1982). Pathogenetic mechanisms of the neurotoxicity of methylmercury. In K. N. Prasad and A. Vernadakis (Eds), *Mechanisms of Actions of Neurotoxic Substances*. New York: Raven Press, 51-66.

Chemical Regulation Reporter (14 March 1986). Health hazards, p. 1598.

Cherry, N., and Waldron, H. A. (Eds) (1983). *The Neuropsychological Effects of Solvent Exposure*. Havant, Hampshire: Colt Foundation.

Cherry, N., Hutchins, H., Pace, T., and Waldron, H. A. (1985). Neurobehavioral effects of repeated occupational exposure to toluene and paint solvents. *British Journal of Industrial Medicine*, **42**, 291-300.

Cherry, N., Rodgers, B., Venables, H., Waldron, H.A., and Wells, G. G. (1981a). Acute behavioral effects of styrene exposure: A further analysis. *British Journal of Industrial Medicine*, **38**, 346–350.

Cherry, N., Venables, H., and Waldron, H. A., (1981b). *A test battery to measure the behavioral effects of neurotoxic substances*. London: TUC Centenary Institute of Occupational Health.

Cherry, N., Venables, H., and Waldron, H. A., (1983). The acute behavioral effects of solvent exposure. *Journal of the Society of Occupational Medicine*, **33**, 13–18.

Chia, L-G., and Chu, F-L., (1985). A clinical and electrophysiological study of patients with polychlorinated biphenyl poisoning. *Journal of Neurology, Neurosurgery, and Psychiatry*, **48**, 894–901.

Chia, L-G., and Chu, F-L. (1984). Neurological studies on polychlorinated biphenyl (PCB)-poisoned patients. In M. Kuratsune and R. Shapiro (Eds), *PCB Poisoning in Japan and Taiwan*. New York: Allan R. Liss, 117–126.

Chmielewski, C., and Golden, C. (1980). Alcoholism and brain damage: An investigation using the Luria–Nebraska neuropsychological battery. *International Journal of Neuroscience*, **10**, 99–105.

Christensen, A. (1975). *Luria's Neuropsychological Investigation*. New York: Spectrum.

Christensen, A. (1984). Neuropsychological investigation with Luria's methods. *Scandinavian Journal of Work Environment and Health*, Suppl. 1, **10**, 33–34.

Christensen, E., Moller, J. E., and Faurbye, A. (1970). Neuropathological investigation of 28 brains from patients with dyskinesia. *Acta Psychiatrica Scandinavica*, **46**, 14–23.

Clark, D. C., Pisani, V. D., Aagesen, C. A., Sellers, D., and Fawcett, J. (1984). Primary affective disorder, drug abuse, and neuropsychological impairment in sober alcoholics. *Alcoholism: Clinical and Experimental Research*, **8**, 399–404.

Clark, G. (1971). Organophosphate insecticides and behavior, a review. *Aerospace Medicine*, **42**, 735–740.

Cohen, N., Modai, D., Golik, A., Pik, A., Weissgarten, J., Sigler, E., and Averbukh, Z. (1986). An esoteric occupational hazard for lead poisoning. *Clinical Toxicology*, **24**, 59–67.

Cohen, S. (1978). An international perspective on solvents and aerosols. In *Solvents, Adhesives and Aerosols*. Addiction Research Foundation of Ontario, 71–79.

Cohen, S. (1980). Adolescence and drug abuse: Biomedical consequences. *National Institute of Drug Abuse Research Monograph Series*, **38**, 104–112.

Cohen, S. (1984). Cocaine: Acute medical and psychiatric complications, *Psychiatric Annals*, **14**, 747–749.

Cohen, S., and Edwards, A. (1969). LSD and organic brain impairment. *Drug Dependence*, **2**, 1–4.

Cohen, W. J. (1974). Lithium carbonate, haloperidol, and irreversible brain damage. *Journal of the American Medical Association*, **230**, 1283–1287.

Cohr, K.-H. (1985). Definition and practical limitation of the concept organic solvents. In Joint WHO/Nordic Council of Ministers Working Group (Eds), *Chronic Effects of Organic Solvents on the Central Nervous System and Diagnostic Criteria*, Document 5. Copenhagen: World Health Organization, Regional Office for Europe.

Cohr, K.-H., and Stokholm, J. (1979). Toluene: A toxicologic review. *Scandinavian Journal of Work Environment and Health*, **5**, 71.

Cook, T. L., Smith, B. A., Starkweather, J. A., Winter, P. M., and Eger, E. S. (1978). Behavioral effects of trace and subanesthetic halothane and nitrous oxide in man. *Anesthesiology*, **49**, 419–424.

Cornelius, J. R., Soloff, P. H., and Reynolds, C. F. (1984). Paranoia, homicidal behavior, and seizures associated with phenylpropanolamine. *American Journal of Psychiatry*, **141**, 120–121.

Coye, M. J., Barnett, P. G., Midtling, J. E., Velasco, A. R., Romero, P., Clements, C. L., O'Malley, M. A., Tobin, M. W., and Lowry, L. (1986). Clinical confirmation of organophosphate poisoning of agricultural workers. *American Journal of Industrial Medicine*, **10**, 399–409.

Cranmer, J. M., and Golberg, L. (Eds) (1986). Proceedings of the workshop on neurobehavioral effects of solvents. *NeuroToxicology*, **7**, 1–95.

Crapper, D. R., and De Boni, U. (1980). Aluminum. In P. S. Spencer and H. H. Schaumburg (Eds), *Experimental and Clinical Neurotoxicology*, Baltimore: Williams and Wilkins, 326–335.

Culver, C., and King, F. (1974). Neuropsychological assessment of undergraduate marijuana and LSD users. *Archives of General Psychiatry*, **31**, 707–711.

Curtis, M. F., and Keller, L. W. (1986). (Co-chairman) Exposure issues in the evaluation of solvent effects. *NeuroToxicology*, **7**, 5–24.

Dackis, C. A., and Gold, M. S. (1985). New concepts in cocaine addiction: The dopamine depletion hypothesis, *Neuroscience and Biobehavioral Review*, **9**, 469–477.

Darley, C. F., Tinklenberg, J. R., Roth, W. T., Hollister, L. E., and Atkinson, R. C. (1973). Influence of marijuana on storage and retrieval processes in memory. *Memory and Cognition*, **1**, 196–200.

Darley, C. F., Tinklenberg, J. R., Roth, W. T., and Atkinson, R. C., (1974). The nature of storage deficits and state dependent retrieval under marijuana. *Psychopharmacologia*, **37**, 139–149.

Darley, C. F., Tinklenberg, J. R., Roth, W. T., Vernon, S., and Koppell, B. S. (1977). Marijuana effects on long-term memory assessment and retrieval. *Psychopharmacologia*, **52**, 239–241.

David, O. J., Hoffman, S. P., Clark, J., Grad, G., and Swerd, J. (1983). The relationship of hyperactivity to moderately elevated lead levels. *Archives of Environmental Health*, **38**, 341–346.

David, O. J., Grad, G., McGann, B., and Kolton, A. (1982). Mental retardation and "nontoxic" lead levels. *American Journal of Psychiatry*, **139**, 806–809.

Dean, A., Pugh, J., Embrey, K. *et al.* (1984). Organophosphate insecticide poisoning among siblings—Mississipi. *Morbidity and Mortality Weekly Report*, **33**, 592–594.

Dempsey, G. M., and Meltzer, H. L. (1977). Lithium toxicity: A review. In L. Roizin, H. Shiraki, and N. Grcevic (Eds), *Neurotoxicology*. New York: Raven Press, 171–183.

Dening, T. R. (1985). Psychiatric aspects of Wilson's disease. *British Journal of Psychiatry*, **147**, 677–682.

DeObaldia, R., Leber, W. R., and Parsons, O. A. (1981). Assessment of neuropsychological functions in chronic alcoholics using a standardized version of Luria's neuropsychological technique. *International Journal of Neuroscience*, **14**, 85–93.

DeRenzi, E., and Vignolo, L. A. (1962). The Token Test: A sensitive test to detect receptive disturbances in aphasics. *Brain*, **85**, 665–678.

Dolcourt, J. L., Hamrick, H. J., O'Tuama, L. A., Wooten, J., and Baker, E. L. (1978). Increased lead burden in children of battery workers: Asymptomatic exposure resulting from contaminated work clothing. *Pediatrics*, **62**, 563–566.

Domino, E. F., and Luby, E. D. (1981). Abnormal mental states induced by phencyclidine as a model of schizophrenia. In E. F. Domino (Ed.), *PCP (Phencyclidine): Historical and Current Perspectives*. Ann Arbor: NPP Books, 401–418.

Donovan, D. M., Kivlahan, D. R., and Walker, D. (1984). Clinical limitations of predicting treatment outcome among alcoholics. *Alcoholism: Clinical and Experimental Research*, **8**, 470–475.

Dornbush, R. L. (1974). Marijuana and memory: Effects of smoking on storage. *Transactions of the New York Academy of Science*, **36**, 94–100.

Dornbush, R. L., Fink, M., and Freedman, A. M. (1976). Marijuana, memory and perception. In E. L. Abel (Ed.), *The Scientific Study of Marijuana*. Chicago: Nelson-Hall, 133–140.

Drejer, K., Theilgaard, A., Teasdale, T. W., Schulsinger, F., and Goodwin, D. W. (1985). A prospective study of young men at high risk for alcoholism: Neuropsychological assessment. *Alcoholism: Clinical and Experimental Research*, **9**, 498–502.

DuBois, K. P. (1971). The toxicity of organophosphorus compounds to mammals. *Bulletin of the World Health Organization*, **44**, 233–240.

Duckett, S., (1986). Abnormal deposits of chromium in the pathological human brain. *Journal of Neurology, Neurosurgery, and Psychiatry*, **49**, 296–301.

Dudek, B. (1985). The effect of perchloroethylene on mental functions. In *Neurobehavioral Methods in Occupational and Environmental Health*. Copenhagen: World Health Organization, Regional Office for Europe, 141–146.

Dudley, A. W. Jr., Chang, L. W., Dudley, M. A., Bowman, R. E., and Katz, J. (1977). Review of effects of chronic exposure to low levels of Halothane. In L. Roizin, H. Shiraki, and N. Grcevic (Eds), *Neurotoxicology*. New York: Raven Press,137–146.

Duffy, F. H., and Burchfiel, J. L. (1980). Long term effects of the organophosphate Sarin on EEGs in monkeys and humans. *NeuroToxicology*, **1**, 667–689.

Duffy, F. H., Burchfiel, J. L., Bartels, P. H., Gaon, M., and Sim, V. M. (1979). Long-term effects of an organophosphate upon the human electroencephalogram. *Toxicology and Applied Pharmacology* **47**, 161–176.

Eckardt, M. J., and Martin, P. R. (1986). Clinical assessment of cognition in alcoholism. *Alcoholism: Clinical and Experimental Research*, **10**, 123–127.

Eckardt, M. J., Ryback, R. S., and Pautler, C. P. (1980). Neuropsychological deficits in alcoholic men in their mid thirties. *American Journal of Psychiatry*, **137**, 932–936.

Eckerman, D. A., Carroll, J. B., Foree, C. M., Gullion, M., Lansman, E. R., Long, E. R., Waller, M. B., and Wallsten, T. S. (1985). An approach to brief testing for neurotoxicity. *Neurobehavioral Toxicology and Teratology*, **7**, 387–394.

Ecobichon, D., and Joy, R. (1982). *Pesticides and Neurological Diseases*, Florida: CRC Press.

Edling, C. (1980). Anesthetic gases as an occupational hazard—a review. *Scandinavian Journal of Work Environment and Health*, **6**, 85–93.

Edling, C. (1985). Nervous system symptoms and signs associated with long-term organic solvent exposure. In *Chronic Effects of Organic Solvents on the Central Nervous System and Diagnostic Criteria*. Copenhagen: World Health Organization, 149–155.

Edling, C., and Ekberg, K. (1985). No acute behavioral effects of exposure to styrene: A safe level of exposure? *British Journal of Industrial Medicine*, **42**, 301–304.

Ekberg, K., Barregard, L., Hagberg, S., and Sallsten, S., (1986). Chronic and acute effects of solvents on central nervous system functions in floorlayers. *British*

Journal of Industrial Medicine, **43**, 101-106.

Elofsson, S., Gamberale, F., Hindmarsh, T., Iregren, A., Isaksson, A., Johnsson, I., Knave, B., Lydahl, E., Mindus, P., Persson, H. E., Philipson, B., Steby, M., Struwe, G., Soderman, E., Wennberg, A., and Widen, L. (1980). Exposure to organic solvents: A cross-sectional epidemiologic investigation on occupationally exposed car and industrial spray painters with special reference to the nervous system. *Scandinavian Journal of Work Environment and Health*, **6**, 239-273.

Engstrom, J., Bjurstrom, R., Astrand, I., and Ovrum, P. (1978). Uptake, distribution and elimination of styrene in man. *Scandinavian Journal of Work Environment and Health*, **4**, 315-323.

Eskelinen, L., Luisto, M., Tenkanen, L., and Mattei, O. (1986). Neuropsychological methods in the differentiation of organic solvent intoxication from certain neurological conditions. *Journal of Clinical and Experimental Neuropsychology*, **8**, 239-256.

Estrin, W. J., Cavalieri, S. A., Wald, P., Becker, C. E., Jones, J. R., and Cone, J. E. (1986). Evidence of neurologic dysfunction related to chronic ethylene oxide exposure. Unpublished manuscript. Available from the first author, Department of Neurology, 4M71, San Francisco General Hospital, 1001 Potrero Avenue, San Francisco, CA 94110.

Evans, R. W., and Gualtieri, C. T. (1985). Carbamazepine: a neuropsychological and psychiatric profile. *Clinical Neuropharmacology*, **8**, 221-241.

Fabian, M. S., Jenkins, R. L., and Parsons, O. A. (1981). Gender, alcoholism, and neuropsychological functioning. *Journal of Consulting and Clinical Psychology*, **49**, 138-140.

Fairchild, E. J. (1974). Welcoming remarks from NIOSH. In C. Xintarus, B. L. Johnson, and I. deGroot (Eds), *Behavioral Toxicology: Early detection of occupational hazards*. Washington, DC: U. S. Department of Health, Education and Welfare (NIOSH) Publication No. 74-126, pp. 3-4.

Fauman, M. A., and Fauman, B. J. (1981). Chronic phencyclidine (PCP) abuse: A psychiatric perspective. In E. F. Domino (Ed.), *PCP (Phencyclidine): historical and current perspectives*. Ann Arbor: NPP Books, 419-436.

Fein, G. G., Schwartz, P. M., Jacobson, S. W., and Jacobson, J. L. (1983). Environmental toxins and behavioral development. A new role for psychological research. *American Psychologist*, 1188-1196.

Feldman, R. G. (1982a). Central and peripheral nervous system effects of metals: A survey. *Acta Neurologica Scandinavica*, Suppl. 92, **66**, 143-166.

Feldman, R. G. (1982b). Neurological manifestations of mercury intoxication. *Acta Neurologica Scandinavica*, Suppl. 92, **66**, 201-209.

Feldman, R. G., Niles, C. A., Kelly-Hayes, M., Sax, D., Dixon, W., Thompson, D. J., and Landau, E. (1979). Peripheral neuropathy in arsenic smelter workers. *Neurology*, **29**, 939-944.

Feldman, R. G., Ricks, N. L., and Baker, E. L. (1980). Neuropsychological effects of industrial toxins: A review. *American Journal of Industrial Medicine*, **1**, 211-227.

Feldman, R. G., White, R. F., Currie, J. N. Travers, P. H., and Lessell, S. (1985). Long-term follow-up after single toxic exposure to trichlorethylene. *American Journal of Industrial Medicine*, **8**, 119-126.

Fernandez, P. G. (1976). Alpha methyldopa and forgetfulness. *Annals of Internal Medicine*, **85**, 128.

Ferraro, D. P. (1980). Acute effects of marijuana on human memory and cognition. *National Institute of Drug Abuse Research Monograph Series*, **31**, 98-119.

Fetzer, J., Kader, G., and Danahy, S. (1981). Lithium encephalopathy: a clinical, psychiatric, and EEG evaluation. *American Journal of Psychiatry*, **138**, 1622–1623.

Fields, S., and Fullerton, J. (1975). Influence of heroin addiction on neuropsychological functioning. *Journal of Consulting and Clinical Psychology*, **43**, 114.

Finelli, P. F., Morgan, T. F., Yaar, I., and Granger, C. V. (1983). Ethylene oxide-induced polyneuropathy. *Archives of Neurology*, **40**, 419–421.

Firth, J. B., and Stuckey, R. E. (1945). Decomposition of trilene in closed circuit anesthesia. *Lancet*, **1**, 814.

Fischman, M. W. (1984). The behavioral pharmacology of cocaine in humans. In J. Grabowski (Ed.), *Cocaine: pharmacology, effects, and treatment of abuse*, NIDA Research Monograph 50, Washington, DC: Department of Health and Human Services, 72–91.

Fisher, D. G., Sweet, J. J., and Pfaelzer-Smith, E. A. (1986). The influence of depression on repeated neuropsychological testing. *The International Journal of Clinical Neuropsychology*, **8**, 14–18.

Fisher, K. (December 1985). Measuring effects of toxic chemicals: a growing role for psychology. *APA Monitor*, 13–14.

Fitzhugh, L. C., Fitzhugh, K. B., and Reitan, R. M. (1960). Adaptive abilities and intellectual functioning in hospitalized alcoholics. *Quarterly Journal of Studies on Alcohol*, **21**, 414–423.

Fitzhugh, L. C., Fitzhugh, K. B., and Reitan, R. M. (1966). Adaptive abilities and intellectual functioning in alcoholics: Further considerations. *Quarterly Journal of Studies on Alcohol*, **26**, 402–411.

Flodin, U., Edling, C., and Axelson, O. (1984). Clinical studies of psychoorganic syndromes among workers with exposure to solvents. *American Journal of Industrial Medicine*, **5**, 287–295.

Foa, V. (1982). Evaluation, limits and perspectives of neurobehavioral toxicology in occupations health. In R. Gilioli, M. G. Cassitto, and V. Foa (Eds), *Neurobehavioral Methods in Occupational Health*. New York: Pergamon Press, 173–176.

Fodor, G. G., and Winneke, G. (1972). Effect of low CO concentrations on resistance to monotony and on psychomotor capacity. *Staub-Reinhalt Luft*, **32**, 46–54.

Fornazzari, L., Wilkinson, D. A., Kapur, B. M., and Carlen, P. L. (1983). Cerebellar, cortical and functional impairment in toluene abusers. *Acta Neurologica Scandinavica*, **67**, 319–329.

Fortemps, E., Amand, G., Bomboir, A., Lauwerys, R., and Laterre, E. C. (1978). Trimethyltin poisoning: report of two cases. *International Archives of Occupational and Environmental Health*, **41**, 1–6.

Franchini, I., Ferri, F., Lommi, G., Lotta, S., Lucertini, S., and Mutti, A. (1982). Brain evoked potentials in solvent exposure. In R. Gilioli, M. G. Cassitto, and V. Foa (Eds), *Neurobehavioral Methods in Occupational Health*. New York: Pergamon Press, 197–204.

Freud, S. (1985). Project for a scientific psychology. In J. Strachey (Ed.), *The Standard Edition of the Complete Psychological Works of Sigmund Freud*, Volume I (reprinted in 1975). London: Hogarth Press, 283–346.

Freud, S. (Letter to Wilhelm Fleiss, 26 October 1896). In J. Masson (Ed.), *The Complete Letters of Sigmund Freud*. Cambridge: Belknap Press, 1985, 201.

Friedman, M. J., Culver, C. M., and Ferrell, R. B. (1977). On the safety of long-term treatment with lithium. *American Journal of Psychiatry*, **134**, 1123–1126.

Frontali, N., Amantini, M. C., Spagnolo, A., Guarcini, A. M., and Saltari, M. C.

(1981). Experimental neurotoxicity and urinary metabolites of the C5–C7 aliphatic hydrocarbons used as glue solvents in shoe manufacture. *Clinical Toxicology*, **18**, 1357–1367.

Fullerton, P. M. (1966). Chronic peripheral neuropathy produced by lead poisoning in guinea pigs. *Journal of Neuropathology and Experimental Neurology*, **25**, 214.

Gade, A., Mortensen, H., and Udesen, H. (1984). The pattern of intellectual impairment in toxic encephalopathy, or a study of the pattern, degree, and validity of intellectual impairment in toxic encephalopathy. Presented at the *International Conference on Organic Solvent Toxicity*, 15–17 October, Stockholm, Sweden.

Gade, A., Mortensen, H., Udesen, H., and Bruhn, P. (1985). On the importance of control data and background variables in the evaluation of neuropsychological aspects of brain functioning. *Neurobehavioral Methods in Occupational and Environmental Health*, Document 3, Copenhagen: World Health Organization, 91–96.

Gallant, D. M. (1986). Hypertension and alcohol consumption. *Alcoholism: Clinical and Experimental Research*, **10**, 358.

Gallant, D. M. (1985). Alcoholism: The most common psychiatric illness. *Alcoholism: Clinical and Experimental Research*, **9**, 297.

Gamberale, F. (1985). Use of behavioral performance tests in the assessment of solvent toxicity. *Scandinavian Journal of Work Environment and Health*, Suppl. 1, **11**, 65–74.

Gamberale, F., and Hultengren, M. (1972). Toluene exposure: II. Psychophysiological functions. *Work Environment and Health*, **9**, 131–139.

Gamberale, F., and Hultengren, M. (1973). Methylchloroform exposure. II. Psychophysiological functions. *Work Environment and Health*, **10**, 82–92.

Gamberale, F., and Kjellberg, A. (1982). Behavioral performance assessment as a biological control of occupational exposure to neurotoxic substances. In R. Gilioli, M. G. Cassitto, and V. Foa (Eds), *Neurobehavioral Methods in Occupational Health*. New York: Pergamon Press, 111–121.

Gamberale, F., Annwall, G., and Hultengren, M. (1978). Exposure to xylene and ethylbenzene: III. Effects on central nervous system functions. *Scandinavian Journal of Work Environment and Health*, **4**, 204–211.

Garland, H., and Pearce, J. (1967). Neurological complications of carbon monoxide poisoning. *Quarterly Journal of Medicine*, **144**, 445–455.

Gawin, F. H., and Kleber, H. D. (1986). Abstinence symptomatology and psychiatric diagnosis in cocaine abusers. *Archives of General Psychiatry*, **43**, 107–113.

Gebhardt, C., Naeser, M., and Butters, N. (1984). Computerized measure of CT scans of alcoholics: Thalamic region related to memory. *Alcohol*, **1**, 133–140.

Gershon, S., and Shaw, F. H. (24 June 1961). Psychiatric sequelae of chronic exposure to organophosphorus insecticides. *Lancet*, 1371–1374.

Geschwind, N., and Behan, P. (1982). Left handedness: Association with immune disease, migraine and developmental learning disorder. *Proceedings of the National Academy of Sciences, USA*, **79**, 5097–5100.

Ghadirian, A. M., Engelsmann, F., and Ananth, J. (1983). Memory functions during lithium therapy. *Journal of Clinical Psychopharmacology*, **3**, 313–315.

Ghosh, S. K. (1976). Methyldopa and forgetfulness. *Lancet*, **1**, 202–203.

Ginsberg, M. (1980). Carbon monoxide. In P. S. Spencer and H. H. Schaumberg (Eds), *Experimental and Clinical Neurotoxicology*. Baltimore: Williams & Wilkins, 374–394.

Giovacchini, R. P. (1985). Abusing the volatile organic chemicals. *Regulatory Toxicology and Pharmacology*, **5**, 18–37.

Girkem, W., Krebs, F. A., and Muller-Oerlinghausen, B. (1975). Effects of lithium on electromyographic recordings in man. *Pharmacopsychiatry*, **10**, 79–82.

Gittelman, R., and Eskenazi, B. (1983). Lead and hyperactivity revisited. An investigation of nondisadvantaged children. *Archives of General Psychiatry*, **40**, 827–833.

Goetz, C. G. (1985). *Neurotoxins in Clinical Practice*. New York: SP Medical and Scientific Books.

Gold, J. H. (1969). Chronic perchloroethylene poisoning. *Canadian Psychiatric Association Journal*, **14**, 627–630.

Gold, M. S., and Verebey, K. (1984). The psychopharmacology of cocaine. *Psychiatric Annals*, **14**, 714–723.

Golden, C. J. (1978). *Diagnosis and Rehabilitation in Clinical Neuropsychology*. Springfield: Charles C. Thomas.

Golden, C. J., Hammeke, T. A., and Purisch, A. D. (1980). *The Luria-Nebraska Neuropsychological Battery: Manual*. Los Angeles: Western Psychological Services.

Golden, C. J., Kane, R., Sweet, J., Moses. J. A., Cardellino, J. P., Templeton, R., Vicente, P., and Graber, B. (1981). Relationship of the Luria-Nebraska to the Halstead-Reitan Neuropsychological Battery. *Journal of Consulting and Clinical Psychology*, **49**, 410–417.

Goldings, A. S., and Stewart, M. (1982). Organic lead encephalopathy: Behavioral change and movement disorder following gasoline inhalation. *Journal of Clinical Psychiatry*, **43**, 70–72.

Goldman, M. S. (1986). Neuropsychological recovery in alcoholics: Endogenous and exogenous processes. *Alcoholism: Clinical and Experimental Research*, **10**, 136–144.

Goldman, M. S. (1983). Cognitive impairment in chronic alcoholics. *American Psychologist*, 1045–1053.

Goldman, M. S., Williams, D. L., and Klisz, D. K. (1983). Recoverability of psychological functioning following alcohol abuse: Prolonged visual-spatial dysfunction in older alcoholics. *Journal of Consulting and Clinical Psychology*, **51**, 370–378.

Goldstein, G., and Shelly, C. (1979). Neuropsychological investigation of brain lesion localization in alcoholism. In H. Begleiter (Ed.), *Biological Effects of Alcoholism*. New York: Plenum Press, 731–743.

Goldwater, L. J. (1972). *Mercury: A history of quicksilver*. Baltimore: York Press.

Gossel, T. A., and Bricker, J. D. (1984). *Principles of Clinical Toxicology*. New York: Raven Press.

Grabski, D. A. (1961). Toluene sniffing producing cerebellar degeneration. *American Journal of Psychiatry*, **118**, 461–462.

Grandjean, E. (1960). Trichloroethylene effects on animal behavior. *Archives of Environmental Health*, **1**, 106–108.

Grandjean, P. (1983). Behavioral toxicity of heavy metals. In P. Zbinden, V. Cuomo, G. Racagni, and B. Weiss (Eds), *Application of Behavioral Pharmacology in Toxicology*. New York: Raven Press, 331–340.

Grandjean, P. (Ed.) (1985). Neurobehavioral methods in occupational and environmental health: Symposium Report Number 6, *World Health Organization*. Regional Office for Europe, Copenhagen.

Grandjean, P., Arnvig, E., and Beckmann, J. (1978). Psychological dysfunctions in lead-exposed workers. *Scandinavian Journal of Work Environment and Health*, **4**, 295–303.

Grandstaff, N. (1973). Carbon monoxide and human functions. In C. Xintaras, B. L. Johnson, and I. deGrott (Eds), *Behavioral Toxicology: Early detection of occupational hazards*. Washington, DC: HEW Publication No. (NIOSH), 74–126, 292–305.

Grant, D. A., and Berg, E. A. (1948). A behavioral analysis of degree of reinforcement and ease of shifting to new responses in Weigl-type card sorting problem. *Journal of Experimental Psychology*, 38, 404–411.

Grant, I. (1987). Alcohol and the brain: Neuropsychological correlates. *Journal of Consulting and Clinical Psychology*, 55, 310–324.

Grant, I., Adams, K. M., Reed, R., and Carlin, A. (1979). Neuropsychological function in young alcoholics and polydrug abusers. *Journal of Clinical Neuropsychology*, 1, 39–47.

Grant, I., Adams, K. M., Carlin, A. S., Rennick, P. M., Judd, L. L., Schooff, K., and Reed, R. (1978). Neuropsychological effects of polydrug abuse. In D. R. Wesson, A. S. Carlin, K. M. Adams, and G. Beschner (Eds), *Polydrug Abuse: The results of a national collaborative study*. New York: Academic Press, 223–261.

Grant, I., Adams, K. M., and Reed, R. (1984). Aging, abstinence, and medical risk factors in the prediction of neuropsychologic deficit among long-term alcoholics. *Archives of General Psychiatry*, 41, 710–718.

Grant, I., and Mohns, L. (1975). Chronic cerebral effects of alcohol and drug abuse. *International Journal of the Addictions*, 883–920.

Grant, I., and Reed, R. (1985). Neuropsychology of alcohol and drug abuse. In A. I. Alterman (ed.), *Substance Abuse and Psychopathology*. New York: Plenum Press, 289–339.

Grant, I., Rochford, J., Fleming, T., and Stunkard, H. (1973). A neuropsychological assessment of the effects of moderate marihuana use. *Journal of Nervous and Mental Disease*, 156, 278–280.

Grcevic, N., Jadro-Santel, D., and Jukic, S. (1977). Cerebral changes in paraquat poisoning. In L. Roizin, H. Shiraki, and N. Grcevic (Eds), *Neurotoxicology*, New York: Raven Press, 469–484.

Greenberg, B. D., Moore, P. A., Letz, R., and Baker, E. L. (1985). Computerized assessment of human neurotoxicity: Sensitivity to nitrous oxide exposure. *Clinical Pharmacology and Therapeutics*, 38, 656–660.

Greenblatt, D. J., and Shader, R. I. (1974). *Benzodiazepines in Clinical Practice*. New York: Raven Press.

Gregersen, P., and Stigsby, B. (1981). Reaction time of industrial workers exposed to organic solvents: Relationship to degree of exposure and psychological performance. *American Journal of Industrial Medicine*, 2, 313–321.

Gregersen, P., Angelso, B., Neilsen, T. E., Norgaard, B., and Uldal, C. (1984). Neurotoxic effects of organic solvents in exposed workers: An occupational, neuropsychological, and neurological investigation. *American Journal of Industrial Medicine*, 5, 201–225.

Griffen, J. W. (1981). Hexacarbon neurotoxicity. *Neurobehavioral Toxicology and Teratology*, 3, 437–444.

Griffiths, R. R., Bigelow, G. E., Stitzer, M. L., and McLeod, D. R. (1983). Behavioral effects of drugs of abuse. In. G. Zbinden, V. Cuomo, G. Racagni, and B. Weiss (Eds), *Applications of Behavioral Pharmacology*. New York: Raven Press, 367–382.

Gross, J. A., Hass, M. L., and Swift, T. R. (1979). Ethylene oxide neurotoxicity: report of four cases and review of the literature. *Neurology*, 29, 978–983.

Guerit, J. M., Meulders, M., Amand, G., Roels, H. A., Buchet, J. P., Lauwerys, R.,

Bruaux, P., Claeys-Thoreau, F., Ducoffre, G., and Lafontaine, A. (1981). Lead neurotoxicity in clinically asymptomatic children living in the vicinity of an ore smelter. *Clinical Toxicology*, 18, 1257-1267.

Gun, R. T., Grysorewicz, C., and Nettelbeck, J. (1978). Choice reaction time in workers using trichloroethylene. *Medical Journal of Australia*, 1, 535-546.

Gustafson, C., and Tagesson, C. (1985). Influence of organic solvent mixtures on biological membranes. *British Journal of Industrial Medicine*, 42, 591-595.

Guthrie, A. (1980). The first year after treatment: Factors affecting time course of reversibility of memory and learning deficits in alcoholism. In H. Begleiter (Ed.), *Biological Effects of Alcohol*. New York: Plenum Press, 757-770.

Halikas, J. A., Weller, R. A., Morse, C. L., and Hoffmann, R. G. (1985). A longitudinal study of marijuana effects. *International Journal of the Addictions*, 20, 701-711.

Hall, R. C. W., and Zisook, S. (1981). Paradoxical reactions to benzodiazepines. *British Journal of Clinical Pharmacology*, 11, Suppl., 99s-104s.

Halstead, W. C. (1947). *Brain and Intelligence*. Chicago: University of Chicago Press.

Hamilton, A. (1985). Forty years in the poisonous trades. *American Journal of Industrial Medicine*, 7, 3-18.

Hamilton, A., and Hardy, H. L. (1974). *Industrial Toxicology*. Acton, Mass,: Publishing Sciences Group, Inc.

Hanakago, R. (1979). Severe polyneuritis showed amyotrophy following gold therapy for bronchial asthma. In L. Manzo (Ed.), *Advances in Neurotoxicology*. New York: Pergamon Press, 391-396.

Hane, M., and Ekberg, K. (1984). Current research in behavioral toxicology. *Scandinavian Journal of Work, Environment and Health*, Suppl. 1, 8-9.

Hane, M., Axelson, O., Blume, J., Hogstedt, C., Sundell, L., and Ydreborg, B. (1977). Psychological function changes among house painters. *Scandinavian Journal of Work Environment and Health*, 3, 91-99.

Hane, M., Hogstedt, C., and Sundell, L. (1980). Neuropsychiatric symptoms among solvent workers—a questionnaire for screening. *Lakartidningen*, 77, 437-439.

Hanin, I., Krigman, M. R., and Mailman, R. B. (1984). Central neurotransmitter effects of organotin compounds: Trials, tribulations and observations. *NeuroToxicology*, 5, 267-278.

Hänninen, H. (1971). Psychological picture of manifest and latent carbon disulphide poisoning. *British Journal of Industrial Medicine*. 28, 374-381.

Hänninen, H. (1982). Behavioral effects of occupational exposure to mercury and lead. *Acta Neurologica Scandinavica*, Suppl. 92, 66, 167-175.

Hänninen, H. (1983). Psychological test batteries: New trends and developments. In R. Gilioli, M. G. Cassitto, and V. Foa (Eds), *Neurobehavioral Methods in Occupational Health*. New York: Pergamon Press, 123-130.

Hänninen, H., and Lindström, K. (1979). *Behavioral test battery for toxic psychological studies*. Helsinki: Institute of Occupational Health.

Hänninen, H., Eskeline, L., Husman, K., and Nurminen, M. (1976). Behavioral effects of long-term exposure to a mixture of organic solvents. *Scandinavian Journal of Work Environment and Health*, 4, 240-255.

Hänninen, H., Hernberg, S., Mantere, P., Vesanto, R., and Jalkanen, M. (1978). Psychological performance of subjects with low exposure to lead. *Journal of Occupational Medicine*, 20, 683-689.

Hänninen, H., Mantere, P., Hernberg, S., Mantere, P., Seppäläinen, A. M., and Kock, B. (1979). Subjective symptoms to low-level exposure to lead.

NeuroToxicology, **1**, 333–347.

Hänninen, H., Nurminen, M., Tolonen, M., and Martelin, T. (1978). Psychological tests as indicators of excessive exposure to carbon disulfide. *Scandinavian Journal of Psychology*, **19**, 163–174.

Hannon, R., Butler, C. P., Day, C. L., Khan, S. A., Quittoriano, L A., Butler, A. M., and Meredith, L. (1985). Alcohol use and cognitive functioning in men and women college students. In M. Galanter (Ed.), *Recent Developments in Alcoholism*, Volume 3: *High risk studies, prostaglandins and leukotrienes, cardiovascular effects, cerebral function in social drinkers*. New York: Plenum Press, 241–252.

Hansen, O. N., Trillingsgaard, A., Beese, I., Lyngbye, T., and Grandjean, P. (1985). Neurobehavioral methods in assessment of children with low-level lead exposure. In *Neurobehavioral Methods in Occupational and Environmental Health*, Document 3, Copenhagen: World Health Organization, 183–187.

Härkönen, H., Lindström, K., Seppäläinen, A. M., Sisko, A., and Hernberg, S. (1978). Exposure–response relationship between styrene exposure and central nervous system functions. *Scandinavian Journal of Work Environment and Health*, **4**, 53–59.

Harper, C. G. (1979). Wernicke's encephalopathy: a more common disease than realized. A neuropathological study of 51 cases. *Journal of Neurology, Neurosurgery, and Psychiatry*, **42**, 226–231.

Harper, C. G. (1983). The incidence of Wernicke's encephalopathy in Australia — a neuropathological study of 131 cases. *Journal of Neurology, Neurosurgery, and Psychiatry*, **46**, 593–598.

Harper, C. G., and Blumbergs, P. C. (1983). Brain weights in alcoholics. *Journal of Neurology, Neurosurgery and Psychiatry*, **45**, 838–840.

Harper, C., and Kril, J. (1985). Brain atrophy in chronic alcoholic patients: a quantitative pathological study. *Journal of Neurology, Neurosurgery, and Psychiatry*, **48**, 211–217.

Harper, C. G., Giles, M., and Finlay-Jones, R. (1986). Clinical signs in the Wernicke–Korsakoff complex: A retrospective analysis of 131 cases diagnosed at necropsy. *Journal of Neurology, Neurosurgery, and Psychiatry*, **49**, 341–345.

Hartitzsch, von B., Hoenich, N. A., Leigh R. J., Wilkinson, R., Frost, T. H. Weddel, A., and Posen, G. A. (1972). Permanent neurological sequelae despite haemodialysis for lithium intoxication. *British Medical Journal*, **4**, 757–759.

Hartlage, L., and Knowles, E. (1986). Reaction time correlates of occasional substance abuse. Presented at the 1986 annual meeting of the National Academy of Neuropsychologists, Las Vegas, Nevada, 27–29 October.

Hartman, D. E. (1986a). On the use of clinical psychology software: practical, legal and ethical concerns. *Professional Psychology: Research and Practice*, **17**, 462–465.

Hartman, D. E. (1986b). Artificial intelligence or artificial psychologist?: conceptual issues in clinical microcomputer use. *Professional Psychology: Research and Practice, 17*, 528–534.

Hartman, D. E. (1987). Neuropsychological toxicology: identification and assessment of neurotoxic syndromes. *Archives of Clinical Neuropsychology*, **2**, 45–65.

Hartman, D. E., Sweet, J. J., and Elvart, A. (1985). Neuropsychological effects of Wernickes encephalopathy as a consequence of hyperemesis gravidarum: a case study. *International Journal of Clinical Neuropsychology*. **7**, 204–207.

Hayes, W. L. (1971). Studies on exposure during the use of anticholinesterase pesticides. *Bulletin of the World Health Organization*, **44**, 277–288.

Heaton, R. K., and Crowley, T. J. (1981). Effects of psychiatric disorders and their somatic treatments on neuropsychological test results. In S. B. Filskov and T. J. Boll (Eds), *Handbook of Clinical Neuropsychology*. New York: John Wiley & Sons, 481–525.

Heimann, H., Reed, C. F., and Witt. P. N. (1968). Some observations suggesting preservation of skilled motor acts despite drug-induced stress. *Psychopharmacologia*, **13**, 287–298.

Hendler, N., Cimini, C., Terrence, M. A., and Long, D. (1980). A comparison of cognitive impairment due to benzodiazepines and to narcotics. *American Journal of Psychiatry*, **137**, 828–830.

Hernberg, S. (1980). Evaluation of epidemiologic studies in assessing the long-term effects of occupational noxious agents. *Scandinavian Journal of Work Environment and Health*, **6**, 163–169.

Hernberg, S. (1983). Does solvent poisoning exist? In N. Cherry and H. A. Waldron (Eds), *The Neuropsychological Effects of Solvent Exposure*. Havant, Hampshire: Colt Foundation, 63–72.

Hill, S. Y. (1980). Comprehensive assessment of brain dysfunction in alcoholic individuals. *Acta Psychiatrica Scandinavica*, Suppl. 286, **62**, 57–75.

Hillbom, M., and Kaste, M. (1983). Ethanol intoxication: a risk factor for ischemic brain infarction. *Stroke*, **14**, 694–695.

Hindmarch, I. (1980). Psychomotor function and psychoactive drugs. *British Journal of Clinical Pharmacology*, **10**, 189–209.

Hindmarch, I., and Gudgeon, A. C. (1980). The effects of clobazam and lorazepam on aspects of psychomotor performance and car handling ability. *British Journal of Clinical Pharmacology*, **10**, 145–150.

Hippolito, R. N. (1980). Xylene poisoning in laboratory workers: case reports and discussion. *Laboratory Medicine*, **11**, 593–595.

Hodgson, M. J., Block, G. D., and Parkinson, D. K. (1986). Organophosphate poisoning in office workers. *Journal of Occupational Medicine*, **28**, 434–437.

Hoffman, P., and Tabakoff, B. (1980). Receptor and neurotransmitter changes produced by chronic alcohol ingestion. In L. Manzo (Ed.), *Advances in Neurotoxicology*. New York: Pergamon Press, 107–116.

Hoffman, R. E., Stehr-Green, P. A., Webb, K. B., Evans, G., Knutsen, A. P., Schramm, W. F., Staake, J. L., Gibson, B. B., and Steinberg, K. K. (1986). Health effects of long-term exposure to 2,3,7,8-tetrachlorodibenzo-*p*-dioxin. *Journal of the American Medical Association*, **255**, 2031–2038.

Hogstedt, C., Hane, M., Agrell, A., and Bodlin, L. (1983). Neuropsychological test results and symptoms among workers with well defined long-term exposure to lead. *British Journal of Industrial Medicine*, **40**, 99–105.

Hogstedt, C., Hane, M., and Axelson, O. (1980). Diagnostic and health care aspects of workers exposed to solvents. In C. Zenz (Ed.), *Developments in Occupational Medicine*. Chicago: Year Book Medical Publishers, 249–258.

Holmes, T. M., Buffler, P. A., Holguin, A. H., and Hsi, B. P. (1986). A mortality study of employees at a synthetic rubber manufacturing plant. *American Journal of Industrial Medicine*, **9**, 355–362.

Hormes, J. T., Filley, C. M., and Rosenberg, N. L. (1986). Neurologic sequelae of chronic solvent vapor abuse. *Neurology*, **36**, 698–702.

Howard, M. L., Hogan, T. P., and Wright, M. W. (1975). The effects of drugs on psychiatric patients' performance on the Halstead–Reitan neuropsychological test battery. *Journal of Nervous and Mental Disease*, **161**, 166–171.

Hunter, J., Urbanowicz, M. A., Yule, W., and Lansdown, R. (1985). Automated testing of reaction time and its association with lead in children. *International Archives of Occupational and Environmental Health*, **57**, 27–34.

Husman, K. (1980). Symptoms of car painters with long-term exposure to a mixture of organic solvents. *Scandinavian Journal of Work Environment and Health*, **6**, 19–32.

Husman, K., and Karli, P. (1980). Clinical neurological findings among car painters exposed to a mixture of organic solvents. *Scandinavian Journal of Work Environment and Health*, **6**, 33–39.

Irons, R., and Rose, P. (1985). Naval biodynamics laboratory computerized cognitive testing. *Neurobehavioral Toxicology and Teratology*, **7**, 395–397.

James, R. C. (1985). Neurotoxicity: toxic effects in the nervous system. In P. L. Williams and J. L. Burson (Eds), *Industrial Toxicology: Safety and health applications in the workplace*. New York: Van Reinhold, 123–137.

Janowsky, D. S., Meacham, M. P., Blaine, J. D., Schoor, M., and Bozzetti, L. P. (1976). Marijuana effects on simulated flying ability. *American Journal of Psychiatry*, **133**, 384–388.

Jellinger, K. (1977). Neuropathologic findings after neuroleptic long-term therapy. In L. Roizin, H. Shiraki, and N. Grcevic (Eds), *Neurotoxicology*. New York: Raven Press.

Johnson, J. L., Adinoff, B., Bisserbe, J-C., Martin, P. R., Rio, D., Rohrbaugh, J. W., Zubovic, E., and Eckardt, M. J. (1986). Assessment of alcoholism-related organic brain syndromes with positron emission tomography. *Alcoholism: Clinical and Experimental Research*, **10**, 237–240.

Johnson, B. L., and Anger, W. K. (1983). Behavioral toxicology. In W. N. Rom (Ed.), *Environmental and Occupational Medicine*. Boston: Little, Brown and Company, 329–350.

Johnson, B. L., Boyd, J., Burg, J. R., Lee, S. T., Xintaras, C., and Albright, B. E. (1983). Effects on the peripheral nervous system of workers' exposure to carbon disulfide. *NeuroToxicology*, **4**, 53–66.

Johnson, B. L., Cohen, A., Struble, R., Selzer, J. V., Anger, W. K., Gutnik, B.D., McDonough, T., and Houser, P. (1974). In C. Xintaras, B. L. Johnson, and I. deGroot (Eds), *Behavioral Toxicology: Early detection of occupational hazards*. Washington. DC: HEW Publication No. (NIOSH) 74–126, 306–328.

Johnson, B. P., Meredith, T. J., and Vale, J. A. (1983). Cerebellar dysfunction after acute carbon tetrachloride poisoning. *Lancet*, Volume II, 968.

Johnson L. D., Bachman, J. G., and O'Malley, P. M. (1979). *Drugs and the Nation's High School Students: Five Year Trends, 1979 Highlights*. Rockville, Md. National Institute on Drug Abuse.

Jones, B. (1971). Verbal and spatial intelligence in short and long term alcoholics. *Journal of Nervous and Mental Disease*, **153**, 292–297.

Jones, B., and Parsons, O. (1971). Impaired abstracting ability in chronic alcoholics. *Archives of General Psychiatry*, **24**, 71–75.

Jones, B., and Parsons, O. (1972). Specific vs. generalized deficits of abstracting ability in chronic alcoholics. *Archives of General Psychiatry*, **26**, 380–384.

Jones, B. M., and Vega, A. (1982). Cognitive performance measured on the ascending limb of the blood alcohol curve. *Psychopharmacologia* (Berlin), **23**, 99–114.

Jones, R. T. (1984). The pharmacology of cocaine. In J. Grabowski (Ed.), *Cocaine: Pharmacology, effects, and treatment of abuse*. NIDA Research Monograph 50, Washington, DC: Department of Health and Human Services, 34–53.

Jorgensen, N. K., and Cohr, K.-H. (1981). *n*-Hexane and its toxicologic effects: A review. *Scandinavian Journal of Work Environment and Health*, 157-168.

Juntunen, J. (1982a). Alcoholism in occupational neurology: Diagnostic difficulties with special reference to the neurological syndromes caused by exposure to organic solvents. *Acta Neurologica Scandinavica*, **66**, 89-108.

Juntunen, J. (1982b). Neurological examination and assessment of the syndromes causes by exposure to neurotoxic agents. In R. Gilioli, M. G. Cassitto, and V. Foa (Eds), *Neurobehavioral Methods in Occupational Health*. New York: Pergamon Press, 3-10.

Juntunen, J., Hupli V., Hernberg, S., and Luisto, M. (1980). Neurological picture of organic solvent poisoning in industry. *International Archives of Occupational and Environmental Health*, **46**, 219-231.

Jusic, A. (1974). Anticholinesterase pesticides of organophosphorus type: Electromyographic, neurological and psychological studies in occupationally exposed workers. In C. Xintaras, B. L. Johnson, and I. deGrott (Eds), *Behavioral Toxicology: Early detection of occupational hazards*. Washington, DC: HEW Publication No. (NIOSH) 74-126, 182-190.

Kardel, T., and Stigsby, B. (1975). Period-amplitude analysis of the electroencephalogram correlated with liver function in patients with cirrhosis of the liver. *Electroencephalopgraphy and Clinical Neurophysiology*, **38**, 605-609.

Kardel, T., Zander Olsen, P., Stigsby, B., and Tonneson, K. (1972). Hepatic encephalopathy evaluated by automatic period analysis of the electroencephalogram during lactulose treatment. *Acta Medica Scandinavica*, **192**, 493-498.

Katz, G. V. (1985). Metals and metalloids other than mercury and lead. In J. L. O'Donoghue (Ed.), *Neurotoxicity of Industrial and Commercial Chemicals*, Volume I. Boca Raton: CRC Press, 171-191.

Kendrick, D. C., and Post, F. (1967). Differences in cognitive status between healthy, psychiatrically ill, and diffusely brain-damaged elderly subjects. *British Journal of Psychiatry*, **113**, 75-81.

Kessler, R. M., Parker, E. S., Clark, C. M., Martin, P. R., George, D. T., Weingartner, H., Sokoloff, L., Ebert, M. H., and Mishkin, M. (1984). Regional cerebral glucose metabolism in patients with alcoholic Korsakoff's syndrome. *Society of Neuroscience Abstracts*, **10**, 541.

Key, M. M., Henschel, A. F., Butler, J., Ligo, Tabershaw, I. R., and Ede, L. (Eds), (1977). *Occupation diseases: A guide to their recognition*. DHEW Publication No. (NIOSH) 77-181, Washington, DC: U.S. Government Printing Office.

Kilburn, K. H., Seidman, B. C., and Warshaw, R. (1985a). Neurobehavioral and respiratory symptoms of formaldehyde and xylene exposure in histology technicians. *Archives of Environmental Health*, **40**, 229-233.

Kilburn, K. H., Warshaw, R., Boylen, C. T., Johnson, S.-J. S., Seidman, B., Sinclair, R., and Takaro, T. (1985b). Pulmonary and neurobehavioral effects of formaldehyde exposure. *Archives of Environmental Health*, **40**, 254-260.

King, M. (1983). Long term neuropsychological effects of solvent abuse. In N. Cherry and H. A. Waldron (Eds), *The Neuropsychological Effects of Solvent Exposure*. Havant, Hampshire: Colt Foundation, 75-84.

Kleinknecht, R. A., and Donaldson, D. (1975). A review of the effects of diazepam on cognitive and psychomotor performance. *Journal of Nervous and Mental Disease*, **161**, 399-411.

Klisz, D., and Parsons, O. A. (1977). Hypothesis testing in younger and older alcoholics. *Journal of Studies on Alcohol*, **38**, 1718-1729.

Knave, B. K., Olson, A., Elofsson, S., Gamberale, F., Isaksson, A., Mindus, P., Persson, H. E., Struwe, G., Wennberg, A., and Westerholm, P. (1978). Long-term exposure to jet fuel. *Scandinavian Journal of Work Environment and Health*, 4, 19–45.

Konietzko, H., Keilbach, J., and Drysch, J. (1980). Cumulative effects of daily toluene exposure. *International Archives of Occupational and Environmental Health*, 46, 53–58.

Konietzko, H., Elster, J., Bencsath, A., Drysch, K., and Weichard, H. (1975). Psychomotor responses under standardized tricholoroethylene load. *Archives of Toxicology*, 33, 129–139.

Korgeski, G. P., and Leon, G. (1983). Correlates of self-reported and objectively determined exposure to Agent Orange. *American Journal of Psychiatry*, 140, 1443–1449.

Korman, M., Matthews, R. W., and Lovitt, R. (1981). Neuropsychological effects of abuse of inhalants. *Perceptual and Motor Skills*, 53, 547–553.

Korsak, R. J., and Sato, M. M. (1977). Effects of chronic organophosphate pesticide exposure on the central nervous system. *Clinical Toxicology*, 11, 83–95.

Krigman, M. R., Bouldin, T. W., and Mushak, P. (1980). Lead. In P. S. Spencer and H. H. Schaumberg (Eds), *Experimental and Clinical Neurotoxicology*. Baltimore: Williams & Wilkins, 490–507.

Kruger, G., Weinhardt, F., and Hoyer, S. (1979). Brain energy metabolism and blood flow in bismuth encephalopathy. In L. Manzo (Ed.), *Advances in Neurotoxicology*. New York: Pergamon Press, 63–68.

Landrigan, P. J. (1983). Toxic exposures and psychiatric disease — lessons from the epidemiology of cancer. *Acta Psychiatrica Scandinavica*, Suppl. 303, 67, 6–15.

Landrigan, P. J., Whitworth, R. H., Baloh, R. W., Staehling, N. W., Barthel, W. F., and Rosenblum, B. F. (1975). Neuropsychological dysfunction in children with chronic low-level lead absorption. *Lancet*, Volume I, 708–712.

Landrigan, P. J., Kreiss, K., Xintaras, C., Feldman, R. G., and Heath Jr, C. W. (1980). Clinical epidemiology of occupational neurotoxic disease. *Neurobehavioral Toxicology*, 2, 43–48.

Langolf, G. D., Chaffin, D. B., Henderson, R., and Whittle, H. P. (1978). Evaluation of workers exposed to elemental mercury using quantitative tests of tremor and neuromuscular functions. *American Industrial Hygiene Association Journal*, 39, 976–984.

Lee, G. P., and DiClimente, C. C. (1985). Age of onset versus duration of problem drinking on the alcohol use inventory. *Journal of Studies on Alcohol*, 46(5), 398–402.

Legg, J. F., and Stiff, M. P. (1976). Drug-related test patterns of depressed patients. *Psychopharmacology*, 50, 205–310.

Le Quesne, P. M. (1979). Neurological disorders due to toxic occupational hazards. *Practitioner*, 223, 40–47.

Le Quesne, P. M. (1982). Metal-induced diseases of the nervous system. *British Journal of Hospital Medicine*, 534–537.

Le Quesne, P. M. (1984). Neuropathy due to drugs. In P. J. Dyck, P. K. Thomas, E. H. Lambert, and R. Bunge (Eds), *Peripheral Neuropathy*, Volume II. Philadelphia: W. B. Saunders, 2162–2179.

Lerman, Y., Hirshberg, A., and Shteger, Z. (1984). Organophosphate and carbamate pesticide poisoning: The usefulness of a computerized clinical information system. *American Journal of Industrial Medicine*, 6, 17–26.

Letz, R., and Singer, R. (1985). Neuropsychological tests. In P. Grandjean (Ed.),

Neurobehavioral Methods in Occupational and Environmental Health. Document 6, Copenhagen: World Health Organization, 17–18.

Levin, H. S. (1973). Behavioral effects of occupational exposure to organophosphorate pesticides. In C. Xintaras, B. L. Johnson, and I. deGroot (Eds), *Behavioral Toxicology: Early detection of occupational hazards.* Washington. DC: HEW Publication No. (NIOSH) 74–126, 154–163.

Levin, H. S., and Rodnitzky, R. L. (1976). Behavioral aspects of organophosphorous pesticides in man. *Clinical Toxicology*, **9**, 391.

Levin, H. S., Rodnitzky, R. L., and Mick, D. L. (1976). Anxiety associated with exposure to organophosphate compounds. *Archives of General Psychiatry*, **33**, 225–228.

Levinson, J. L. (1985). Neuroleptic malignant syndrome. *American Journal of Psychiatry*, **142**, 1137–1144.

Lewis, J. E., and Hordan, R. B. (1986). Neuropsychological assessment of phencyclidine abusers. In D. H. Clouet (Ed.), *Phencyclidine: an update.* NIDA Research Monograph 64, Washington, DC: Department of Health and Human Services, 190–208.

Lezak, M. D. (1984). Neuropsychological assessment in behavioral toxicology — developing techniques and interpretive issues. *Scandinavian Journal of Work Environment and Health*, Suppl. 1, **10**, 25–29.

Lilis, R. A., Fischbein, A., Diamond, S., Anderson, H. A., Selikoff, I. J., Blumberg, W. E., and Eisinger, J. (1977). Lead effects among secondary lead smelter workers with blood lead levels below 80 ug/100 ml. *Archives of Environmental Health*, **32**, 256–266.

Liljequist, R., Linnoila, M., and Mattila, M. J. (1974). Effect of two weeks' treatment with chlorimipramine and nortriptyline, alone or in combination with, on learning and memory, *Psychopharmacologia*, **39**, 181–186.

Lindberg, N., Basch, K. E., and Lindberg, E. (1982). Psychotherapeutic examination of patients with suspected chronic solvent intoxication. An overview. *Psychotherapy and Psychosomatics*, **37**, 36–63.

Lindström, K. (1980). Changes in psychological performance of solvent-poisoned and solvent-exposed workers. *American Journal of Industrial Medicine*, **1**, 69–84.

Lindström, K. (1981). Behavioral changes after long-term exposure to organic solvents and their mixtures. *Scandinavian Journal of Work Environment and Health*, Suppl. 4, **7**, 48–53.

Lindström, K. (1982). Behavioral effects of long-term exposure to solvents. *Acta Neurologica Scandinavica*, Suppl. 92, **66**, 131–141.

Lindström, K. (1984). The Rorschach test in behavioral toxicology. *Scandinavian Journal of Work Environment and Health*, Suppl. 1, **10**, 20–23.

Lindström, J., and Wickstrom, G. (1983). Psychological function changes among maintenance house painters exposed to low levels of organic solvent mixtures. *Acta Psychiatrica Scandinavica*, Suppl. 303, **67**, 81–91.

Lindström, K., Antti-Poika, M., Tolla, S., and Hyytianinen, A. (1982). Psychological prognosis of diagnosed organic solvent intoxication. *Neurobehavioral Toxicology and Teratology*, **4**, 581–588.

Lindström, K., Härkönen, H., and Hernberg, S. (1976). Disturbances in psychological functions of workers occupationally exposed to styrene. *Scandinavian Journal of Work Environment and Health*, **3**, 129–139.

Lindström, K., Riihimaki, H., and Hänninen, K. (1984). Occupational solvent exposure and neuropsychiatric disorders. *Scandinavian Journal of Work Environment and Health*, **10**, 321–323.

Linz, D. H., deGarmo, P. L., Morton, W. E., Weins, A. N., Coull, B. M., and Maricle, R. A. (1986). Organic solvent-induced encephalopathy in industrial painters. *Journal of Occupational Medicine*, **28**, 119–125.

Lishman, W. A. (1978). *Organic Psychiatry: The psychological consequences of cerebral disorder*. Oxford: Blackwell Scientific Publications.

Lister, R. G. (1985). The amnesic action of benzodiazepines in man. *Neuroscience and Biobehavioral Review*, **9**, 87–94.

Løberg, T. (1978). Neuropsychological deficits in alcoholics: Lack of personality (MMPI) correlates. In H. Begleiter (Ed.), *Biological Effects of Alcoholism*. New York: Plenum Press, 797–808.

Løberg, T. (1986). Neuropsychological findings in the early and middle phases of alcoholism. In I. Grant, and K. M. Adams (Eds), *Neuropsychological Assessment of Neuropsychiatric Disorders*. New York: Oxford University Press, 441–477.

London, W. P. (1985). Treatment outcome of left-handed versus right-handed alcoholic men. *Alcoholism: Clinical and Experimental Research*, **9**, 503–504.

Long, J. A., and McLachlan, J. F. C. (1974). Abstract reasoning and perceptual-motor efficiency in alcoholics: Impairment and reversibility. *Quarterly Journal of Studies on Alcohol*, **35**, 1220–1229.

Longstreth, W. T., Rosenstock, L., and Heyer, N. J. (1985). Potroom palsy? Neurologic disorder in three aluminum smelter workers. *Archives of Internal Medicine*, **145**, 1972–1975.

Lu, Y-C., and Wong, P-N. (1984). Dermatological, medical and laboratory findings of patients in Taiwan and their treatments. In M. Kuratsune and R. Shapiro (Eds), *PCB Poisoning in Japan and Taiwan*. New York: Alan. R. Liss, 81–116.

Lubit, R., and Russett, B. (1984). The effects of drugs on decision-making. *Journal of Conflict Resolution*, **28**, 85–102.

Lucki, I., Rickels, K., and Geller, A. M. (1986). Chronic use of benzodiazepines and psychomotor and cognitive test performance. *Psychopharmacology*, **88**, 426–433.

Lund, Y., Nissen, M., and Rafaelsen, O. J. (1982). Long-term lithium treatment and psychological functions *Acta Psychiatrica Scandinavica*, **65**, 233–244.

Luria, A. (1973). *The Working Brain*. New York: Basic Books.

Lusins, J., Zimberg, S., Smokler, H., and Gurley, K. (1980). Alcoholism and cerebral atrophy: a study of 50 patients with CT scan and psychologic testing. *Alcoholism: Clinical and Experimental Research*, **4**, 406–410.

MacFarland, H. N. (1986). Toxicology of solvents. *Journal of the American Industrial Hygiene Association*, **47**, 704–707.

Mackay, C. J., Campbell, L., Samuel, A. M., Alderman, K. J., Idzikowski, C., Wilson, H. K., and Gompertz, D. (1987). Behavioral changes during exposure to 1,1,1-trichlorothane: Time-course and relationship to blood solvent levels. *American Journal of Industrial Medicine*, **11**, 223–239.

Maddox, V. H. (1981). The historical development of phencyclidine. In E. F. Domino (Ed.), *PCP (Phencyclidine): Historical and current perspectives*. Ann Arbor: NPP Books, 1–8.

Mahaffey, K. R., Annest, J. L., Roberts, J., and Murphy, R. S. (1982). National estimates of blood lead levels: United States 1976–1980: Association with selected demographic and socioeconomic factors. *New England Journal of Medicine*, **307**, 573–579.

Mantere, P., Hänninen, H., Hernberg, S., and Luukkonen, R. (1984). A prospective followup study on psychological effects in workers exposed to low levels of organic solvent mixtures. *Scandinavian Journal of Work Environment and Health*, **10**, 43–50.

Marecek, J., Shapiro, I. M., Burke, A., Katz, S. H., and Hediger, M. L. (1983). Low-level lead exposure in childhood influences neuropsychological performance. *Archives of Environmental Health*, **38**, 355-359.

Marks, G., and Beatty, W. K. (1975). *The Precious Metals of Medicine*. New York: Charles Scribner's Sons.

Marlowe, M., Stellern, J., Errera, J., and Moon, C. (1985). Main and interaction effects of metal pollutants on visual-motor performance. *Archives of Environmental Health*, **40**, 221-224.

Maroni, M., Bulgheroni, C., Cassitto, M. G., Merluzzi, F., Gilioli, R., and Foa, V. (1977). A clinical, neurophysiological and behavioral study of female workers exposed to 1,1,1-trichloroethane. *Scandinavian Journal of Work Environment and Health*, **3**, 16-22.

Maizlish, N. A., Langolf, G. D., Whitehead, L. W., Fine. L. J., Albers, J. W., Goldberg, J., and Smith, P. (1985). Behavioural evaluation of workers exposed to mixtures of organic solvents. *British Journal of Industrial Medicine*, **42**, 579-590.

Matarazzo, J. D. (1985). Clinical psychological test interpretations by computer: Hardware outpaces software, *Computers in Human Behavior*, **1**, 235-253.

Matikainen, E., and Juntunen, J. (1985). Examination of the peripheral autonomic nervous system in occupational neurology. In *Neurobehavioral Methods in Occupational and Environmental Health*, Document 3, Copenhagen: World Health Organization, 57-60.

McCrady, B. S., and Smith, D. E. (1986). Implications of cognitive impairment for the treatment of alcoholism. *Alcoholism: Clinical and Experimental Research*, **10**, 145-149.

McGlaughlin, A. I. G., Kazantzis, G., King, E., Teare, D., Porter, R. J., and Owens, R. (1962). Pulmonary fibrosis and encephalopathy associated with the inhalation of aluminium dust. *British Journal of Industrial Medicine*, **19**, 253.

McGlothlin, W., Arnold, D., and Freedman, D. (1969). Organicity measures following repeated LSD ingestion. *Archives of General Psychiatry*, **21**, 704-709.

McLaughlin, D. R. C., and DeBoni, U. (1980). Aluminum in human brain disease — an overview. *NeuroToxicology*, **1**, 3-16.

McNair, D. M., Lorr, M., and Droppleman, L. F. (1971). *EITS Manual — Profile of Mood States*. San Diego: Educational and Industrial Testing Service.

Melamed, J. I., and Bleiberg, J. (1986). Neuropsychological deficits in freebase cocaine abusers after cessation of use. Paper presented at the 93rd annual convention of the American Psychological Association, Washington, DC, 23 August.

Melgaard, B., Arlien-Søborg, P., and Brulin, P. Chronic toxic encephalopathy in styrene exposed workers. Unpublished manuscript, Department of Neurology, Rigshospitalet, Copenhagen, Denmark.

Melgaard, B., Danielsen, U. T., Sorensen, H., and Ahlgren, P. (1986). The severity of alcoholism and its relation to intellectual impairment and cerebral atrophy. *British Journal of Addiction*, **81**, 77-80.

Melges, F. T., Tinklenberg, J. R., Hollister, L. E., and Gillespie, H. K. (1970a). Marihuana and temporal disintegration. *Science*, **168**, 1118-1120.

Melges, F. T., Tinklenberg, J. R., Hollister, L. E., and Gillespie, H. K. (1970b). Temporal disintegration and depersonalization during marihuana intoxication. *Archives of General Psychiatry*, **23**, 204-210.

Messite, J., and Bond, M. B. (1980). Occupational health considerations for women at work. In C. Zenz (Ed.), *Developments in Occupational Medicine*. Chicago: Year Book Medical Publishers, 43-57.

Metcalf, D. R., and Holmes, J. H. (1969). EEG, psychological and neurological alteration in humans with organophosphorous exposure. *Annals of the New York Academy of Science*, **160**, 357.

Mihevic, P. M., Gliner, J. A., and Horvath, S. M. (1983). Carbon monoxide exposure and information processing during perceptual-motor performance. *International Archives of Occupational and Environmental Health*, **51**, 355-363.

Mikkelsen, S. (1980). A cohort study of disability pension and death among painters with special regard to disabling presenile dementia as an occupational disease. *Scandinavian Journal of Social Medicine*, Suppl. 16, 34-43.

Mikkelsen, S., Browne, E., Jorgensen, M., and Gyldensted, C. (1985). Association of symptoms of dementia with neuropsychological diagnosis of dementia and cerebral atrophy. In *Chronic Effects of Organic Solvents on the Central Nervous System and Diagnostic Criteria*. Copenhagen: World Health Organization, 166-184.

Miller, L. (1985). Neuropsychological assessment of substance abusers: Review and recommendations. *Journal of Substance Abuse Treatment*, **2**, 5-17.

Miller, L. L., Cornett, T. L., Brightwell, D. R., McFarland, D. J., Drew, W. G., and Wikler, A. (1977). Marijuana: Effects on storage and retrieval of prose material. *Psychopharmacology*, **51**, 311-316.

Miller, L., Drew, W. G., and Kiplinger, G. C. (1976). Effects of marijuana on recall of narrative material and Stroop color-word performance. In E. L. Abel (Ed.), *The Scientific Study of Marijuana*. Chicago: Nelson-Hall, 117-120.

Min, S. K. (1986). A brain syndrome associated with delayed neuropsychiatric sequelae following acute carbon monoxide intoxication. *Acta Psychiatrica Scandinavica*, **73**, 80-86.

Minocha, A., Barth, J. T., Roberson, D. G., Herold, D. A., and Spyker, D. A. (1985). Impairment of cognitive and psychomotor function by enthanol in social drinkers. *Veterinary and Human Toxicology*, **27**, 533-536.

Mitchell, M. C. (1985). Alcohol-induced impairment of central nervous system function: Behavioral skills involved in driving. *Journal of Studies on Alcohol*, **10**, 109-116.

Money, J., Alexander, D., and Walker, H. T. (1965). *Manual for a Standardized Road-map Test of Direction Sense*. Baltimore: Johns Hopkins University Press.

Moreau, A., Jones, B. D., and Bano, V. (1986). Chronic central anticholinergic toxicity in manic depressive illness mimicking dementia. *NeuroToxicology*, **31**, 339-341.

Morgan, B. B. Jr, and Repko, J. D. (1974). Evaluation of behavioral functions in workers exposed to lead. In C. Xintaras, B. L. Johnson, and I. deGroot (Eds), *Behavioral Toxicology: Early detection of occupational hazards*. Washington, DC: Department of Health, Education, and Welfare Publication No. (NIOSH) 74-126, 248-265.

Morgan, D. P. (1982). Pesticide toxicology. In A. T. Yu (Ed.), *Survey of Contemporary Toxicology*. New York: John Wiley and Sons, 1-36.

Morley, R., Eccleston, D. W., Douglas, C. P., Greville, W. E. J., Scott, D. J., and Anderson, J. (1970). Xylene poisoning — A report on one fatal case and two cases of recovery after prolonged unconsciousness. *British Medical Journal* **3**, 442-443.

Morris, R. A., and Sonderegger, T. B. (1984). Legal applications and implications for neurotoxin research of the developing organism. *Neurobehavioral Toxicology and Teratology*, **6**, 303-306.

Moses, M. (1983). Pesticides. In W. Rom (Ed.), *Environmental and Occupational Medicine*. Boston: Little, Brown and Co., 547-571.

Muijser, H., Juntunen, J., Matikainen, E., and Seppäläinen, A. M. (1985).

Neurophysiological tests of the peripheral nervous system (PNS). In *Neurobehavioral Methods in Occupational and Environmental Health*, Document 6, Copenhagen: World Health Organization, 23–25.

Mulé, S. J. (1984). The pharmacodynamics of cocaine abuse. *Psychiatric Annals*, **14**, 724–727.

Muller, K. E., Barton, C. N., and Benignus, V. A. (1984). Recommendations for appropriate statistical practice in toxicologic experiments. *NeuroToxicology*, **5**, 113–126.

Murphy, L. R., and Colligan, M. J. (1979). Mass psychogenic illness in a shoe factory. A case report. *International Archives of Occupational and Environmental Health*, **44**, 133–138.

Murray, J. B. (1986). Marijuana's effects on human cognitive functions, psychomotor functions, and personality. *Journal of General Psychology*, **113**, 23–55.

Mutti, A., Mazzucchi, A., Frigeri, G., Falzoi, M., Arfini, G., and Franchini, I. (1983). In A. Gilioli, M. A. Cassitto, and V. Foa, (Eds), *Neurobehavioral Methods in Occupational Health*. New York: Pergamon Press, 271–281.

Mutti, A., Mazzucchi, A., Rustichelli, P., Frigeri, G., Arfini, G., and Franchini, I. (1984). Exposure-effect and exposure-response relationships between occupational exposure to styrene and neuropsychological functions. *American Journal of Industrial Medicine*, **5**, 275–286.

Namba, T. (1971). Cholinesterase inhibition by organophosphorus compounds and its clinical effects. *Bulletin of the World Health Organization*, **44**, 289–307.

National Academy of Science (1973). *Medical and Biological Effects of Environmental Pollutants: Manganese*. Washington, D.C.

National Institute for Occupational Safety and Health (1973). *Criteria for a Recommended Standard: Occupational exposure to toluene*. HEW Publication No. (NIOSH) 73–11023, Washington, DC: Department of Health, Education, and Welfare.

National Institute for Occupational Safety and Health (1975a). *Criteria for a Recommended Standard: Occupational exposure to arsenic, new criteria*. HEW Publication No. (NIOSH) 75–149. Washington, DC.

National Institute for Occupational Safety and Health (1975b). *Criteria for a Recommended Standard: Occupational exposure to xylene*. HEW Publication No. (NIOSH) 75–168. Washington, DC.

National Institute for Occupational Safety and Health (1977). *Behavioral and Neurological Effects of Methyl Chloride*. DHEW (NIOSH) Publication No. 77–125.

National Institute for Occupational Safety and Health (1978). *Special Occupational Hazard Review of Trichloroethylene*. DHEW (NIOSH) Publication No. 78–130.

Needleman, H. L. (1982). The neurobehavioral consequences of low lead exposure in childhood. *Neurobehavioral Toxicology and Teratology*, **4**, 729–732.

Needleman, H. L. (1983). Lead at low dose and the behavior of children. *Acta Psychiatrica Scandinavica*, Suppl. 303, **67**, 26–37.

Needleman, H. L., Gunnoe, C., Leviton, A., Reed, R., Peresie, H., Maher, C., and Barrett, P. (1979). Deficits in psychologic and classroom performance of children with elevated dentine lead levels. *New England Journal of Medicine*, **300**, 689–695.

Neurobehavioral Methods in Occupational and Environmental Health (1985). Document 3, Copenhagen: World Health Organization, Regional Office for Europe.

Neurobehavioral Methods in Occupational and Environmental Health (1985).

Document 6, Copenhagen: World Health Organization, Regional Office for Europe.

Newman, P. J., and Sweet, J. J. (1986). The effects of clinical depression on the Luria–Nebraska neuropsychological battery. *Clinical Neuropsychology*, **8**, 109–114.

Nicholi, A. M. (1984). Cocaine use among the college age group: Biological and psychological effects—clinical and laboratory research findings. *Journal of American College Health*, **32**, 258–261.

Niklowitz, W. J. (1979). Neurotoxicology of lead. In L. Manzo (ed.), *Advances in Neurotoxicology*. New York: Pergamon Press, 27–34.

Niklowitz, W. J., and Mandybur, T. I. (1975). Neurofibrillary changes following childhood lead encephalopathy. *Journal of Neuropathology and Experimental Neurology*, **34**, 445–455.

NIOSH (1987). Current Intelligence Bulletin 48, *Organic Solvent Neurotoxicity*. Department of Health and Human Services (NIOSH) Publication No. 87-104.

NIOSH Pocket Guide to Chemical Hazards (1985).Cincinnati: DHHS (NIOSH) Publication No. 85-114.

Noonberg, A., Goldstein, G., and Page. H. A. (1985). Premature aging in male alcoholics: "Accelerating aging" or "increased vulnerability"? *Alcoholism: Clinical and Experimental Research*, **9**, 334–338.

Nordberg, G. F. (1976). Effects and dose–response levels of toxic metals. *Scandinavian Journal of Work Environment and Health*, **2**, 37–43.

Nordberg, G. F. (1979). Neurotoxic effect of metals and their compounds. In L. Manzo (ed.), *Advances in Neurotoxicology*. New York: Pergamon Press, 3–15.

Oberg, R. C. E., Udeson, H., Thomsen, A. M., Gade, A., and Mortensen, E. L. (1985). Psychogenic behavioral impairments in patients exposed to neurotoxins. Neuropsychological assessments in differential diagnosis. In *Neurobehavioral Methods in Occupational and Environmental Health,* Document 3, World Health Organization, 130–135.

Occupational Exposure to Styrene (1983). U.S. Department of Health and Human Services. DHHS (NIOSH) Publication No. 83-119.

O'Donoghue, J. L. (1985). Carbon monoxide, inorganic nitrogenous compounds and phosphorus. In J. L. O'Donoghue (Ed.), *Neurotoxicity of Industrial and Commercial Chemicals*, Volume I. Boca Raton: CRC Press, 193–203.

O'Donoghue, J. L. (1985). Aromatic hydrocarbons. In J. L. O'Donoghue (Ed.), *Neurotoxicity of Industrial and Commercial Chemicals*, Volume II. Boca Raton, CRC Press, 127–136.

Oliver, T. (1901). *Dangerous Trades*. London: Murray.

Olsen, J., and Sabroe, S. (1980). A case-referent study of neuropsychiatric disorders among workers exposed to solvents in the Danish wood and furniture industry. *Scandinavian Journal of Social Medicine*, Suppl. 16, 44–49.

Olson, B. A., Gamberale, F., and Iregren, A. (1985). Co-exposure to toluene and *p*-xylene in man: Central nervous functions. *British Journal of Industrial Medicine*, **42**, 117–122.

Olson, B. B. (1982). Effects of organic solvents on behavioral performance of workers in the paint industry. *Neurobehavioral Toxicology and Teratology*, **4**, 703–708.

O'Malley, P. M., Johnston, L. D., and Bachman, J. G. (1985). Cocaine use among American adolescents and young adults. *Cocaine Use in America: Epidemiologic and clinical perspectives*. National Institute on Drug Abuse Research Monograph **61**, Washington, DC: Superintendent of Documents, U.S. Government Printing

Office, 50–273.

Orbaek, P., Risberg, J., Rosen, I., Haeger-Aronson, B., Hagstadius, S., Hjortsberg, U., Regnell, G., Rehnstrom, S., Svensson, K., and Welinder, H. (1985). Effects of long-term exposure to solvents in the paint industry. *Scandinavian Journal of Work Environment and Health*, Suppl. 2, **11**, 1–28.

Organic Solvents and the Central Nervous System (1985). Copenhagen: World Health Organization.

Osterrieth, P. A. (1944). Le test de copie d'une figure complexe. *Archives de Psychologie*, **30**, 206–356.

Otto, D. (1983a). Computer based behavioural test batteries. In N. Cherry and H. A. Waldron (Eds), *The Neuropsychological Effects of Solvent Exposure*. Havant, Hampshire: Colt Foundation, 130–135.

Otto, D. (1983b). Event-related brain potentials: An alternative methodology for neurotoxicological research. In N. Cherry, and H. A. Waldron (Eds), *The Neuropsychological Effects of Solvent Exposure*. Havant, Hampshire: Colt Foundation, 33–40.

Otto, D., Benignus, V., Muller, K., Barton, C., and Mushak, P. (1982). Event-related slow brain potential changes in asymptomatic children with secondary exposure to lead. In. R. Gilioli, M. G. Cassitto, and V. Foa (Eds), *Neurobehavioral Methods in Occupational Health*, 295–300.

Otto, D., Benignus, V., Muller, K., Barton, C., Seiple, K., Prah, J., and Schroeder, S. (1982). Effects of low to moderate lead exposure on slow cortical potentials in young children: Two year follow-up study. *Neurobehavioral Toxicology and Teratology*, **4**, 733–737.

Oxford English Dictionary — Compact Edition (1971). New York: Oxford University Press.

Parker, E. S., and Noble, E. P. (1977). Alcohol consumption and cognitive function in social drinkers. *Journal of Studies on Alcohol*, **38**, 1224–1232.

Parsons, O. A. (1986). Cognitive functioning in sober social drinkers: A review and critique. *Journal of Studies on Alcohol*, **47**, 101–114.

Parsons, O. A., and Farr, S. P. (1981). The neuropsychology of drug and alcohol abuse. In S. B. Filskov and T. J. Boll (Eds), *Handbook of Clinical Neuropsychology*. New York: John Wiley & Sons, 320–365.

Parsons, O. A., Tarter, R. E., and Edelberg, R. (1972). Altered motor control in chronic alcoholics. *Journal of Abnormal Psychology*, **72**, 308–314.

Patterson, W. B., Craven, D. E., Schwartz, D. A., Nardell, E. A., Kasmer, J., and Noble, J. (1985). Occupational hazards to hospital personnel. *Annals of Internal Medicine*, **102**, 658–680.

Paulson, G. W. (1983). Steroid-sensitive dementia. *American Journal of Psychiatry*, **140**, 1031–1033.

Pelham, R. W., Marquis, J. K., Kugelmann, K., and Munsat, T. L. (1980). Prolonged ethanol consumption produces persistent alterations of cholinergic function in rat brain. *Alcoholism: Clinical and Experimental Research*, **4**, 282–287.

Pennsylvania Department of Labor and Industry (1938). Survey of carbon disulphide and hydrogen sulphide hazards in the viscose rayon industry, Bulletin No. 46.

Pearlson, G. D., Garbacz, D. J., Tomkins, R. H., Ahn, H. S., Gutterman, D. F. Veroff, A. E., and De Paulo J. R. (1984). Clinical correlates of lateral ventricular enlargement in bipolar affective disorder. *American Journal of Psychiatry*, **141**, 253–256.

Peoples, S. A., Maddy, K. T., and Thomas, W. (1976). *Occupational Health Hazards of Exposure to 1,3-Dichloropropene*. California Department of Agriculture,

Publication No. ACF 59-241.

Perbellini, L., Brugnone, F., and Gaffuri, E. (1981). Neurotoxic metabolites of "commercial hexane" in the urine of shoe factory workers. *Clinical Toxicology*, **18**, 1377-1385.

Perlick, D., Stastny, P., Katz, I., Mayer, M., and Mattis, S. (1986). Memory deficits and anticholinergic levels in chronic schizophrenia. *American Journal of Psychiatry*, **143**, 230-232.

Peterson, C. D. (1981). Seizures induced by acute loxapine overdose. *American Journal of Psychiatry*, **138**, 1089-1091.

Piikivi, L., Hänninen, H., Martelin, T., and Mantere, P. (1984). Psychological performance and long-term exposure to mercury vapors. *Scandinavian Journal of Work Environment and Health*, **10**, 35-41.

Pishkin, V., Lovallo, W. R., and Bourne, L. E. (1985). Chronic alcoholism in males: Cognitive deficit as a function of age of onset, age, and duration. *Alcoholism: Clinical and Experimental Research*, **9**, 400-406.

Platt, J. E., Campbell, M., Green, W. H., and Grega, D. M. (1984). Cognitive effects of lithium carbonate and haloperidol in treatment-resistant aggressive children. *Archives of General Psychiatry*, **41**, 657-662.

Poklis, A., and Burkett, C. D. (1977). Gasoline sniffing: A review. *Clinical Toxicology*, **11**, 35-41.

Politis, M. J., Schaumberg, H. H., and Spencer, P. S. (1980). Neurotoxicity of selected chemicals. In P. S. Spencer and H. H. Schaumberg (Eds), *Experimental and Clinical Neurotoxicology*. Baltimore: Williams & Wilkins, 613-630.

Pomes, A., Frustace, S., Cattaino, G., De Grandis, D., Bongiovanni, L. G., Tumolo, S., and Quadu, G. (1986). Local neurotoxicity of Cisplatin after intra-arterial chemotherapy. *Acta Neurologica Scandinavica*, **73**, 302-303.

Pope, H. G., Jonas, J. M., Hudson, J. I., and Kafka, M. P. (1985). Toxic reactions to the combination of monoamine oxidase inhibitors and tryptophan. *American Journal of Psychiatry*, **142**, 491-492.

Prakash, R., Kelwala, S., and Ban, T. A., (1982). Neurotoxicity with combined administration of lithium and a neuroleptic. *Comprehensive Psychiatry*, **23**, 567-571.

Press, R. J. (1983). *The Neuropsychological Effects of Chronic Cocaine and Opiate Use*. Ann Arbor: University Microfilms International.

Prigatano, G. P. (1977). Neuropsychological functioning in recidivist alcoholics treated with disulfiram. *Alcoholism: Clinical and Experimental Research*, **1**, 81-86.

Purisch, A. D., and Sbordone, R. J. (1986). The Luria–Nebraska neuropsychological battery. In G. Goldstein and R. E. Tarter (Eds), *Advances in Clinical Neuropsychology*, Volume 3. New York: Plenum Press, 291-316.

Putz-Anderson, V., Albright, B. E., Lee, S. T., Johnson, B. L., Chrislip, D. W., Taylor, B. J., Brightwell, W. S., Dickerson, N., Culver, M., Zentmeyer, D., and Smith, P. (1983). A behavioral examination of workers exposed to carbon disulfide. *NeuroToxicology*, **4**, 67-78.

Ramsey, J. M., (1972). Carbon monoxide, tissue hypoxia and sensory psychomotor response in hypoxemia. *Clinical Science*, **42**, 619-625.

Raneletti, A. (1931). Die beruflichen Schwefelkohlenstoffvergiftungen (in Italian). *Arch. Gewerbepathol. Gewebehyg*, **2**, 664-676.

Rasmussen, H., Olsen, J., and Lauritsen, J. Risk of encephalopathia among retired solvent-exposed workers. (1985). *Journal of Occupational Medicine*, **27**, 561-566.

Ratner, D., Oren, B., and Vigder, K. (1983). Chronic dietary anticholinesterase poisoning. *Israeli Journal of Medical Science*, **19**, 810–814.

Rawat, A. K. (1979). Neurotoxic effects of maternal alcoholism on the developing fetus and newborn. In L. Manzo (Ed.), *Advances in Neurotoxicology*. New York: Pergamon Press, 155–164.

Rebeta, J. L., McAllister, D. A., Gange, J. J., Jordan, R. C., and Riley, A. L. (1986). The relationship between alcohol-related variables and Luria-Nebraska Neuropsychological Battery performance in a cross-sectional V.A. population. Paper presented at the sixth annual meeting of the National Academy of Neuropsychologists, 27–29 October, Las Vegas, Nevada.

Reggiani, G., and Bruppacher, R., (1985). Symptoms, signs and findings in humans exposed to PCBs and their derivatives. *Environmental Health Perspectives*, **60**, 225–232.

Reichert, E. R., Yauger, W. L., Rashad, M. N., and Klemmer, H. W. (1977). Diazinon poisoning in eight members of related households. *Clinical Toxicology*, **11**, 5–11.

Reitan, R. M. (1966). Problems and prospects in studying the psychological correlates of brain lesions. *Cortex*, **2**, 127–154.

Reitan, R. M., and Wolfson, D. (1985). *The Halstead-Reitan Neuropsychological Battery. Theory and clinical interpretation*. Tucson, Arizona: Neuropsychology Press.

Reiter, L. W. (1985). Introductory remarks to workshop on neurotoxicity testing in human populations. *Neurobehavioral Toxicology and Teratology*, **7**, 287–288.

Reiter, L. W., and Ruppert, P. H. (1984). Behavioral toxicity of trialkyltin compounds: A review. *NeuroToxicology*, **5**, 177–186.

Repko, J. D. (1981). Neurotoxicity of methyl chloride. *Neurobehavioral Toxicology and Teratology*, **3**, 425–429.

Repko, J. D., Corum, C. R., Jones, P. D., and Garcia, L. S. (1978). The effects of inorganic lead on behavioral and neurologic function. Final report USDHEW (NIOSH). Publication No. 78-128, Washington, DC.

Repko, J. D., Jones, P. D., Garcia, L. S., Scheider, E. J., Roseman, E., and Corum, C. R. (1976). *Final Report of the Behavioral and Neurological Evaluation of Workers Exposed to Solvents: methyl chloride*. DHEW Publications N. (NIOSH) 77-125, Washington DC: U.S. Government Printing Office.

Reuhl, K. R., and Cranmer, J. M. (1984). Developmental neuropathology of organotin compounds. *NeuroToxicology*, **5**, 187–204.

Rey, A. (1959). Sollicitation del la memoire de fixation par des mots et des objets presentes simultanement. *Archives de Psychologie*, **37**, 126–139.

Reynolds, E. H., and Trimble, M. R. (1985). Adverse neuropsychiatric effects of anticonvulsant drugs. *Drugs*, **29**, 570–581.

Richardson, E. P., and Adams, R. D. (1977). Degenerative diseases of the nervous system. In G. W. Thorn, R. D. Adams, E. Braunwald, K. J. Isselbacher, and R. G. Petersdorf (Eds), *Harrison's Principles of Internal Medicine*, eighth edition. New York: McGraw-Hill, 1919–1934.

Richelle, M. (1983). New approaches and neglected areas. In G. Zbinden, V. Cuomo, G. Racagni and B. Weiss (Eds), *Applications of Behavioral Pharmacology in Toxicology*. New York: Raven Press, 127–140.

Rickles, W. H., Jr, Cohen, M. J., Whitaker, C. A., and McIntyre, K. E., (1973). Marijuana induced state-dependent verbal learning. *Psychopharmacologia*, **30**, 349–354.

Riege, W. H., Tomaszewski, R., Lanto, A., and Metter, E. J. (1984). Age and alcoholism: Independent memory decrements. *Alcoholism: Clinical and*

Experimental Research, **8**, 42–47.

Riley, J. N., and Walker, D. W. (1978). Morphological alterations in hippocampus after long-term alcohol consumption in mice. *Science*, **201**, 646–648.

Risberg, J., and Hagstadius, S. (1983). Effects on the regional cerebral blood flow of long-term exposure to organic solvents. *Acta Psychiatrica Scandinavica*, Suppl. 303, **67**, 92–99.

Rochford, J., Grant, I., and LaVigne, G. (1977). Medical students and drugs. Neuropsychological and use pattern considerations. *International Journal of the Addictions*, **12**, 1057–1065.

Rodepierre, J. J., Truhaut, J., Alizon, J., and Champion, Y. (1955). The possible etiological role of methyl chloride in an obscure syndrome. *Society of Medical, Legal and Criminal Police Science Toxicology*, **35**, 80.

Rodier, J. (1955). Manganese poisoning in Moroccan miners. *British Journal of Industrial Medicine*, **12**, 21–35.

Rodnitzky, R. L. (1973). Neurological and behavioral aspects of occupational exposure to organophosphate pesticides. In C. Xintaras, B. L. Johnson, and I. deGroot (Eds), *Behavioral Toxicology: Early detection of occupational hazards*. Washington, DC: HEW Publication No. (NIOSH) 74–126, 165–173.

Ron, M. A. (1983). The alcoholic brain: CT scan and psychological findings. *Psychological Medicine*, Monograph Supplement 3. New York: Cambridge University Press, 1–33.

Rosati, G., De Bastiani, P., Gilli, P., and Paolino, E. (1980). Oral aluminum and neuropsychological functioning. *Journal of Neurology*, **223**, 251–257.

Rosen, I., Haeger-Aronsen, B., Rehnstrom, S., and Welinder, H. (1978). Neurophysiological observations after chronic styrene exposure. *Scandinavian Journal of Work Environment and Health*, Suppl. 2, **4**, 184–194.

Rosengren, L. E., Wronski.A., Briving, C., and Haglid, K. G. (1985). Long lasting changes in gerbil brain after chronic ethanol exposure: A quantitative study of the glial cell marker S-100 and DNA. *Alcoholism*, **9**, 109–113.

Rosenstock, H. A., Simons, D. G., and Meyer, J. S. (1971). Chronic manganism. Neurologic and laboratory studies during treatment with levodopa. *Journal of the American Medical Association*, **217**, 1354–1358.

Ross, W. D., Emmett, E. A., Steiner, J., and Tureen, R. (1981). Neurotoxic effects of occupational exposure to organotins. *American Journal of Psychiatry*, **138**, 1092–1095.

Ross, W. D., and Sholiton, M. C. (1983). Specificity of psychiatric manifestations in relation to neurotoxic chemicals. *Acta Psychiatrica Scandinavica*, Suppl. 303, **67**, 100–104.

Rosselli, M., Lorenzana, R., Rosselli, A., and Vergara, I. (1987). Wilson's Disease, a reversible dementia: Case report. *Journal of Clinical and Experimental Neuropsychology*, **9**, 399–406.

Rothke, S., and Bush, D. (1986). Neuropsychological sequelae of neuroleptic malignant syndrome. *Biological Psychiatry*, 838–841.

Rounsaville, B. J., Jones, C., Novelly, R. A., and Kleber, H. (1982). Neuropsychological functioning in opiate addicts. *Journal of Nervous and Mental Disease*, **170**, 209–216.

Ryan, C., and Butters, N. (1980). Learning and memory impairments in young and old alcoholics: Evidence for the premature-aging hypothesis. *Alcoholism: Clinical and Experimental Research*, 288–293.

Ryan, C., Butters, N., and Montgomery, K. (1980). Memory deficits in chronic alcoholics: Continuities between the "intact" alcoholic and the alcoholic

Korsakoff patient. In H. Begleiter (Ed.), *Biological Effects of Alcoholism.* New York: Plenum Press, 683–699.

Ryan, C. M., Morrow, L. A., Bromet, E. J., and Parkinson, D. K. (1986). The assessment of neuropsychological dysfunction in the workplace: Normative data from the Pittsburgh Occupational Exposures Test Battery. Unpublished manuscript. Available from the first author, Western Psychiatric Institute and Clinic, University of Pittsburgh School of Medicine, 3811 O'Hara Street, Pittsburgh, PA 15213.

Ryback, R. S. (1971). The continuum and specificity of the effects of alcohol on memory: A review. *Quarterly Journal of Studies on Alcohol*, **32**, 995–1016.

Rylander, R., and Vesterlund, J. (1981). Carbon monoxide criteria. *Scandinavian Journal of Work Environment and Health.* Suppl. 1, **1**, 20–39.

Russell, E. W. (1975). A multiple scoring method for assessment of complex memory functions. *Journal of Consulting and Clinical Psychology*, **43**, 800–809.

Russell, E. W., Neuringer, P., and Goldstein, G. (1970). *Assessment of brain damage: A neuropsychological key approach.* New York: Wiley and Sons.

Russell, P. R. (1983). Neuropsychological effects of individuals exposed to Telone (1,3-dichloropropene). Presented at the American Psychological Association Convention, Anaheim, Ca.

Rutter, M. (1980). Raised lead levels and impaired cognitive/behavioral functioning: A review of the evidence. *Developmental Medicine and Child Neurology*, Suppl. 1, **22**, 1–26.

Salvini, M., Binaschi, S., and Riva, M. (1971a). Evaluation of the psychophysiological functions in humans exposed to the threshold limit value of 1,1,1-trichloroethane. *British Journal of Industrial Medicine*, **28**, 256–292.

Salvini, M., Binaschi, S., and Riva, M. (1971b). Evaluation of the psychophysiological functions of humans exposed to trichloroethylene. *British Journal of Industrial Medicine*, **28**, 293–295.

Sansone, M. E., and Ziegler, D. K. (1985). Lithium, toxicity: A review of neurologic complications. *Clinical Neuropharmacology*, **8**, 242–248.

Savage, E. P., Keefe, T. J., Mounce, L. M., Lewis, J. A., Heaton, R. K., and Parks, L. H. (1980). *Chronic neurological sequelae of acute organophosphate pesticide poisoning: A case-control study.* (Available from the Epidemiologic Studies Program, Health Effects Branch, Hazard Evaluation Division of the U.S. Environmental Protection Agency, Washington, DC.

Savard, R. J., Rey, A. C., and Post, R. M. (1980). Halstead–Reitan Category Test in bipolar and unipolar affective disorders. Relationship to age and phase of illness. *Journal of Nervous and Mental Disease*, **118**, 297–304.

Savolainen, H. (1982). Toxicological mechanisms in acute and chronic nervous system degeneration. *Acta Neurologica Scandinavica*, Suppl. 92, **66**, 23–35.

Savolainen, H., and Pfaffli, P. (1977). Effects of chronic styrene inhalation on rat brain protein metabolism. *Acta Neuropathologica* (Berlin), **40**, 237–241.

Savolainen, K., Riihimaki, V., Laine, A., and Kekoni, J. (1981). Short term exposure of human subjects to m-xylene and 1,1,1-trichloroethane. *International Archives of Occupational and Environmental Health*, **49**, 89–98.

Savolainen, K., Riihimaki, V., and Linnoila, M. (1979). Effects of short-term xylene exposure on psychophysiological functions in man. *International Archives of Occupational and Environmental Health*, **44**, 201–211.

Scelsi, R., Poggi, P., Fera, L., and Gonella, G. (1981). Industrial neuropathy due to *n*-hexane. Clinical and morphological findings in three cases. *Clinical Toxicology*, **18**, 1387–1393.

Schaeffer, J., Andrysiak, T., and Ungerleider, J. T. (1981). Cognition and long-term use of ganja (cannabis). *Science*, **213**, 465–466.

Schaeffer, K. W., Parsons, O. A., and Yohman, J. R. (1984). Neuropsychological differences between male familial and nonfamilial alcoholics and nonalcoholics. *Alcoholism: Clinical and Experimental Research*, **8**, 347–351.

Schaumburg, H. H., and Spencer, P. S. (1984). Human toxic neuropathy due to industrial agents. In P. J. Dyck, P. K. Thomas, E. H. Lambert, and R. Bunge (Eds), *Peripheral Neuropathy*, Volume II. Philadelphia: W. B. Saunders, 2115–2132.

Schaumberg, H. H., Spencer, P. S., and Thomas. P. (1983). *Disorders of Peripheral Nerves*. Philadelphia: F. A. Davis.

Schinka, J. A. (1984). *Personal Problems Checklist for Adults*. Odessa, Florida: Psychological Assessment Resources, Inc.

Schoenberg, B. S. (1982). Analytic, experimental, and theoretical neuroepidemiology: Applications to occupational neurology. *Acta Neurologica Scandinavica*, Suppl. 92, **66**, 11–22.

Schottenfeld, R. S., and Cullen, M. R. (1984). Organic affective illness associated with lead intoxication. *American Journal of Psychiatry*, **41**, 1423–1426.

Sedman, A. B., Wilkening, G. N., Warady, B. A., Lum. G. M., and Alfrey, A. C. (1984). Clinical and laboratory observations: Encephalopathy in childhood secondary to aluminum toxicity. *Journal of Pediatrics*, **105**, 836–838.

Selected Petroleum Products (1982). Geneva: World Health Organization.

Seppäläinen, A. M. (1973). Neurotoxic effects of industrial solvents. *Electroencephalography and Clinical Neurophysiology*, **34**, 702–703.

Seppäläinen, A. M. (1978). Neurotoxicity of styrene in occupational and experimental exposure. *Scandinavian Journal of Work, Environment and Health*, Suppl. 2, **4**, 181–183.

Seppäläinen, A. M. (1985). Neurophysiological aspects of the toxicity of organic solvents. *Scandinavian Journal of Work, Environment and Health*, Suppl. 1, **11**, 61–64.

Seppäläinen, A. M. (1982a). The use of EMG techniques in solvent exposure. In R. Gilioli, M. G. Cassitto, and V. Foa (Eds), *Neurobehavioral Methods in Occupational Health*, New York: Pergamon Press, 177–182.

Seppäläinen, A. M. (1982b). Neurophysiological findings among workers exposed to organic solvents. *Acta Neurologica Scandinavica*, Suppl. 92, **66**, 106–116.

Seppäläinen, A. M., and Antti-Poika, M. (1983). Time course of electrophysiological findings for patients with solvent poisoning: A descriptive study. *Scandinavian Journal of Work Environment and Health*, **9**, 15–24.

Seppäläinen, A. M., and Lindström, K. (1982). Neurophysiological findings among house painters exposed to solvents. *Scandinavian Journal of Work, Environment and Health*, Suppl. 1, **8**, 131–135.

Seppäläinen, A. M., Hernberg, S., Vesanto, R., and Kock, B. (1983). Early neurotoxic effects of occupational lead exposure: A prospective study. *NeuroToxicology*, **4**, 181–192.

Seppäläinen, A. M., Husman, K., and Mattenson, G. (1978). Neurophysiological effects of long-term exposure to a mixture of organic solvents. *Scandinavian Journal of Work, Environment and Health*, **4**, 304–314.

Seppäläinen, A. M., Lindström, K., and Martelin, T. (1980). Neurophysiological and psychological picture of solvent poisoning. *American Journal of Industrial Medicine*, **1**, 31–42.

Seppäläinen, A. M., Tolonen, M., Karli, P., Hänninen, H., and Hernberg, S. (1972).

Neurophysiological findings in chronic carbon disulfide poisoning: A descriptive study. *Scandinavian Journal of Work, Environment and Health*, **9**, 71-75.

Seshia, S. S., Rajani, K. R., Boeckx, R. L., and Chow, P. N. (1978). The neurological manifestations of chronic inhalation of leaded gasoline. *Developmental Medicine and Child Neurology*, **20**, 323-334.

Shalev, A., and Munitz, H. (1986). The neuroleptic malignant syndrome: Agent and host interaction. *Acta Psychiatrica Scandinavica*, **73**, 337-347.

Shephard, R. J. (1983). *Carbon Monoxide*. Springfield: Charles C. Thomas.

Shindell, S., and Stack. U. (1985). A cohort study of employees of a manufacturing plant using trichlorolethylene. *Journal of Occupational Medicine*, **27**, 577-579.

Shoemaker, W. J. (1981). The neurotoxicity of alcohols. *Neurobehavioral Toxicology and Teratology*, **3**, 431-436.

Shore, D., and Wyatt, R. J. (1983). Aluminum and Alzheimer's disease. *Journal of Nervous and Mental Disease*, **171**, 553-558.

Siegel, R. K. (1982). Cocaine smoking. *Journal of Psychoactive Drugs*, **14**, 321-337.

Silbergeld, E. K. (1983). Indirectly acting neurotoxins. *Acta Psychiatrica Scandinavica*, Suppl. 303, **67**, 16-25.

Silbergeld, E. K. (1982). Neurochemical and ionic mechanisms of lead neurotoxicity. In K. N. Prasad and A. Vernadakis (Eds), *Mechanisms of Actions of Neurotoxic Substances*. New York: Raven Press.

Silberstein, J. A., and Parsons, O. A. (1979). Neuropsychological impairment in female alcoholics. *Currents in Alcoholism*, **7**, 481-495.

Small, I. F., Small, J. G., Milstein, V., and Moore, J. E. (1972). Neuropsychological observations with psychosis and somatic treatment. *Journal of Nervous and Mental Disease*, **155**, 6-13.

Smigan, L., and Perris, C. (1983). Memory functions and prophylactic treatment with lithium. *Psychological Medicine*, **13**, 529-536.

Smith, G., and Shirley, W. A. (1977). Failure to demonstrate effect of trace concentrations of nitrous oxide and halothane on psychomotor performance. *British Journal of Anaesthiology*, **48**, 65-70.

Smith, J. W., Burt, D. W., and Chapman, R. F. (1973). Intelligence and brain damage in alcoholics: A study in patients of middle and upper social class. *Quarterly Journal of Studies on Alcoholism*, **34**, 414-422.

Smith, M. J., Colligan, M. J., and Hurrell, J. J. (1978). Three incidents of mass psychogenic illness: A preliminary report. *Journal of Occupational Medicine*, **20**, 399-400.

Smith, P. J., and Langolf, G. D. (1981). The use of Sternberg's memory scanning paradigm in assessing effects of chemical exposure. *Human Factors*, **23**, 701-708.

Solomon, S., Hotchkiss, E., Saraway, S. M., Bayer, C., Ramsey, P., and Blum, R. S. (1983). Impairment of memory function by antihypertensive medication. *Archives of General Psychiatry*, **40**, 1109-1112.

Solvent neurotoxicity (1985). *British Journal of Industrial Medicine*, **42**, 433-434.

Spake, A. (1985 March). A new American nightmare? *Ms.* 35-42, 93-95.

Spencer, P. S., and Schaumburg, H. H. (1985). Organic solvent neurotoxicity. Facts and research needs. *Scandinavian Journal of Work Environment and Health*, Suppl. 1, 53-60.

Spencer, P. S., Arezzo, J., and Schaumburg, H. (1985). Chemicals causing disease of neurons and their processes. In J. L. O'Donoghue (Ed.), *Neurotoxicity of Industrial and Commercial Chemicals*, Volume I. Boca Raton: CRC Press, 1-14.

Spencer, P. S., Couri, D., and Schaumburg, H. H. (1980). *N*-hexane and methyl *n*-butyl ketone. In P. S. Spencer and H. H. Schaumberg (Eds), *Experimental and*

Clinical Neurotoxicology. Baltimore: Williams & Wilkins, 456–475.

Spyker, D. A. Gallanose, A. G., and Suratt, P. M. (1982). Health effects of acute carbon disulfide exposure. *Journal of Toxicology—Clinical Toxicology,* **19,** 87–93.

Squire, L. R., Lewis, L. L., Janowsky, D. S., and Huey, L. Y. (1980). Effects of lithium carbonate on memory and other cognitive functions. *American Journal of Psychiatry,* **137,** 1042–1046.

Stahl, S. M., and Lebedun, M. (1974). Mystery gas: An analysis of epidemic hysteria and social sanction. *Journal of Health and Social Behavior,* **15,** 44–50.

Stalberg, E., Hilton-Brown, P., Kolmodin-Hedman, B., Holmstedt, B., and Augustinsson, K.-B. (1978). Effect of occupational exposure to organophosphorus insecticides on neuromuscular function. *Scandinavian Journal of Work Environment and Health,* **4,** 255–261.

Steinberg, W. (1981). Residual neuropsychological effects following exposure to trichloroethylene (TCE): A case study. *Clinical Neuropsychology,* **2(3),** 1–4.

Sterman, A. B., and Schaumberg, H. H., (1980). Neurotoxicity of selected drugs. In P. S. Spencer and H. H. Schaumburg (Eds), *Experimental and Clinical Neurotoxicology.* Baltimore: Williams & Wilkins, 593–613.

Sternberg, D. E. (1986). The neuroleptic malignant syndrome: The pendulum swings. *American Journal of Psychiatry,* **143,** 1273–1275.

Sternberg, D. E., and Jarvik, M. E. (1976). Memory functions in depression: Improvement with antidepressant medications. *Archives of General Psychiatry,* **33,** 219–224.

Steru, L., and Simon, P. (1983). Behavioral toxicology of psychotropic drugs from animal to man. In G. Zbinden, V. Cuomo, G. Racagni, and B. Weiss (Eds), *Application of Behavioral Pharmacology in Toxicology.* New York: Raven Press, 353–366.

Stewart, R. D., Gay, H. H., Schaffer, A. W., Erley, D. S., and Rowe, V. K. (1969). Experimental human exposure to methyl chloroform vapor. *Archives of Environmental Health,* **19,** 467–472.

Stewart, R. D., Peterson, J. E., Bachand, R. T. *et al.* (1970). Experimental human exposure to carbon monoxide. *Archives of Environmental Health,* **21,** 154–164.

Stillman, R. C., Weingartner, H., Wyatt, R. J., Gillin, J. C., and Eich, J. (1974). State-dependent (dissociative) effects of marihuana on human memory. *Archives of General Psychiatry,* **31,** 81–85.

Stoller, A., Krupinski, J., Christophers, A. J., and Blansk, G. K. (1965). Organophosphorus insecticides and major mental illness. *Lancet,* Volume I, 1387–1388.

Stopford, W. (1985). The toxic effects of pesticides. In P. L. Williams and J. L. Burson (Eds), *Industrial Toxicology: Safety and health applications in the workplace.* New York: Van Nostrand Reinhold, 211–229.

Strassman, R. J. (1984). Adverse reactions to psychedelic drugs: A review of the literature. *Journal of Nervous and Mental Disease,* **172,** 577–595.

Strauss, M. E., Lew, M. F., Coyle, J. T., and Tune, L. E. (1985). Psychopharmacologic and clinical correlates of attention in chronic schizophrenia. *American Journal of Psychiatry,* **142,** 497–499.

Streicher, H. Z., Gabow, P. A., Moss, A. H., Kono, D., and Kaehny, W. D. (1981). Syndromes of toluene sniffing in adults. *Annals of Internal Medicine,* **94,** 758–762.

Strub, R. L., and Black, W. F. (1981). *Organic Brain Syndromes.* Philadelphia: Davis and Company.

Struve, F.A., and Willner, A. E. (1983). Cognitive dysfunction and tardive dyskinesia. *British Journal of Psychiatry,* **143,** 597–600.

Struwe, G., and Wennberg, A. (1983). Psychiatric and neurological symptoms in workers occupationally exposed to organic solvents—results of a differential epidemiological study. *Acta Psychiatrica Scandinavica*, Suppl. 303, **67**, 68–80.

Struwe, G., Knave, B., and Mindus, P. (1983). Neuropsychiatric symptoms in workers occupationally exposed to jet fuel—a combined epidemiological and casuistic study. *Acta Psychiatrica Scandinavica*, Suppl. 303, **67**, 55–67.

Struwe, G., Mindus, P., and Jonsson, B. (1980). Psychiatric ratings in occupational health research: A study of mental symptoms in lacquerers. *American Journal of Industrial Medicine*, **1**, 23–30.

Styrene (1983). Geneva: World Health Organization.

Summerfield, A. (1978). Behavioral toxicology—the psychology of pollution. *Journal of Biosocial Science*, **10**, 335–345.

Summerfield, A. (1982). Psychological viewpoint. In N. Cherry and H. A. Waldron (Eds), *The Neuropsychological Effects of Solvent Exposure*. Havant, Hampshire: Colt Foundation, 168–173.

Svanum, S., and Schladenhauffen, J. (1986). Lifetime and recent alcohol consumption among male alcoholics. *Journal of Nervous and Mental Disease*, **174**, 214–220.

Taft, R. Jr. (1974). Federal commitment to occupational safety and health. In C. Xintarus, B. L. Johnson, and I. deGroot (Eds), *Behavioral Toxicology: Early detection of occupational hazards*. Washington, DC: U.S. Department of Health, Education and Welfare (NIOSH) Publication No. 74–126.

Takeuchi, T., Eto, N., and Eto, K. (1979). Neuropathology of childhood cases of methylmercury poisoning (Minamata disease) with prolonged symptoms, with particular reference to the decortication syndrome. *NeuroToxicology*, **1**, 1–20.

Tarbox, A. R., Connors, G. J., and McLaughlin, E. J. (1986). Effects of drinking pattern on neuropsychological performance among alcohol misusers. *Journal of Studies on Alcohol*, **47**, 176–179.

Tarter, R. E., and Edwards, K. L. (1986). Multifactorial etiology of neuropsychological impairment in alcoholics. *Alcohol: Clinical and Experimental Research*, **10**, 128–135.

Tarter, R. E., Hegedus, A. M., Gavaler, J. S. J., Schade, R. R., Van Thiel, D. H., and Starzl, T. E. (1983). Cognitive and psychiatric impairments associated with alcoholic and nonalcoholic cirrhosis: Compared and contrasted. (Abstract) *Hepatology*, **3**, 830.

Tarter, R. E., Hegedus, A. M., Goldstein, G., Shelly, C., and Alterman, A. (1984). Adolescent sons of alcoholics: Neuropsychological and personality characteristics. *Alcohol: Clinical and Experimental Research*, **8**, 216–222.

Tarter, R. E., Hegedus, A. M., Van Thiel, D. H., Gavaler, B. S., and Schade, R. R. (1986). Hepatic dysfunction and neuropsychological test performance in alcoholics with cirrhosis. *Journal of Studies on Alcohol*. **47**, 74–77.

Tarter, R. E., Jones, B. M., Simpson, C. D., and Vega, A. (1971). Effects of task complexity and practice on performance during acute alcohol intoxication. *Perceptual and Motor Skills*, **33**, 307–318.

Taylor, J. R. (1982). Neurological manifestations in humans exposed to chlordecone and follow-up results. *NeuroToxicology*, **3**, 9–16.

Taylor, J. R., Selhorst, J. B., and Calabrese, V. P. (1980). Chlordecone. In. P. S. Spencer and H. H. Schaumburg (Eds), *Experimental and Clinical Neurotoxicology*. Baltimore: Williams & Wilkins, 407–421.

Thompson, P. J., and Trimble, M.R. (1982). Anticonvulsant drugs and cognitive functions. *Epilepsia*, **23**, 531–544.

Thompson, P. J., and Trimble, M. R. (1983). Anticonvulsant serum levels: Relationship to impairments of cognitive function. *Journal of Neurology, Neurosurgery and Psychiatry*, **46**, 227–233.

Thompson, P. J., Huppert, F. A., and Trimble, M.R. (1981). Phenytoin and cognitive functions: Effects on normal volunteers and implications for epilepsy. *British Journal of Clinical Pharmacology*, **20**, 155–161.

Thorne, D. R., Genser, S.G., Sing. H. C., and Hegge, F. W. (1985). The Walter Reed performance assessment battery. *Neurobehavioral Toxicology and Teratology*, **7**, 415–418.

Tilson, H. A. (1981). The neurotoxicity of acrylamide: An overview. *Neurobehavioral Toxicology and Teratology*, **3**, 445–461.

Tolonen, M. (1975). Vascular effects of carbon disulfide. A review. *Scandinavian Journal of Work Environment and Health*, **1**, 63–77.

Tonge, J. I., Burry, A. F., and Saal, J. R. (1977). Cerebellar calcification: A possible marker of lead poisoning. *Pathology*, **9**, 289–300.

Triebig, G., and Schaller, K.-H. (1982). Neurotoxic effects in mercury exposed workers. *Neurobehavioral Toxicology and Teratology*, **4**, 717–720.

Triebig, G., Schaller, K. H., Erzigkeit, H., and Valentin, H. (1977). Biochemical investigations and psychological studies of persons chronically exposed to trichloroethylene with regard to non-exposure intervals (original in German). *International Archives of Environmental Health*, Volume 38, 149–162.

Tsushima, W. T., and Towne, W. S. (1977). Effects of paint sniffing on neuropsychological test performance. *Journal of Abnormal Psychology*, **86**, 402–407.

Tune, L. E., Strauss, M. E., Lew, M. F., Breitlinger, E., and Coyle, J. T. (1982). Serum levels of anticholinergic drugs and impaired recent memory in chronic schizophrenic patients. *American Journal of Psychiatry*, **139**, 1460–1461.

Tuttle, T. C., Wood, G. D., and Grether, C. B. (1977). *A behavioral and neurological evaluation of dry cleaners exposed to perchlorethylene*. Cinncinnati: NIOSH.

Tuttle, T. C., Wood, G. D., and Grether, C. B. (1976). *Behavioral and neurological evaluation of workers exposed to carbon disulfide (CS₂)*. Washington, DC: USDHEW (NIOSH) Publication, 77–128.

Uzzell, B., and Oler, J. (1986). Chronic low-level mercury exposure and neuropsychological functioning. *Journal of Clinical and Experimental Neuropsychology*, **8**, 581–593.

Vainio, H. (1982). Inhalation anesthetics, anticancer drugs and sterilants as chemical hazards in hospitals. *Scandinavian Journal of Work Environment and Health*, **8**, 94–107.

Valciukas, J. A. (1984). A decade of behavioral toxicology: Impressions of a NIOSH/ WHO workshop in Cincinnati, May 1983. *American Journal of Industrial Medicine*, **5**, 405–406.

Valciukas, J. A., and Lilis, R. (1980). Psychometric techniques in environmental research. *Environmental Research*, **21**, 275–297.

Valciukas, J. A., Lilis, R., Singer, R. M., Glickman, L. and Nicholson, W. J. (1985). Neurobehavioral changes among shipyard painters exposed to solvents. *Archives of Environmental Health*, **40**, 47–52.

Valciukas, J. A., Lilis, R., Singer, R., Fischbein, A., and Anderson, H. A. (1980). Lead exposure and behavioral changes: Comparisons of four occupational groups with different levels of lead absorption. *American Journal of Industrial Medicine*, **1**, 421–426.

Vandekar, M., Plestina, R., and Wilhelm, K. (1971). Toxicity of carbamates for mammals. *Bulletin of the World Health Organization*, **44**, 241–249.

Varney, N. R., Alexander, B., and MacIndoe, J. H. (1984). Reversible steroid dementia in patients without steroid psychosis. *American Journal of Psychiatry*, **141**, 369–372.

Vernon, R. J., and Ferguson, R. K. (1969). Effects of trichloroethylene on visual-motor performance. *Archives of Environment and Health*. **18**, 895–900.

Vicente, P. J. (1980). Neuropsychological assessment and management of a carbon monoxide intoxication patient with consequent sleep apnea: A longitudinal case report. *Clinical Neuropsychology*, **2**, 91–94.

Victor, M., Adams, R. D., and Collins, G. H. (1971). *The Wernicke-Korsakoff Syndrome*. Philadelphia: F. A. Davis.

Vining, E. P. G., Mellits, E. D., Cataldo, M. F., Dorsen, M. M., Spielberg, S. P., and Freeman, J. M. (1983). Effects of phenobarbital and sodium valproate on neuropsychological function and behavior. *Annals of Neurology*, **14**, 360.

Walker, D. W., Hunter, B. E., and Abraham, W. C. (1981). Neuroanatomical and functional deficits subsequent to chronic ethanol administration in animals. *Alcoholism: Clinical and Experimental Research*, **5**, 267–282.

Walsh, K.W. (1978). *Neuropsychology: A clinical approach*. New York: Churchill Livingstone.

Walsh, K. W. (1985). *Understanding Brain Damage: A primer of neuropsychological evaluation*. New York: Churchill Livingstone.

Walsh, T. J., Clark, A. W., Parhad, I. M., and Green, W. R. (1982). Neurotoxic effects of cisplatin therapy. *Archives of Neurology*, **39**, 719–720.

Ward, A. A. (1972). Topical convulsant metals. In D. Purpura, J. Penny, D. Tower, D. Woodbury, and R. Walter (Eds), *Experimental Models of Epilepsy — A manual for laboratory workers*. New York: Raven Press, 13.

Washton, A. M., and Gold, M. S. (1984). Chronic cocaine abuse: Evidence for adverse effects on health and functioning. *Psychiatric Annals*, 733–743.

Washton, A. M., and Tatarsky, A. (1984). Adverse effects of cocaine abuse. *National Institute on Drug Abuse: Research Monograph Series*, **49**, 247–254.

Watanabe, I. (1980). Organotins (triethyltin). In P. S. Spencer, and H. H. Schaumburg (Eds), *Experimental and Clinical Neurotoxicology*. Baltimore: Williams & Wilkins, 545–557.

Wedeen, R. P. (1984). *Poison in the Pot: The legacy of lead*. Carbondale: Southern Illinois University Press.

Weingartner, H., Rudorfer, M. V., and Linnoila, M. (1985). Cognitive effects of lithium treatment in normal volunteers. *Psychopharmacology*, **86**, 472–474.

Weiss, B. (1978). The behavioral toxicology of metals. *Federation Proceedings*, **37**, 22–27.

Weiss, B. (1983).Behavioral toxicology and environmental health science. *American Psychologist*, November, 1174–1187.

Weiss, B., and Laties, V. (Eds) (1975). *Behavioral Toxicology*. New York: Plenum Press.

Wennberg, A., and Otto, D. (1985). Neurophysiological tests of the central nervous system (CNS). In P. Grandjean (Ed.), *Neurobehavioral Methods in Occupational and Environmental Health*. Document 6, Copenhagen: World Health Organization, 19–22.

Wesson, D. R., Grant, I., Carlin, A. A., Adams, K., and Harris, C. (1978). Neuropsychological impairment and psychopathology. In D.R. Wesson, A. S. Carlin, K. M. Adams, and G. Beschner (Eds), *Polydrug Abuse: The results of a national collaborative study*. New York: Academic Press, 263–272.

Whorton, M. D., and Obrinsky, D. L. (1983). Persistence of symptoms after mild to moderate acute organophosphate poisoning among 19 farm field workers. *Journal of Toxicology and Environmental Health*, 11, 347-354.

Wilkinson, D. A., and Carlen, P. L. (1980a). Neuropsychological and neurological assessment of alcoholism. *Journal of Studies on Alcohol*, 41, 129-139.

Wilkinson, D. A., and Carlen, P. L. (1980b). Relation of neuropsychological test performance in alcoholics to brain morphology measured by computed tomography. In H. Begleiter (Ed.), *Biological Effects of Alcoholism*. New York: Plenum Press, 683-699.

Wilkinson, D.A., and Carlen, L. (1980c). Relationship of neuropsychological test performance to brain morphology in amnesic and non-amnesic chronic alcoholics. *Acta Psychiatrica Scandinavica*, Suppl. 286, 62, 89-101.

Williams, P. L., and Burson, J. L. (Eds) (1985). *Industrial Toxicology: Safety and health applications in the workplace*. New York: Van Nostrand Reinhold.

Williamson, A. M., and Teo, R. K. C. (1986). Neurobehavioral effects of occupational exposure to lead. *British Journal of Industrial Medicine*, 43, 374-380.

Williamson, A. M., Teo, R. K. C., and Sanderson, J. (1982). Occupational mercury exposure and its consequences for behaviour. *International Archives of Occupational and Environmental Health*, 50, 273-286.

Wills, M. R., and Savory, J. (1983, July 2). Aluminium poisoning: Dialysis encephalopathy, ostomalacia and anaemia. *Lancet*, 2, 29-34.

Windebank, A. J., McCall, J. T., and Dyck, P. J. (1984). Metal neuropathy. In P. J. Dyck, P. K. Thomas, E. H. Lambert, and R. Bunge (Eds), *Peripheral Neuropathy*, Volume II. Philadelphia: W. B. Saunders, 2133-2161.

Winneke, G. (182). Acute behavioral effects of exposure to some organic solvents—Psychophysiological aspects. *Acta Neurologica Scandinavica*, Suppl. 92, 66, 117-129.

Winneke, G., and Collet, W. (1985). Components of test batteries for the detection of neuropsychological dysfunction in children. In *Neurobehavioral Methods in Occupational and Environmental Health*. Document 3, Copenhagen: World Health Organization, 44-48.

Winneke, G., and Kraemer, U. (1984). Neuropsychological effects of lead in children: Interactions with social background variables. *Neuropsychobiology*, 11, 195-202.

Winneke, G., Hrdina, K.-G., and Brockhaus, A. (1982). Neuropsychological studies in children with elevated tooth-lead concentrations. 1. Pilot study. *International Archives of Occupational and Environmental Health*, 51, 169-183.

Winneke, G., Kraemer, U., Brockhaus, A., Ewers, U., Kujanek, G., Lechner, H., and Janke, W. (1983). Neuropsychological studies in children with elevated tooth-lead concentrations. II. Extended study. *International Archives of Occupational and Environmental Health*, 51, 231-252.

Wise, R. A. (1984). Neural mechanisms of the reinforcing action of cocaine. In J. Grabowski (Ed.), *Cocaine: Pharmacology, effects, and treatment of abuse*. NIDA Research Monograph 50. Washington, DC: Department of Health and Human Services, 15-33.

Wittenborn, J. R. (1980). Behavioral toxicity of psychotropic drugs. *Journal of Nervous and Mental Disease*, 168, 171-176.

Wolff, M., Osborne, J. W., and Hanson, A. L. (1983). Mercury toxicity and dental amalgam. *Neurotoxicology*, 4, 201-204.

Wolkowitz, O. W., Weingartner, H., Thompson, K., Pickar, D., Paul, S. M., and Hommer, D. W. (1987). Diazepam-induced amnesia: A neuropharmacological model of an "organic amnestic syndrome". *American Journal of Psychiatry*, 144,

25-29.

Wood, R. (1981). Neurobehavioral toxicity of carbon disulfide. *Neurobehavioral Toxicology and Teratology 3*, 397-405.

World Health Organization (1976). *Mercury,* Geneva: WHO.

World Health Organization (1979a). *Carbon Disulfide.* Geneva: WHO.

World Health Organization (1979b). *Carbon Monoxide.* Geneva: WHO.

Wright, M., and Hogan, T. P. (1972). Repeated LSD ingestion and performance on neuropsychological tests. *Journal of Nervous and Mental Disease,* **154,** 432-438.

Wyse, D. G. (1973). Deliberate inhalation of volatile hydrocarbons: A review. *Canadian Medical Association Journal,* **108,** 71-74.

Wysocki, J. J., and Sweet, J. J. (1985). Identification of brain damage, schizophrenic, and normal medical patients using a brief neuropsychological screening battery. *International Journal of Clinical Neuropsychology,* **7,** 40-44.

Yesavage, J. A., Leirer, V. O., Denari, M., and Hollister, L. E. (1985). Carry-over effects of marijuana intoxication on aircraft pilot performance: A preliminary report. *American Journal of Psychiatry,* **142,** 1325-1329.

Yohman, J. R., Parsons, O. A., and Leber, W. R. (1985). Lack of recovery in male alcoholics' neuropsychological performance one year after treatment. *Alcoholism Clinical and Experimental Research,* **9,** 114-117.

Yule, W., Lansdown, R., Millar, I. B., and Urbanowicz, M. A. (1981). The relationship between blood lead concentrations, intelligence and attainment in a school population: A pilot study. *Developmental Medicine and Child Neurology,* **23,** 567-576.

Zbinden, G. (1983). Definition of adverse behavioral effects. In G. Zbinden, V. Cuomo, G. Racagni, and, B. Weiss (Eds), *Applications of Behavioral Pharmacology in Toxicology.* New York: Raven Press, 1-14.

Zillmer, E. A., Lucci, K-A., Barth, J. T., Peake, T. H., and Spyker, D. A. (1986). Neurobehavioral sequelae of subcutaneous injection with metallic mercury. *Clinical Toxicology,* **24,** 91-110.

Ziporyn, T. (1986). A growing industry and menace: Makeshift laboratory's designer drugs. *Journal of the American Medical Association,* **256,** 3061-3063.

Zorick, T. R., Sicklesteel, J., and Stepanski, E. (1981). Effects of benzodiazepines on sleep and wakefulness. *British Journal of Clinical Pharmacology,* Suppl. **11,** 31s-35s.

Index

About the Author

David E. Hartman, Ph.D., received his doctorate in clinical psychology from the University of Illinois, an M.A. at Princeton University, and his A.B. from Vassar College. He is currently Director of Neuropsychology and Adult Testing, as well as Adult Coordinator of the clinical psychology internship program at Cook County Hospital, Chicago, Illinois.

Dr. Hartman is Adjunct Assistant Professor of Psychology, Department of Psychiatry, at the University of Illinois College of Medicine at Chicago. He teaches graduate seminars in neuropsychology and psychotherapy at Chicago-area universities and hospitals, and his research interests include the effects of neurotoxins on neuropsychological function, and the ethics of microcomputer use by mental health professions.

Dr. Hartman is a past Clinical Section Chairman of the Illinois Psychological Association and is on the editorial board of the *Archives of Clinical Neuropsychology*. He maintains an active private practice in Chicago, specializing in neuropsychology and psychotherapy.